CYTOLOGY AND EVOLUTION

H.S. BHAMRAH
&
KAVITA JUNEJA

ANMOL PUBLICATIONS PVT LTD
New Delhi-110 002

ANMOL PUBLICATIONS PVT LTD
4374/4B, Ansari Road
Daryaganj, New Delhi-110 002

First Edition 1993

ISBN 81-7041-819-4

PRINTED IN INDIA

Published by J.L. Kumar for Anmol Publications Pvt. Ltd., New Delhi and Printed at Nav Prabhat Printing Press.

Preface

There is a paradox in the growth of scientific knowledge. As information accumulates in ever more intimidating quantities, disconnected facts and imperetrable mysteries give way to rational explanation, and simplicity emerges from chao. Gradually the essential principles of a subject come into focus. This is true of cell biology today. This is true that cell is a vital unit of organism and it can be considered as the anatomic and physiologic substrate of biologic phenomena. Most of the Indian Universities have recognised the importance of cell in due time and have incorporated the Cell Biology, Molecular Biology, Genetics, and Evolution in their syllabi.

This book is principally for students taking a first course in cell biology, be they undergraduates, graduate students, or medical students. Although we assure that most readers have had at least an introductory biology course, we have attempted to write the book so that even a stranger to this branch could follow it by starting at the beginning. Most of the chapters have been updated to give the reader a current view.

It has been the constant endeavour of the authors to furnish maximum substance, keeping in view the limitations of size of the volume. Efforts have been made to condense the matter as far as practicable. It is hoped that this book will not only meet the requirement of Indian students but will also be useful as a guideline to the teachers in their teaching.

There can be no claim to originality except in the manner of treatment and much of the information has been obtained from the books and scientific journals available in the different libraries.

The authors express their thanks to their friends and colleagues whose continue inspirations have initiated them to bring out this book.

The authors are painfully aware of the shortcomings, errors and misprints that have crept in, and shall be grateful to receive suggestion for improvement of the next edition from all the readers.

Authors

Preface

There is a paradox in the growth of scientific knowledge. As information accumulates in ever more intimidating quantities, disconnected facts and impenetrable mysteries give way to rational explanation and simplicity emerges from chaos. Gradually the essential principles of a subject come into focus. This is true of cell biology today. This is true that cell is a vital unit of organism and it can be considered as the anatomical and physiological unit of biologic phenomena. Most of the Indian Universities have recognised the importance of cell in due time and have incorporated the Cell Biology, Molecular Biology, Genetics, and Evolution in their syllabi.

This book is principally for students taking a first course in cell biology, be they undergraduates, graduate students, or medical students. Although we assume that most readers have had at least an introductory biology course, we have attempted to write the book so that even a stranger to this subject could follow it by starting at the beginning. Most of the chapters have been updated to give the reader a current view.

It has been the constant endeavour of the authors to furnish maximum substance, keeping in view the limitations of size of the volume. Efforts have been made to condense the matter as far as practicable. It is hoped that this book will not only meet the requirement of Indian students but will also be useful as a guideline to the teachers in their teaching.

There can be no claim to originality except in the manner of treatment and much of the information has been obtained from the books and scientific journals available in the different libraries.

The authors express their thanks to their friends and colleagues whose continue inspirations have initiated them to bring out this book.

The authors are painfully aware of the shortcomings, errors and misprints that have crept in and shall be grateful to receive suggestion for improvement of the next edition from all the readers.

Authors

Contents

Section I : Cell Biology

1. **Structure of a Cell** 1 - 18
Prokaryotic cells, Eukaryotic cells, Morphology of Eukaryotic cell, Shape, Number, Size, Structure, Electron microscopic structure of a Typical cell, Plasma membrane, Mitochondria, Golgi body, Lysosomes, Endoplasmic Reticulum, Plastid, Ribosome, Peroxisomes, Cilia and Flagells, Vacuoles, Nucleus, Cytosol, Comparison between Plant and Animal cells, Function of cellular organelles.

2. **Plasma Membrane** 19 - 41
Chemical composition, Lipids, Carbohydrates, Proteins, Molecular structure of Plasma membrane, The lipid bilayer, Sandiwich model, Robert son's unit membrance model, Fluid mosaic model, Pores in plasma membrane, Specialization or Modifications, Permeability of membranes, Diffusion, Osmosis, Active transport, Origin of Plasma membrane.

3. **Mitochondria** 42 - 62
Distribution, Morphology, Shape, Size, Number, Structure, Mitochondrial cristae, Mitochondrial particle, Biochemistry of mitochondria Functions, Origin of mitochondria.

4. **Golgi Complex** 63 - 76
Occurrence, Morphology of Golgi Complex, Shape, Number, Size, Position, Detailed Structure of Golgi Complex, Chemical composition, Functions of Golgi complex, Origin of Golgi complex.

5. **Lysosomes** 77 - 70
Occurrence, Morphology, Shape, Size, Structure, Permeability of lysosomal membrane, Polymorphism, Chemistry of lysosome, Different Nomenclature, Functions of lysosomes, Origin of lysosomes.

6. **Endoplasmic Reticulum** **91 - 103**
Occurrence, Morphology, Ultra Structure of Endoplasmic Reticulum, Types of Endoplasmic Reticulus, Modifications of Endoplasmic Reticulus, Origin of Endoplasmic Reticulus, Enzymes of the ER membrane, Functions.

7. **Ribosomes** **104 - 114**
Occurrence, Distribution, Number, Ribosomal Sub-units, Ribsomal RNA, Types of ribosomes, Chemical Composition, Protein, Ribosomal enzymes protein, Functions of Ribosomes.

8. **Plastids** **115 - 135**
Various types of Plastids, Chromoplasts, Leucoplasts, Chloroplast, Distribution and Orientation, Morphology, Shape, Size, Number and Chemical composition, Structure, Quantosome Concept, Functions of the Chloroplast, Photosynthesis, Origin of the plastids.

9. **Nucleus** **136 - 153**
Significance of Nucleus, Hammerling's experiment, Morphology, Shape, Position, Size, Number, Nuclear envelope, Pore complex, Permeability of the nuclear envelope, Origin of nuclear membrane, Chemical composition of nucleus, Nucleoproteins, Nucleic acids, Nuclear enzymes, Nuclear lipids, Nuclecolus, Fine Structure of nucleolus, Chemistry, Biosynthesis of nucleolus or nucleolar cycle, Functions.

Section II : Molecular Biology

1. **Nucleic Acids** **155 - 175**
Deoxyribonucleic acid or DNA, Physical Structure of DNA, Molecular Structure of DNA, Nucleosides and nucleotides, Structural Variation in DNA, Z-DNA or left handed DNA, Biological replacation of DNA, Mechanism of replication, Enzymes for DNA Synthesis, Types of replications, Evidences in Support of Semiconservative replication of DNA, Biological Significance of DNA.

2. **Ribonucleic Acids (RNA)** 176 - 190
Primary structure of RNA, Secondary Structure of Ribonucleic acid, Types of Ribonucleic acids, mRNA, Informosomes, RNA, unusual bases, RNA, Replication of Ribonucleic acid, Comparison of different types of RNA.

3. **Protein Synthesis** 191 - 206
Central dogmas and Reverse Central dogma, Role of amino acids, Role of mRNA during synthesis of protein, Role of tRNA, Poly ribosomes and their role in Protein Synthesis, Polyribosome cycle and association and dissociation of subunits, Role of Subunits in Protein Synthesis, Mechanism of Protein Synthesis, Transcription, Translation, Inhibit of Protein Synthesis.

4. **Regulation of Gene Action or Protein Synthesis** 207 - 213
Induction or Repression, Operon hypothesis, Structural Gene, Promoter Gene, Regulator Gene, Feedback inhibition, Regulation of cyclic AMP.

5. **Genetic Code** 214 - 225
The Genetic Code of a triplet code, Properties of Genetic code, Genetic code is non-overlapping, Genetic code is degenerate, Genetic code is commaless, Universality of the code, The code has polarity, Initiation code, Nonsense Codons, Deciphering or cracking of Genetic code, Wobbel Hypothesis, Contribution of Khorana.

Section III : Evolution

1. **Origin of Life** 1 - 16
Special creation theory, Theory of spontaneous generation, Theory of eternity of life, Cosmozoic theory, Theory of catastropnism, Modern concept on the origin of life, Life on other planets.

2. **Evidences in favour of Organic Evolution** 17 - 47
Evidences from taxonomy, Evidences from comparative anatomy, Evidences from embryology, Evidences from comparative physiology and biochemistry, Evidences from Palaeotology, Evidences from geographical

distribution, Evidences from cytology, Evidences from genetics.

3. **Lamarckism** 48 - 55
Lamarckism, Analysis of Lamarck's theory, Criticism of Lamarckism, Neo-Lamarckism.

4. **Theory of Natural Selection** 56 - 64
Origin of New Species, Criticism and objections to Darwinism, Neo-Darwinism.

5. **Mutation Theory** 65 - 72
Criticism of mutation theory, Causes of mutations, Mutagenic agents, Significance of mutations.

6. **Isolation** 73 - 82
Isolating mechanism, Genetic of Isolating mechanism, Origin of reproductive isolation, Role of isolation in evolution.

7. **Adaptations** 83 - 108
Cursorial adaptations, Fossoreal adaptations, Aquatic adaptations, Scansorial adaptations, Volant adaptations, Cave adaptations, Deep Sea adaptations.

8. **Variations** 109 - 114
Kinds of variations, Sources of variation, Significance of variation.

9. **Species and Origin of Species** 115 - 121
Phylatic species, Sub-Species, Clins, Race, Supra-species, Clone, Linage, Origin of species.

10. **Zoogeographical Distribution** 122 - 147
Palearctic region, Nearctic region, Ethiopian region, Neotropical region, Australian region, Oriental region, Zoogeography of Indian Sub-region, Wallace's line, Weber's line.

11. **Geological Distribution** 148 - 166
Geological time scale, Eras, Periods, Epochs.

12. **Evolution of Horse** 167 - 174
Place of Origin, Horses of Eocene, Horses of Oligocene, Horses of Miocene, Horses of Pliocene.

13. **Evolution of Man** 175 - 186
Ancestral apes, Origin of man, Fossil men, Races of modern man.

Cell Biology

1

STRUCTURE OF A CELL

The cell is a unit of biological activity delimited by a semipermeable membrane and capable of self reproduction in a suitable non living medium. The body of all living organisms (bacteria, blue green algae, plants and animals) except viruses has cellular organization and may contain one or many cells. The organisms with only one cell in their body are called *unicellular organisms* (e.g. bacteria, blue green algae, some algae, protozoan, etc.). The organisms having many cells in their body are called *multicellular organisms* (e.g., most plants and animals). Any cellular organism may contain only one type of cells—Prokaryotic cells, or Eukaryotic cells.

It was *Robert Hooke* who first of all in 1665 observed under a microscope certain honeycomb like structure in cork, and he applied the term *'cell'* (L., *cella*; Small room) for the same. Previously it was believed that there was only one component of the cell which was the cell wall. But in 1831, one more peculiar structure was observed by *Robert Brown*. He gave the name *'nucleus'*. Later on, in 1835, the word *'sarcode'* was proposed for the jelly like material present inside the cell by *Dujardin*. In 1840 *Purkinje* replaced the word sarcode by *protoplasm* which is now used universally.

PROKARYOTIC CELLS

The prokaryotic (Gr., *pro*; primitive, *Karyon*; nucleus) cells are the most primitive cells from morphological point of view. They occur in bacteria and blue green algae. Prokaryotes are small, single cell organism, usually less than a micrometer (abbreviated µm; 1000 µm = 1 millimeter, abbreviated mm) are generally not longer than µm. Their structural organization is more simple than that of the eukaryotes. They do not have a distinct nucleus, and they are lacking in many membranous structures found in the more complex cell types. The hereditary information is contained in a single circular structure that lacks many of the molecular components of the eukaryotic hereditary structure called the *chromosome.* In addition, the prokaryotes seem to lack any kind of special apparatus for cells division, that is why they divide amitotically or by fission.

The prokaryotes are characterized by:

(i) the absence of a membrane around the nuclear material,
(ii) the absence of clearly defined membrane-limited organelles like mitochondria, chloroplasts, Golgi body and lysosomes,
(iii) the genetic material is located on a single chromosome which consists of a circular double strand of DNA,
(iv) the basic protein, histones, which are one of the most important constituents of chromosomes of eukaryotic cells, are absent in prokaryotic chromosomes,

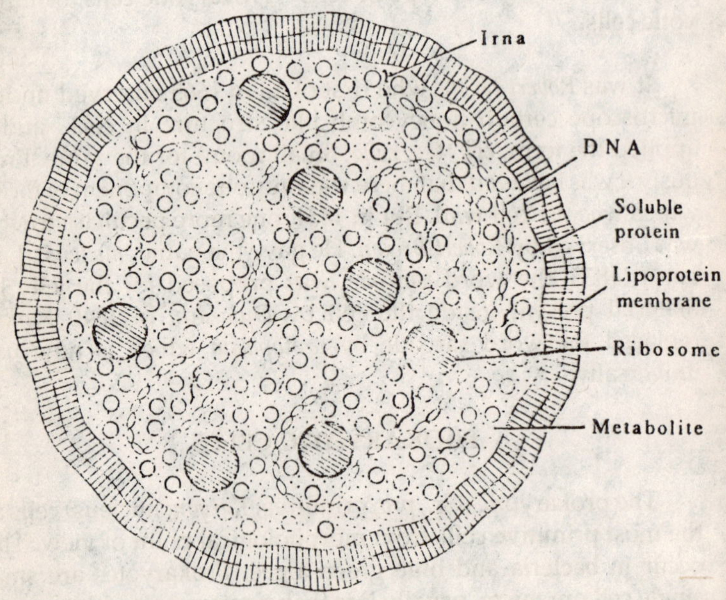

Fig. 1.1 A prokaryotic cell.

(v) the absence of nucleolus and mitotic apparatus,

(vi) the cell wall in non-cellulosic, being formed of carbohydrates and amino acids,

(vii) the plasma membrane which lies below the cell wall is produced into the cytoplasm and acts as the mitochondrial membrane carrying respiratory enzymes, and

(viii) the cytoplasm neither exhibits streaming nor the amoeboid movement.

The prokaryotes include bacteria, blue green algae, spirochaete, *Mycoplasma* or pleuropneumonia like org-nism (PPLO).

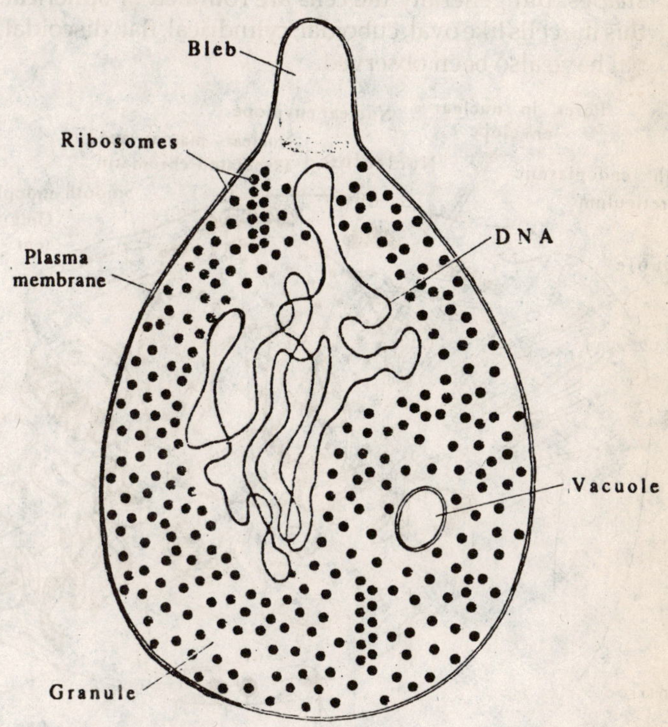

Fig. 1.2 Diagram of a Mycoplasma

EUKARYOTIC CELLS

Eukaryotic cells may be unicellular organisms, such as protozoans and unicellular algae, or they may be cells that make up the tissue and organs of multicellular organisms. Though the eukaryotic cells have different shape, size, and physiology yet all the cells are typically composed of plasma membrane, cytoplasm and its organelles, viz., mitochondria, endoplasmic reticulum, ribosomes, Golgi complex, etc., and a true nucleus.

MORPHOLOGY OF EUKARYOTIC CELL

Shape. Cell shapes are almost as numerous as cell types; there is no typical shape. The cells of certain unicellular forms, such as *Amoeba, Diatoms, Acetabularia* and bacteria exhibit a number of shapes. But generally the cells are rounded or spherical. Besides this the cells like oval, cuboidal, cylindrical, flat, discoidal, polygonal have also been observed.

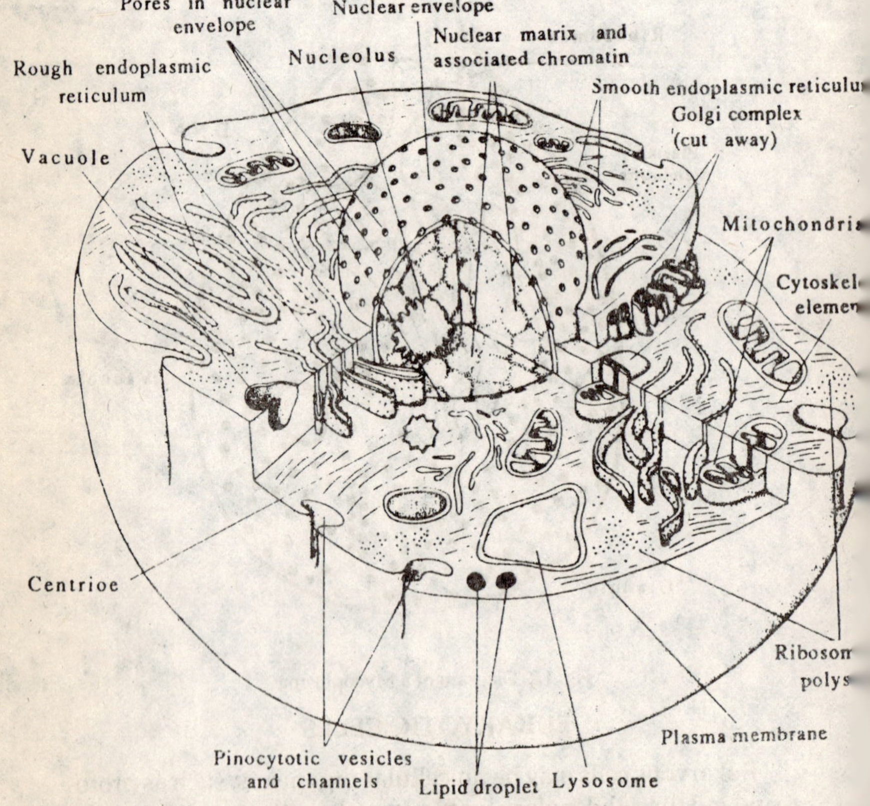

Fig. 1.3. A three dimensional view of a typical animal cell

The shape of cells depends mainly on functional adaptations and partly on the surface tension and viscosity of the protoplasm, the mechanical action exerted by the adjoining cells and the rigidity of the cell membrane. Some cells, such as *Amoeba* and *leucocytes*, can change their body shape very frequently.

Number. Some organisms like protozoans are single celled and others are multicellular. The body of human being is composed of about 26 trillions of cells. In human blood the number of erythrocytes is about five million per cubic ml of blood. About 10 billion neurons constitute the nervous system in human being.

Size. The size of different cells ranges within broad limits. Some plant and animal cells are visible to the naked eye, such as eggs of certain birds have a diameter of several centimeters. But the great majority of cells are visible only under a microscope. The smallest living cells are found among bacteria and viruses where the size ranges 0.1μ to 1μ (1μ = 0.001 mm). Organisms like Pleuropneumonia, so called "elementary bodies" have been observed with diameters of 100 μ. These appear to be a resting from of the bacteria which may grow into bodies of 250 μ in diameter during the active metabolism of the organism. It would seem that 200-250 mμ in diameter is the lower limit for the sizeof inactive, living cells. This lower limit may be set by the minimum number and size of the component necessary for independent cellular existance.

Usually the vast majority of cells lie in the range of .5 to 20μ in diameter. The length of unicellular diatoms is about 100μ. And the size of *Amoeba proteus* is 1 m.m. (1000μ) in length. The size of human R.B.C., is 7-8μ in diameter.

The long nerve is also an example of the extremes in cell sizes, the range of which is quite remarkable in the living world.

Factors Restriciting Cell size

In general, the size of the cell is correlated with its function. In no way is it associated with the size of the organism. For instance, a microscopic cell of bread mould can be seveal metres long, whereas cells in the body of whale or elephant may be as small as 10μ. Two major factors seem to restrict cell size:

1. *The nucleocytoplasmic ratio.* The nucleus controls activities of the cell by protein synthesis through RNA synthesis. In a large cell cytoplasm requires more proteins and consequently more RNA. The DNA content of a cell is constant, which can control the activities of the cell upto a specific size, beyond which proper control is not possible. For this reason a cell after attaining a specific size stops growing.
2. *The surface area.* As shown in fig, the small cells have more surface area per unit volume and with an increase in size, this ratio between surface area and volume gradually decreases. However, a large cell naturally requires more nutrients and oxygen for its metabolism, which diffuse into the cell through its surface. It means, the surface area of a cell affects its ability to exchange materials with its environment and puts a check on cell volume. For this reason, the cells that are metabolically more active are small in size.

Similarly, large cells face problems in the diffusion of excretory products from cell cytoplasm to the exterior.

STRUCTURE OF FIXED CELLS

Examination of the living cell is limited to light microscopy and is based mainly on the differencess in refractive index of the different cell components. Sometimes the use of stains that act on the living organism (vital staining) facilitates observation of the living cell. However, more important in the morphologic study of the cell are methods of fixation, by which cell death results in such a way that physiologic structure and chemical composition are preserved as much as possible.

The complexity of the structural organization in a cell of the higher plants and animals is most impressive. Although there are great differences between the primitive forms of life, and the higher plant and animal cells, the similarities between primitive and advanced cells are also notable. Eukaryotic cells are characterized by a true nucleus with a nuclear membrane or envelop which divides the cell into two main compartments: nucleus and cytoplasm. The cytoplasm in turn is limited by the plasma membrane. In a plant, cell the plasma membrane is covered and protected on the ouside by a thicker cell wall through which there are tunnels, the *plamodesmta*, by which the cell intercommunicates with neighbouring cells via fine cell process. In animal cells, parts of the plasma membrane are covered by a thin layer of material, which is generally described as the extraneous coat of the plasma membrane. The so-called *basement membranes* correspond to this extraneous coat.

In every stained cell usually one nucleus is present. It is central organelle of cell and is the main site of hereditary material. The nucleus is surrounded by a nuclear membrane. Within the nucleus a single nucleolus and network of chromatin is present. These two materials remain suspended in the nucleoplasm.

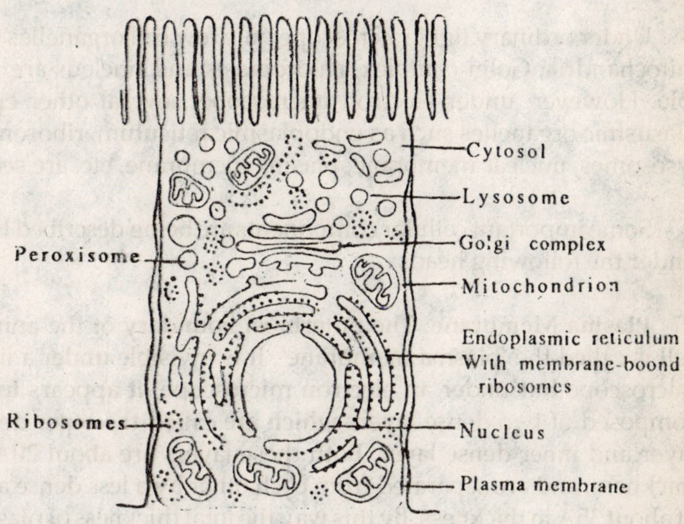

Fig. 1.4. A typical animal cell

A small cytoplasmic organoid 'centriole' is present in the majority of animal cells and in some cells of the lower plants. The position is generally fixed for each type of cell. Generally the cell centre or centriole occupies an axial position behind the nucleus. In some cells, it has the tendency to occupy the geometrical centre i.e., in leucocytes it occupies this position within the nucleus which is horseshoe shaped. The morphology of centriole changes with the functional state of the cell.

In the cytoplasm of the cell, there are several organelles; out of them, only mitochondira and Golgi bodies are visible under light microscope. Mitochandria or chondriosomes are scattered in the cytoplasm of all kinds of cells. Their shape in fixed cells depends upon the fixation and handling of the tissues. Before preparation they may appear as long rods, short rods or as small granules. Golgi material appears in its very prominent form in nervous and secretory cells in animals. Plastids are cytoplasmic organelles of plant cells may or may not contain pigments. In green plants chlorophyll is present in these organelles and thus termed as chloroplasts.

ELECTRON MICROSCOPIC STRUCTURE OF A TYPICAL CELL

Under ordinary light microscope only few cell organelles like mitochandria, Golgi complex, chloroplasts and nucleus are visible. However, under electron microscope, several other cytoplasusmic organelles such as endoplasmic reticulum, ribosomes, lysosomes, nuclear membrane, plasma membrane, etc. are seen.

Some important cellular components are being described here under the following heads:

Plasma Membrane: The outermost boundary of the animal cell is called the 'plasma membrane'. It is invisible under a light microscope but under an electron microscope, it appears to be composed of two dense layers which are called the outer dense layer and inner dense layer. Both these layers are about 20Å in thickness, and are separated from each other by a less dense area of about 35Å in thickness. By this way the total thickness of plasma membrane is about 75Å. Before the advance of electron microscope people used to think of the plasma membrane as stretched tightly over the cell. But now we know that a single plasma membrane can have as many as 3000 microvilli. Another peculiarity of the structure of the membrane is that it remains connected with the endoplasmic reticulum.

Plasma membrane is lipo-protein in composition.

Functions

(1) Gives an identity to the cell.
(2) Protects the cell organelles.
(3) Helps in digestion through phagocytosis and pinocytosis.
(4) Being permeable to water, water can pass through it.
(5) Helps in the transport of ions.
(6) Helps in the formation of cytoplasmic organelles.

Mitochondria : The term mitochondria was for the first time used by *Benda* (1902) to designate the filamentous and granular structure of cell cytoplasm. Most of the knowledge related to mitochondrial fine structure is due to the studies of *Palade* (1952, 55, 56) and *Sjostrand* (1955). Due to these studies, now mitochondria are defined as the double walled structures of cell organelles within which the membranous structures called *Cristae* are present. The outer chamber of mitochondria is made up of two dense layers and a less dense layer having the total thickness of 140Å to 180Å while the outer and inner dense layers vary in their measurements from 35Å to 60Å in thickness depending upon the physiological state of the cell. The less dense layer is 40-70 A° in thickness.

The matrix of the mitochondria may have some fine opaque granules of various sizes. *David E. Green* (1964) observed in a very highly magnified electron microscope that the inside of the inner membrane and the outside of outer membrane are covered with very small particles. They measure about 90-100A° in diameter. The particles on the outer membrane differ from those on the inner membrane. The former generally appear as simple spheres packed closely together which give to the surface of the mitochondrion, a rough or pimped appearance. The particle on the inside of the inner membrane has the more complex configuration. In some cells, but not all, this particle is seen to have a base, a stalk and a spherical head. Mitochondria represent the power generating centres of the cell. They can bring about oxidation of the intermediates of carbohydrates, fat and amino acid metabolism in the presence of O_2 releasing energy. The released energy is trapped in the form of adenosine triphosphate (ATP).

Golgi bodies : Golgi bodies have probably been first observed earlier in 1867 by *La. Vallete St. George*, but anyhow credit goes to

Camillo Golgi (1898) who described it as internal 'reticulate apparatus' and after it, was named Golgi apparatus. It is variously called Golgi element, Golgi complex, Dalton's complex etc. Each Golgi complex is composed of many lamella, tubules, vesicles and vacuoles. The membranes of Golgi complex are of lipoproteins and these are supposed to be originated from the membranes of endoplasmic reticulum. The function of the Golgi complex is storage of proteins and enzymes which are synthesized by ribosomes and transported by endoplasmic reticulum to them. Further the Golgi complex has most important secretory function. It secretes many secretory granules and lysosomes. In plant cells the Golgi complex is known as dictyosome and secretes necessary materials for cell wall formation during cell division.

Lysosomes : The lysosomes (*Gr. lyso; digestive + some;* body) are also found scattered in the cytoplasm. By gently centrifuging lysosomes can be separated from other cell organelles. They are usually spherical but may be irregular in shape, covered with a membrane of lipoprotein. Inside structure is always variable. Lysosomes contain hydrolysing enzymes, such as acid phosphatase, acid ribonuclease, acid deoxyribonuclease and cathespins. But they do not have oxidative enzymes. This property distinguishes them from the mitochondira. Lysosomes are polymorphic in nature and are commonly known as suicide bags and are responsible for postmortem changes in cells.

Endoplasmic Reticulum : The term "Microsome" was introduced to the modern cytology of *Claude* (1943) to represent one of the submicroscopic cellular components isolated by centrifugation. These are now known to be the broken parts of the endoplasmic reticulum after the studies of *Kollman* (1953). *Porter* (1945) was the first man to describe their electron microscopic structure in cultured cells. He described them as lace like reticulum. There are membrane bounded sacs in the form of double membrane or cisternae. The term cisternae was introduced by *Sjostrand* (1953) to describe long or elongated rod like parts of the endoplasmic reticulum measuring 50-200Å. *Wiess* (1953) described the vesicles of the endoplasmic reticulum which usually has a diameter of 25-500 Å while *Bradfield* (1913) came across another type of endoplasmic reticulum termed them as tubules; they measure from 50 to 100 Å in diameter.

On the basis of presence or absence of ribosomes or RNP particles the endoplasmic reticulum (E.R.) is distinguished in two varieties. The *rough walled endoplasmic reticulum, and smooth walled endoplasmic reticulum*. They are also know as granular or X-B of endoplasmic reticulum.

Rough Walled Endoplasmic Reticulum. Rough walled endoplasmic reticulum (R.E.R.) is that variety which bears the ribosomes at the external surface of the cisternae. The distribution of the ribosomes can be circular, spiral, or rosette type. These particles may be induced to leave the surface of the cisternae without damaging the structure of the cisternae or the capacity to associate again with the particles. Usually the rough walled endoplasmic reticulum richly distributed in those cells which are engaged in the synthesis of the protein.

Smooth Walled Endoplasmic Reticulum. The other large division of the system owes its identity in parts to the absence of the particles and therefore commonly referred to as the smooth surfaced agranular form. Like the R.E.R., the S.E.R. shows a characteristic morphology which is tubular rather than cisternae. The tubules have the diameter nearly of 50-100 mu. As studied by *Fawcett* (1960) S.E.R. are richly distributed in those cells which are engaged in the synthesis of steroids.

Continuity between the S.E.R. of a particular cell type possesses a characteristic pattern of structure. Thus it is typical for rat liver cells to show groups of eight or ten slender profiles in parallel array.

Plastids. Plastids are present only in plant cells (not in animal cells). These are double-membrane structure relatively larger than the mitochondria. Some of the plastids are colourless and store starch (leucoplasts). Others contain various pigments and impart different colours (red, brown, yellow, etc.) to different parts of the plant. These are collectively called chromoplasts. Those containing green pigment — cholorophyll—are called choloroplasts. These contain several enzymes in their matrix necessary for photosynthesis. The chloroplasts capture light energy of the sun and convert it into the chemical energy — ATP—which is used in the biosynthesis of glucose from CO_2 and H_2O.

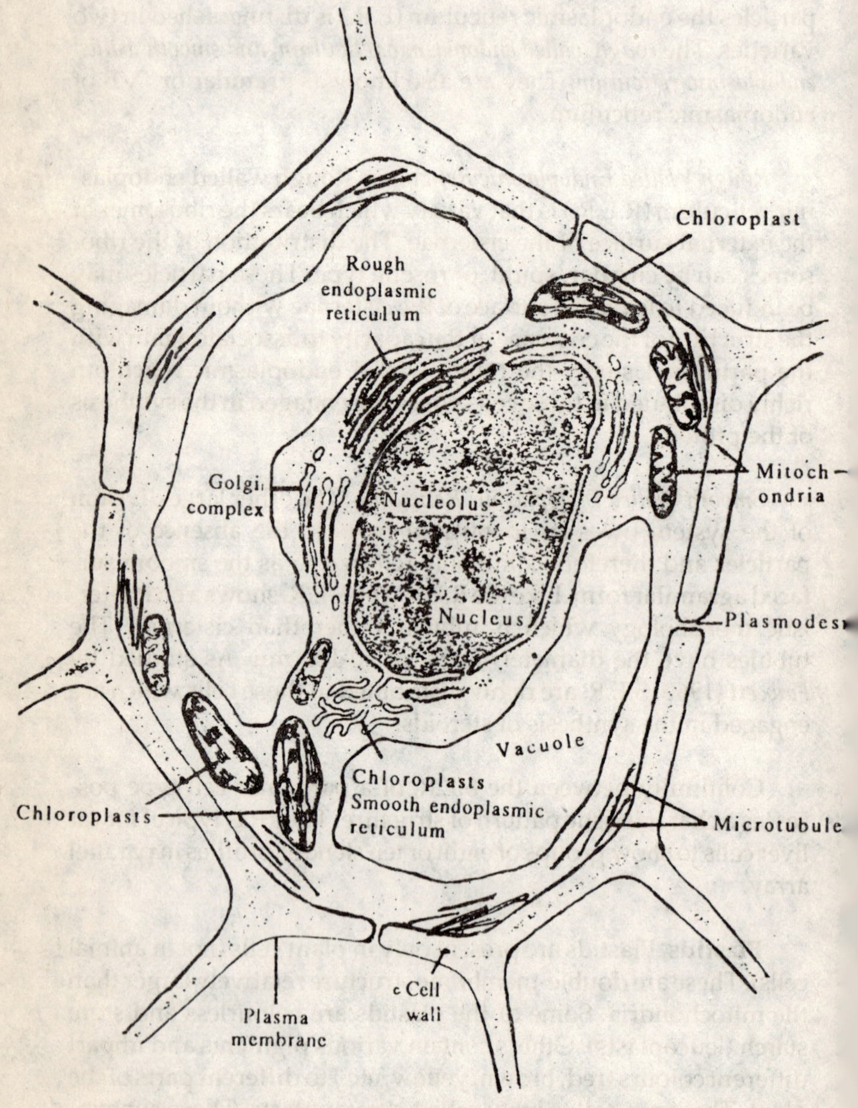

Fig. 1.5 A typical plant cell

Ribosomes : Many minute, spherical structures known as ribosomes remain attached with the membrane of endoplasmic reticulum and forms granular or rough type of E.R. The ribosomes are originated in the nucleolus and consist of mainly the ribonucleic acids (RNA) and proteins. Each ribosome is composed of two structural units, smaller subunit known as 40 S subunit and a larger subunit known as 60 S subunit. The ribosomes remain attached with the membranes of endoplasmic reticulum by the 60 S subunits. The 40 S subunits occur on the larger sub unit and form a cap-like structure. The ribosomes consists of 3 types of RNA's known as ribosomal RNA's or rRNA, viz., 5 S, 18 S and 28 S rRNA's. The 28 S and 5 S rRNA's occur in large (60 S) subunit, while 18 S rRNA occur in the smaller ribosomal subunit. The ribosomes also occur freely in the cytoplasm. They are the sites of protein synthesis.

Peroxisomes : These are also bounded by a single membrane. These contain enzymes for the breakdown of hydrogen peroxide to from water and oxygen. These are protective organelles of the cell.

Cilia and Flagella : The cells of many unicellular organisms and ciliated epithelium of multicellular organisms consists of some hair-like cytoplasmic projections outside the surface of the cell. These are known as cilia or flagella. They help in locomotion of the cell. The cilia and flagella consist of nine outer fibrils around two large central fibrils. Each outer fibrils consists of two microtubules. The two microtubules of each peripheral pair or *doublet* remain morphologically distinct. The central fibril are separate but remain enveloped in a common *central sheath*. Cilia and flagella are involved in locomotion, feeding, cleansing etc.

Vacuoles : These structures are fluid-filled "bubbles" found in the cytoplasm. Vacuoles are bound by a membrane, called *tonoplast*, which is structurally similar to, if not identical with, a cell-membrane. Inside the vacuoles, food materials or wastes are found.

Vacuoles are conspicuous in plant-cells but they are found less in animal cells. Vacuoles are absent in actively dividing cells. In a young plant-cell, there are many vacuoles but, when a cell matures, they unite to form a single, large, central vacuole.

Guilliermond (1941) was of the opinion that vacuoles are colloidal with a strong imbibing capacity. Vacuoles arise *denovo* i.e., spontaneously formed from pre-existing vacuole.

In many protozoan, vacuoles are formed at the bottom of the gullet. In these vacuoles, food-materials, such as bacteria, are collected. Some vacuoles are formed by cell-drinking. This type of vacuoles are called *pinosomes*. Food-vacuoles formed by evagination of cell-membrane surrounding food-particles with some fluid, are called *phagosomes*. In animals cells, the vacuoles are bound by a lipoprotein membrane that helps in storage and transport of materials and in the maintenance of internal pressure of the cell.

Vacuoles are not a living part of the protoplasm but are a storing place of reserve materials and waste products.

Crystals and oil droplets : In certain plant cells the food or waste material is found deposited in the form of crystals. The oils droplets are round in both plant and animal cells, which appear as tiny glistening white spheres. These serve as a reserve supply of energy-rich fuel.

Nucleus : It is the most vital part of cell which is invariably present in all the cells of higher animals and plants. Normally one nucleus is present in a cell but more than one may be present in certain cells.

Structurally it is enveloped by a porous *nuclear membrane* that separates it from the surrounding cytoplasm. It has the characteristic permeability. During cell division, it breaks up and soon after mitosis it is reconstituted. The inside of nucleus is filled with *nuclear sap or karyolymph*. In nuclear sap remain embedded other nuclear constituents. The *chromatin* is the Feulgen positive material in the interphase nucleus which during division becomes the definite chromosomes. In short it represents the chromosome substance. The sex-chromatin are the specific heterochromatic bodies, found generally near the periphery of the nucleus. In nucleus usually one sex chromatin body is found but more than one can also be observed. *Nucleolus* is relatively large, generally spherical ball like body. It has a high concentration of RNA and thus is an important structure involved in protein synthesis. Its number in a nucleus vary in structure involved in protein synthesis. Its number in a nucleus vary in different cells and depend on either the species or the sets of chromosomes.

The nucleus coordinates the many cell activities. DNA molecules are the source of coded instructions, which pass to RNA molecule which then act as messenger, moving out of the nucleus to one of the various structures of the cytoplasm. It also controls the cell reproduction. Here too, DNA is the source of coded instruction.

The Cytosol, Hyaloplasm or Ground Substance. The material that remains suspended under conditions sufficient to sediment even the ribosomes is referred to by biochemists as the *soluble fraction* or *cytosol*. This fraction usually contains some material lost from the organelles in the course of homogenization and centrifugation. However, it also contains other molecules, including some enzymes, that are not known to be part of the intracellular structure identifiable in the microscope. Such molecules are usually thought to derive from the hyaloplasm (also called ground substance, cell matrix, or cell sap), which was originally defined by microscopists as the apparently structureless medium that occupies the space between the visible organelles. As will be evident in subsequent chapters, with the improved techniques less and less of the cell appears structureless. Most investigators continue to believe that there does exist in the cytoplasm a "soluble phase"—a soluble containing inorganic ions and small molecules, materials in transit from one cell region to another and dissolved or suspended enzymes that function as individual molecules or perhaps as parts of small groups of molecules rather than as components of large, microscopically recognizable organelles. But there is a lively debate going on over proposals that many components once thought to be suspended in this solution are actually bound, perhaps loosely, in structured arrangements that do not survive the disruption involved in cell fractionation.

Table 3-1 The Relative Volumes Occupied by the Major Intracellular Compartments in a Typical Liver Cell (Hepatocyte)

Intracellular Compartment	*Per cent of Total Cell volume*	*Approximate Number per Cell*
Cytosol	54	1
Mitochondria	22	1700
Rough endoplasmic reticulum cisternae	9	1
Smooth endoplasmic reticulum cisternae plus Gogi cisternae	6	
Nucleus	6	1
Peroxisomes	1	400
Lysosomes	1	300

Table 3.2. Comparison of Prokarytoic and Eukaryotic Organisms

	Prokaryotes	*Eukaryotes*
Organism	becteria and cyanobacteria	protists, fungi, plants, and animals
Cell Size	generally 1 to 10 um in linear dimension	generally 10 to 100 um in linear dimension
Metabolism	anaerobic or aerobic	aerobic
Organelles	few or none	nucleus , mitochondria, chloroplasts, endoplasmic reticulum, etc.
DNA	circulars DNA in cytoplasm	very long DNA containing many noncoding regions; organized into chromosomes and bounded by nuclear envelope
RNA and protein	RNA and protein synthesized in same compartment	RNA synthesized and processed in nucleus; proteins synthesized in cytoplasm
Cytoplasm	no cytoskeleton, cytoplasmic streaming, endocytosis, or exocytosis	cytoskeleton composed of protein filaments; cytoplasmic steaming; endocytosis and exocytosis
Cell division	by binary fission	by mitosis (or meiosis)
Cellular organization	mainly unicellular	mainly multicellular, with differentiation of cells

Table 3.3. Comparison of Plant and Animal Cells

Plant cell	*Animal cell*
1. Generally larger than the animal cell	1. Usually smaller than the plant cell.
2. Plant cells are surrounded by a rigid cellulose wall.	2. Cellulose wall is not found in animal cell.
3. Majority of the mature plant cells have a large central sap vacuole	3. Vacuoles in animal cells are small
4. Plastids, especially choloroplasts are found usually in cells of green plants.	4. Choloroplast is not found in animal cell except in some Protozoa.
5. In the cell division, the division of cytoplasm of plant cells take place by formation of a partition called cell plate.	5. Animal cells divide by a constriction during cell division.

Table 3.4 Functions of Cellular Organells

Cell Organelles	*Functions*
Cells or Plasma membrane	Serves as a differentially permeable membrane through which extra-cellular substances may be selectively sampled and cell products may be liberated. Gives external form. Provides mechanical support and thus protects the cell.
Cell Wall (in plants)	Thick cellulose wall around the cell membrane gives strength and rigidity of the cells.
Cytoplasm	Provides greatly expanded surface Endoplasmic reticulum area for various biochemical reactions which normally take place at or across membrane surface.
Ribosomes	Sites of protein synthesis and known as "Protein factories on the cell".
Mitochondria	Oxidation of food substances, changes potential energy into a form of energy to be used by cell. Energy production (Krebs' cycle, electron transport chain, beta oxidation of fatty acids etc.). Power house of cell.
Centrioles (usually not seen in plant cells)	Form poles for the cell division Capable of replication usually.

Golgi body or apparatus	Produce cellular secretions known as dictyosomes in plants.
Lysosome (in animals)	Produce intracellular digestive enzymes which help in disposal of bacteria and other foreign bodies. If ruptured, may cause cell destruction.
Plastids (in plants)	Serve for storage of starch, pigments and other cellular products. Photosynthesis takes place in chloroplasts.
Vacuoles	Store excess water, waste products, soluble pigments etc.
Hyaloplasm	Contains enzymes for glycolysis and structural materials, viz, sugars, amino acids, water, vitamins, nucleotides etc.
Cilia and flagella	Serve to move the animals or to move the material.
Nucleus Nuclear membrane	Provides selective continuity between nuclear and cytoplasmic materials.
Nucleoplasm	Contain materials, for building DNA and messenger molecules which serve as intermediates between nucleus and cytoplasm.
Nucleolus	May synthesize ribosomes. Disappears during cellular replication. Function uncertain.
Chromosomes	Bearers of heriditary instructions. Regulation of cellular processes (evident only during nuclear division). Control the nucleus and metabolism.

2

PLASMA MEMBRANE

The outer most limit of a cell is composed of living or non-living materials or both. Whatever their chemical constitution and structural organization, their function includes regulation of the flow of materials into and out of the cell and they provide some degree of support and maintenance of cell shape and cell size. Plasma membrane is variously called as *cell membrane, plasmalemma, plasma membrane* etc. The term plasma membrane was given by *Nageli* in 1855. On account of the technical difficulties it is not possible to investigate the structure of plasma membrane in every kind of cell. Most of the informations on the subject has accumulated through the study of mammalian R.B.C. and the myelin sheath of the nerve fibres.

This membrane is so thin that it cannot be resolved with the light microscope, but in some cells it is covered by thicker protective layers that are within the limits of microscopic resolution. For example, most plant cells have a thick cellulose wall that covers and protects the true plasma membrane. Some animal cells are surrounded by cement-like substances that constitute visible cell walls. Such layers, also called extraneous coats, generally play no role in permeability, but do have other important functions.

For the study of their structure, chemical composition and for knowing the physiological and biochemical nature of the plasma membrane or any other cytoplasmic organelle the first thing which we face is their isolation in pure state.

CHEMICAL COMPOSITION

The plasma membrane is composed mainly of protein, lipid, and a small percentage (1 to 5 per cent) of oligosaccharides that may be attached to either the lipids (glycolipids) or the proteins (glycoproteins). There is a wide variation in the lipid protein ratio between different cell membranes. Myelin is an exception, in the sense that the lipid predominates; in the other cell membranes there is higher protein/lipid ratio. In myelin the area occupied by the protein is insufficient to cover that of the lipids, whereas in a red cell ghost the opposite situation is found.

Lipids : The main lipid components of the plasma membrane are the phospholipids, cholesterol and galactolipids; their proportion varies in different cell membranes. Myelin differs, with regard to lipid composition, from other cell membrane found in the brain. The major proportion of membrane phospholipids is represented by phosphatidylcholine, phosphatidylethanolamine, and sphingiomyelin, all of which have no net charge at neutral pH (i.e. neutral phospholipids) and tend to pack tightly in the bilayer. This property is also shared by cholesterol. Five to 20 per cent of the phospholipids are acidic, including: phosphatidylinositol, phosphatidylserine, cardiolipin phosphatidylglycerol, and sulfolipids. Acid phospholipids are negatively charged and in the membrane are associated principally with proteins by way of lipid-protein interactions.

Recent studies demostrate that there is an asymmetry in the erythrocyte membrane regarding not only the protein, but also the phospholipids. There are more choline phospholipids and glycolipids in the external half of the bilayer and more amino phospholipids in the inner, or cytoplasmic, half of the bilayer. It is assumed that this asymmetry is rather stable and that there is no exchange of lipids across the bilayer.

Carbohydrates : In red cell ghosts hexose, hexosamine fucose, and sialic acid are bound mainly to protein; the same is true of carbohydrates in liver membranes. Sialic acid is sensitive to neuraminidase and is attached to protein by N-acetylgalactosamine on the outer surface of the membrane.

Because of the presence of sialic acid residues, as well as carboxyl and phosphate groups, the outer surface of the membrane is negatively charged; consequently, positively charges may be bound by electrostatic interactions to the plasma membrane, Only a small amout of sialic acid exists in the form of gangliosides (i.e., glycolipids) in the plasma membrane of liver. However, gangliosides are important constituents of the neuronal surface and are probably involved in ion transfers. The preferential localization of gangliosids in the acetylcholinesterase rich nerve-ending membranes has been demonstrated.

Proteins : Proteins represent the main component of most biological membranes. They play an important role not only in the mechanical structure of the membrane, but also as carriers or channels, serving for transport : they may also be involved in regulatory or ligand-recognition properties. In addition, numerous enzymes, antigens and various kinds of receptor molecules are present in plasma membrane.

Membrane contains three different classes of proteins, structural proteins, enzymes and carrier proteins. *Stuctural proteins* form the 'back-bone' of the cell membrane. They have little catalytic activity and are extremely lipophilic. Their amino acid compostion is nearly the same. The plasma membrane consists largely of structural proteins. The average molecular weight of structural proteins is $3x10^4$. Enzymes form the major component of many membranes and are catalytic proteins. The endoplasmic reticulum, mitochondria, and plasma membrane contain many enzymes. The structure of the enzymes varies from membrane to membrane. Some 30 enzymes have been detected in isolated plasma membranes. Those most constantly found are 5" nucleotidase, Mg + ATPase, Na + —K + activated -Mg2 + ATPase, alkaline phosphatase, adenyl cyclase, acid phosphomonoesterase, and RNAse.

Some enzymes have a preferential localization; for example, alkaline phosphate and ATPase are more abundant at the bile capillaries, while disaccharidases are present in microvillae of the intestine. A specific localization with a mosaic arrangement has been postulated for some of these enzymes. Disaccharidase forms 5 to 6 nm globular units coating the membrane of the microvillae. The plasma membrane lacks the respiratory chain and glycolytic activity.

Of all the enzymes mentioned, Na + - K + activated - Mg2 + ATPase is one of the most important because of its role in ion transfer across the plasma membrane. The enzymes are dependent on the presence of lipids and are inactivated when all lipids are extracted.

Carrier proteins or permeases transport substances cross the membrane against the concentration gradient. The molecular weight of structural and carrier proteins are rather similar.

The amount of protein varies in different cell membranes. Myelin contains only 20 per cent protein, plasma membranes about 50% and the inner mitochondrial membrane 75 per cent.

The plasma membrane proteins fall in two main categories, *intrinsic* or *integral proteins* and *extrinsic* or *peripheral proteins*. The former are firmly associated with the membrane, while the latter have a weaker association and are bound by electrostatic interaction. Human erythrocyte glycoproteins consist of three chemically distinct regions: (1) N-terminal part external to the membrane and containing all the carbohydrates, (2) a middle hydrophobic region located within the membrane and (3) a hydrophilic C-terminal portion, rich in proline but lacking carbohydrate, on the internal side of the membrane. The middle intramembranous part appears to be intimately associated with the membrane phospholipids.

The glycoprotein of human erythrocyte membrane has a polypeptide backbone to which are attached two types of oligosaccharide chains, straight chain and a longer brached one at about 10 sites.

MOLECULAR STRUCTURE OF PLASMA MEMBRANE

All biological membranes, including the plasma membrane and the internal membranes of eukaryotic cells, have a common overall structure: they are assemblies of lipid and protein molecules held together by noncovalent interactions. The lipid molecules are arranged as a continuous double layer 4 to 5 nm thick. This lipid bilayer provides the basic structure of the membrane and serves as a relatively impermeable barrier to the flow of most water-soluble molecules. The protein molecules are "dissolved" in the lipid bilayer and mediate the various functions of the membrane; some serve to transport specific molecules into or out of the cell; others are enzymes that catalyze membrane-associated reactions; and still others serve as structural links between the cell's cytoskeleton and the extracellular matrix, or as receptors for receiving and transducing chemical signals from the cell's environment.

All cell membranes are dynamic, fluid structures: most of their lipid and protein molecules are able to move about rapidly in the plane of the membranes. Membrane are also asymmetrical structures: the lipid and protein compositions of the two faces differ from one another in ways that reflect the different functions performed at the two surfaces.

Although the specific lipid and protein components vary greatly from one type of membrane to another, most of the basic structural and functional concepts discussed in this chapter are applicable to intracellular membranes as well as to plasma membranes. After considering the structure and organization of the main constituents of biological membranes — the lipids, proteins, and carbohydrates—we will discuss the mechanisms cells employ to transport small molecules across their plasma membranes and the very different mechanisms they use to transfer macromolecules and larger particles across this membrane.

The Lipid Bilayer: The first indication that the lipid molecules in biological membranes are organized in a bilayer came from an experiment performed in 1925. Lipids from red blood cell membranes were extracted with acetone and floated on the surface of water. The area they occupied was then decreased by means of a movable barrier until a monomolecular film (a monolayer) was formed. This monolayer occupied a final area about twice the surface area of the original red blood cells. Because the only membrane in a red blood cell is the plasma membrane, the experimenters concluded that the lipid molecules in the membrane must be arranged as a continuous bilayer. The conclusion was right, but it turned out to be based on two wrong assumptions that fortuitously compensated for each other. On the one hand, the acetone did not extract all of the lipid. On the other, the surface area calculated for the red blood cells was based on dried preparations and was substantially less than the true value seen in wet preparations. None the less, the conclusions drawn from this experiment has a profound influence on cell biology; as a result, the lipid bilayer became an accepted part of most models of membrane structure, long before its existence was actually established.

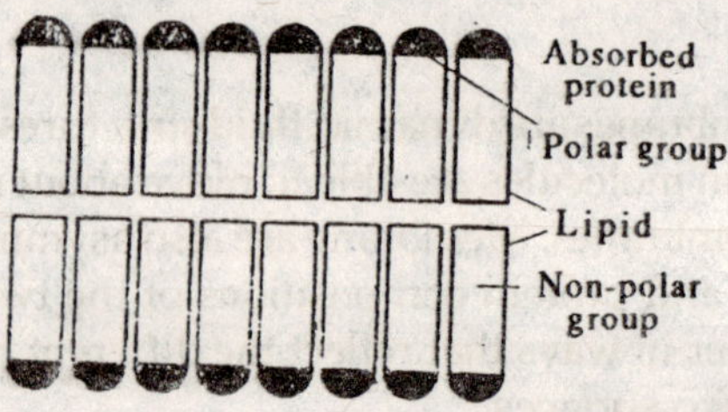

Fig. 2.1. The lipid membrane, of *Gorter* and *Grendel* (1925).

Danielli-Davson Model or Protein-lipid or Sandwich Model:

Harvey and *Cole* (1931) indicated the existence of protein by studying the surface tension of cells. This led them to propose a lipo-protein model of the cell membrane. According to this model the plasma membrane consists of two layers of lipid molecules as shown in the lipid bilayer model. The lipid molecules have their polar regions on the outer side. Globulin proteins are thought to be associated with the polar groups of the lipids. The non-polar hydrophobic ends of the two layers of lipids face each other, whereas their polar hydrophilic ends are associated with protein molecules by electrostatic interation. Protein-linked polar pores are present in the membrane. These pores are formed by periodic continuity of outer and inner layers of proteins of plasma membrane.

Several modifications of the above arrangement have been described:

(A) Some plasma membrane have folded b-chain of proteins on both the surface of lipid bilayer.
(B) Coiled l-chains of helical protein on the surface of lipid bilayer.
(C) With globular proteins on both the surfaces.

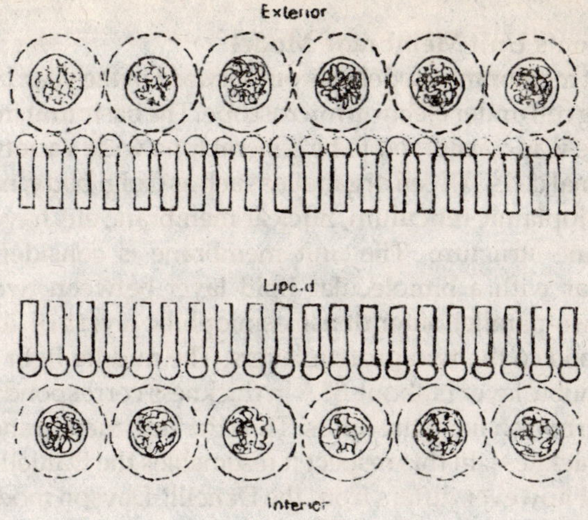

Fig 2.2. The Original Davson-Danielli model

(D) With folded proteins on both the surfaces and helical proteins extending into the pores.

(E) With folded b-chain protein on one side and globular protein on the other side.

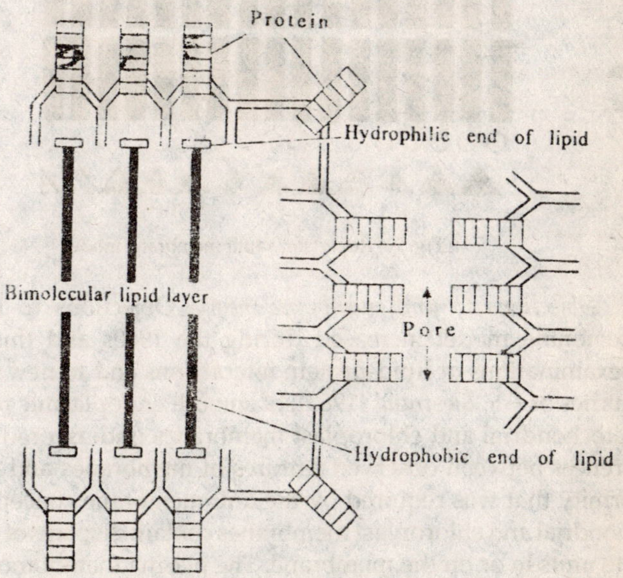

Fig. 2.3. The cell membrane with protein lined pores.

Robertson's Unit Membrane Model

Unit membrane model was put forward in the year 1953 while studying cell under electron microscope. The basic unit membrane structure was considered to be general for a wide variety of plant and animal cells. All cell organelles such as Golgi body, mirochondria, endoplamic reticulum, nuclear membrane etc. have the unit membrane structure. The unit membrane is considered to be trilaminar with a bimolecular lipid layer between two protein layer. Two parallel outer dense osmiophilic layers of 20Å which correspond to the two protein layers. The middle light coloured osmiophobic layer is about 35Å in thickness corresponding to the hydrocarbon chain of the lipids. Thus the unit membrane is about 7A° in thickness. In this respect it resemables the Danielli-Davson model, it however differs from the Daneilli-Davson model in that the protein is asymmetrical. On the outer surface is mucoprotein, while on the inner surface is non-mucoid protein.

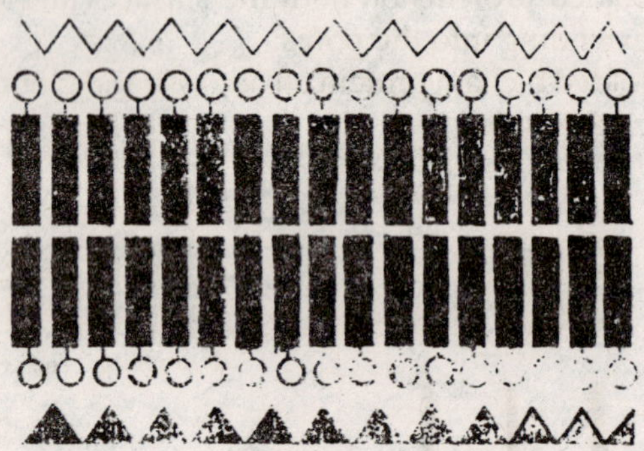

Fig. 2.4 Robertson's unit membrane model

Objections to unit membrane theory. Objections to the unit membrane model increased during the 1960s and this led to reexaminations of lipid-protein interactions and to new models. Studies of *F.S. Sjostrand* (1963), of smooth endoplasmic reticular, mitochondrial and chloroplast membranes underscored the differences between observed features of membranes and the uniformity that was required by the unit membrane concept. Mitochondrial and chloroplast membranes contain displays of particulate units in or on the membrane. The plasma membrane did not present the same appearance as mitochondrial or chloroplast membranes. It seemed that different models might be needed to describe different functional types. This unsuitable approach became unnecessary when a mosaic membrane model was proposed.

Fluid Mosaic Model

This model was proposed by *Singer* and *Nicolson* (1972). According to this concept, the lipid molecules are arranged to form a rather continuous bilayer that forms the structural framework of plasma membrane. The protein molecules are arranged in two different manners. Some proteins are located exclusively adjacent to the outer and inner surfaces of lipid bilayer and are called *extrinsic proteins*. Other proteins penetrate lipid bilayer partially or wholly and form *integral* or *intrinsic proteins*.

The lipids and integral proteins of plasma membrane are *amphipatic* in nature. The term amphipaty was coined by *Hartley*, (1936) for those molecules which have both hydrophobic and hydrophilic groups. The amphipatic molecules tend to constitute liquid crystalline aggregates in which hydrophobic or non-polar groups are situated inside the bilayer, and hydrophilic groups are directed towards the water phase. Therefore, the lipid molecules form a rather continuous bilayer. The integral proteins are intercalated in the lipid bilayer, with their polar regions protruding from the surface and non-polar regions embedded in the lipid bilayer. This arrangement explains why the active sites of enzymes and antigenic glycoproteins are exposed to the outer surface of the membranes. The quasifluid structure of plasma membrane explains the movement of cluster of protein molecules of considerable size across the membrane.

Pores in Plasma Membrane : Plasma membrane is perforated by pores. These have a diameter of about 0.35 nm (nanometer), slightly larger than the sodium ions. Less than 0.1 per cent of the plasma membrane is perforated by pores while 99.9 percent of the cell surface is impenetrable for ions. Several models of structures of pores have been proposed. Some of them are:

1. *Structural pores*: These are permanent cylindrical holes that interrupt the otherwise continuous bilayer sheet.

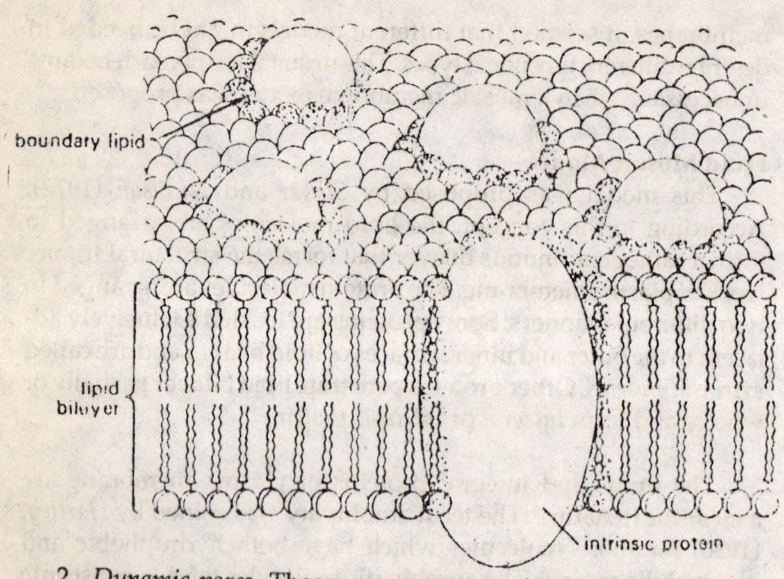

2. *Dynamic pores.* These pores are transient cylindrical holes rather than being permanent. These appear only at the time of intake.
3. *Paving block pores.* According to this concept the pores are regarded to be the corners of the closely filled nearly hexagonal paving blocks of lipid and protein subunits.
4. *Protein channel pores.* These pores are considered to be parts of the lipid-globular protein mosaic model. These form small channels of specific proteins embedded in the membrane through which ions and small molecules can diffuse.
5. *Ionophore.* The ionophores are small polypeptides whose one end is hydrophobic and other hydrophilic. The hydrophobic (outer) end dissolves in the membrane while the hydrophilic end (inner side) picks up ions or water-soluble materials and dumps them on the other side. The ionophores help in exchange of substances from or into the cells.

SPECIALIZATION OR MODIFICATIONS

With the increased resolution of the electron microscope numerous specialization of cell surface have been recognized (*Sjostrand* 1956; *Fawcett* 1958). Following description of *Fawcett*

(1958) deals with the various specializations of plasma membrane studied topographically.

Microvilli: In the intestinal epithelium microvilli are very prominent and form a compact structure that appears under the light microscope as a striated border. These microvilli, which are 0.6 to 0.8 um long and 0.1 um in diameter, represent cytoplasmic process covered by the plasma membrane. Within the cytoplasm core fine microfilaments are observed which in the subjacent cytoplasm form a terminal web. The outer surface of the microvilli covered by a coat of filamentous material (fuzzy coat) composed glycoprotein macro-molecules. Microvilli increase the effective surface of absorption. For example a single cell may have as many as 300 microvilli, and in a square millimetrer of intestine there may be 200,000,000. The narrow spaces between the microvilli form a kind of sieve through which substances must pass during absorption.

Numerous other cells, in addition to intestinal epithelium, have microvilli, although fewer in number. They have been found in mesothelial cells, in the epithelial cells of the gall-bladder, uterus, and yoik sac, in hepatic cells, and so forth.

The brush border of the kidney tubule is similar to the striated border, although it is larger in dimensions. An amorphous substance between the microvilli gives a periodic acid-Schiff reaction for polusaccharides. Between the microvilli, at the base, the cell membrane invaginates into the apical cytoplasm. These invaginations are apparently pathways by which large quantities of flow enter by a process similar to pinocytosis.

Desmosomes or Macula Adhaerens : Desmosomes are cell junctions found mainly in the cell of simple columnar epithelium. These occur as specialized areas along the contact surface. Under light microscope the desmosomes are seen as darkly stained bodies. Under electron microscope these appear as button-like thickenings on the inner surface of plasma membranes of adjacent cells at the point of contact.

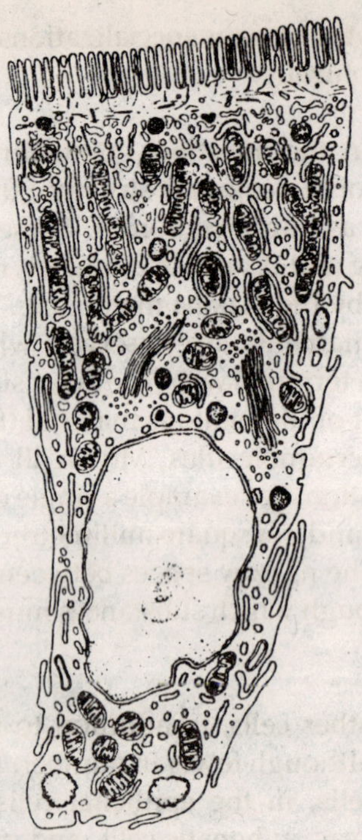

Fig. 2.6 An epithelial cell with microvilli.

The thickenings are traversed by fine cytoplasmic fibrils called *tonofibrils*, which form a kind of loop in a wide arc. These filaments stabilise the junction and act as anchoring sites for the cytoplasmic structures.

The plasma membranes of adjoining cells in the regions of desmosomes are separated by an intercellular space about 30-35 nm. It is filled with intervening dense coating material that forms a dark line in the middle. It is formed of mucopolysaccharides and proteins.

The desmosomes are primarily concerned with cell adhesion, but also help in maintaining cell-shape, providing it rigidity and cellular support. The former is brought about by the intercellular coating substance and the latter by the tonofibrils.

Plasmodesmata : Sometimes, the cells are joined by bridges of cytoplasm passing between pores of cell wall or plasma membrane between the adjacent cells, such connections are called plasmodesmata. They are usually simple but anastomosing phasmodesmata may also be found. Their distribution and number may also very considerably. They were discovered by *Tangl* (1879) and were named as such by *Strasburger* (1882). Endoplasmic reticulum often is closely associated with the cell surface, at the point where plasmodesmata are present. Through them cytoplasmic continuity is often maintained among the adjacent cells. They provide a mean for interaction between adjacent cells which are separated in other regions. Through them the material can pass from cell to cell.

It is not known whether all plasmodesmata are similar to each other. There exist some differences because they are not only produced at the time when cell divides but also formed spontaneously between cells that have grown into contact with one another, e.g. tyloses in xylem vessel elements. They may occur singly or they can be aggregated into groups. In many primary walls, the plasmodesmata are usually associated with a reduced deposition of wall material, and the area then is known as primary pit or field.

Hemidesmosomes: These are found in the basal surface of some epithelial cells. Their structure is similar to desmosomes but these are represented by one half; their counterpart is usually represented by collagen fibrils.

Terminal bars : The terminal bars are also known as intermediary junction or *zonula adhaerens*. The terminal bars are similar to desmosomes except they lack in the tonofibrils. In terminal bar the plasma membrane is thickened and the cytoplasm of thickened area is dense. The terminal bars occur in the intermediary portion of the plasma membrane of columnar cells just below the surface. The correct identity of zonula adhaerens is still questionable (*J.P. Trinkaus*, 1969).

Membrane Interactions: Another aspect of cell membranes that deserve discussion is the interaction between membranes of different cells. Intercellular communication is important in many cell function and especially during development of the organism, when cells are constantly interacting with other cells. The nature of membrane interaction may vary from complete cytoplasmic bridges between cells as localized areas of membrane junctions that may involve an area of contact as small as a few angstroms or as large as several micrometers. The structural nature of the actual contact generally falls into one of three categories: gap junctions, tight junctions, and septate junctions.

Gap junctions appear as multilayered structures when observed with the electron microscope. They appear to be two unit membrane closely apposed to each other with a 20 to 40 Å gap between. The total thickness of the entire gap junction is 170 to 190Å, and they are found in both vertebrates and invertebrates. They are not found in skeletal muscle fibres or red blood cells.

Tight junctions are found only in vertebrates and occur in cells such as epithelial cells. These junctions appear to be true fusions between the two membranes, and they are 100 to 140 Å thick.

Septate junctions have been found only in invertebrates. They are much larger than the other types of junctions and are characterized by electron-dense cross bridges that extend between the two cell membranes.

PERMEABILITY OF MEMBRANES

The membranes of a cell pass small ions and molecules through them. The passage of ions or molecules may occur as passive diffusion, or active transport evolving the expenditure of energy. In passive diffusion, membranes may be classed according to their degree of permeability.

(1) *Impermeable.* A membrane of this kind allows nothing to pass through it. Certain unfertilized fish eggs, such as trout, are permeable only to gases, water labelled with deuterium does not penetrate the egg.
(2) *Semipermeable.* No cell membranes are in this category. A model membrane may be constructed to allow passage of water molecules, but no solute particles.
(3) *Selectively permeable.* Most membranes of the cell belong to

this category. Such membranes allow water and certain selected ions and small molecules to pass through, but prohibit other ions as well as small and large molecules.

(4) *Dialyzing membrane.* The endothelial cells and their basement membranes of the capillaries and nephron can act as a dialyzer. In this way hydrostatic pressure forces water molecules and crystalloids across the membrane down their concentration gradients while restricting the passage of colloids.

Membrane Function : In order to survive, the cell must exchange with its environment. Metabolic essentials, such as oxygen salts, and nutrients, must get into the cell, and waste products, such as carbon dioxide and other metabolites, must pass out of the cell. All of these exchanges take place across the cell membrane by a variety of processes. Although it is really not possible to present one unifying concept of membrane transport, it is reasonable to group the membrane transport phenomena by the type of molecule being regulated.

Passive Diffusion. Passive diffusion is straight diffusion of water, O_2, or CO_2 through the cell membrane from an area of greater concentration to an area of lower concentration. The rate and speed of the diffusion is generally proportional to the difference in concentration of the substance between the two regions. When the concentration in both regions becomes equal, net diffusion ceases.

Free Diffusion : According to a large number of evidences, many substances move though membranes at rates of free diffusion that are directly proportional to their solubility in lipid. Water molecules are a notable exception to this rule, since they freely diffuse through membranes regularly and rapidly. It has been suggested that membranes contain 1 nm-wide pores that are lined by hydrophilic residues. Such openings would be large enough for water molecules but would hardly accommodate other water-soluble substances to pass through the narrow passageway. The suggestion is quite logical to explain diffusion of water through membranes, but there is little direct evidence to support the concept.

Free diffusion along a concentration gradient could be maintained for entry and exit of metabolites and waste products as long as substances were changed or washed away to keep one end of the gradient lower in concentration. If metabolites are chemically changed on entering the cell, then the concentration of the metabolite remain high outside the cell and is kept low inside the cell if it is not retained in its original form. Similarly, wastes leaving the cell could continue to move from the higher concentration inside as long as these substances were washed away or removed somehow from the immediate vicinity of the cell.

Facilitated Diffusion. Certain substances, such as glucose and amino acids, also move acros the membrane as a function of a concentration differential. However, these substances do so only up to a certain concentration level. When the concentration of glucose outside the cell surpasses a certain level, the rate of diffusion no longer increases. It has been suggested that this is because certain specific reactive sites on the cell surface and saturated with the glucose molecules. This theory proposes that there are specific membrane-associated carrier molecules that complex with the glucose and "facilitate" its diffusion into the cell.

Active Transport. Active transport often involves charged ions, such as Na + and K +, and electrolytes. These substances do not necessarily move across the cell membrane in response to a concentration differential. In fact, active transport is a mechanism that promotes the movement against a concentration gradient and results in the buildup of a marked concentration differential. Because active transport is a process that works against a concentration gradient, it is not surprising to learn that it requires the expenditure of energy. The process involves the use of carrier molecules within the cell membrane proper. These molecules apparently shuttle back and forth between the inner and outer cell membrane surfaces and either pick up to release the particular molecule being regulated. This entire process involves the expenditure of energy according to the equation ATP —> ADP + P_1 + energy.

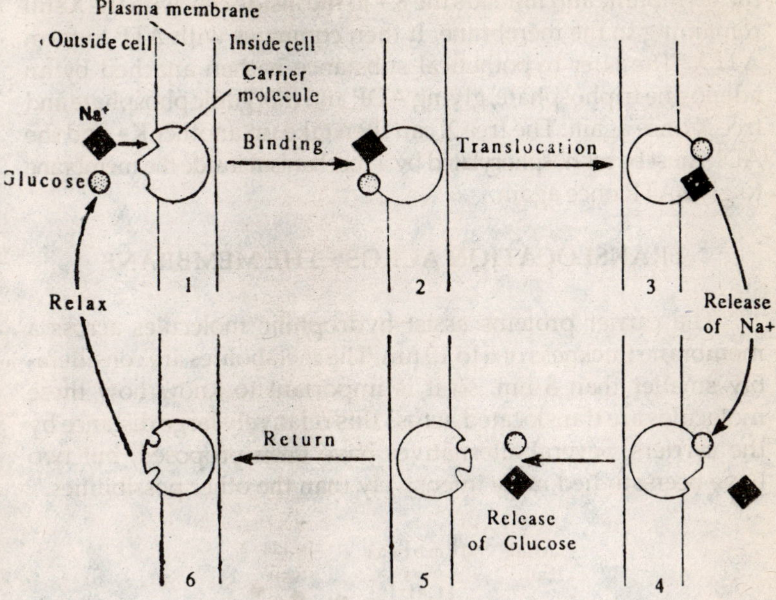

Fig. 2.7. Sodium Pump

Ion Pump. Potassium ions, often, suggest that there must be energy available for such a "pumping" mechanism. *Hepel* observed in 1939 that in animls fed with potassium-deficient diet, the muscle cells exchange almost 50 per cent of their K + by sodium (Na) even though under normal circumstances, these cells are practically impermeable to sodium ion. The passage of Na + could be carried out exclusively by an active process, which is sometimes called the "sodium pump". Because there is a good evidence that other ions may be transported by a similar mechanism. We can speak in general of an "ion pump". Such a mechanism was postualated by *Hober* in 1911 under the name of "Physiological permeability". There is a carrier molecule `X'.

What this carrier X might be is unknown, but in the case of Na+ and K+ transport, it is now thought possibly to be ATP itself or an ATPX compound. The entire mechanism could work as shown in the figure 2.7.

K+ combines with X to form K+-X, which then moves across the membrane and unloads the K+ to the inside cell, with the X still remaining in the membrane. It then combines with ATP to form ATPX. The later hypothetical substance is then attached by an adenosine triphosphate, giving ADP and inorganic phosphate and free X once again. The free X can then take up another K+ and the ADP must be rephosphorylated by a mechanism inside the membrane to give ATP once again.

TRANSLOCATION ACROSS THE MEMBRANE

The carrier proteins assist hydrophilic molecules across a membrane thickness of 6 to 10 nm. The metabolites are considerably smaller than 6 nm, so it is important to know how these molecules are translocated across this relatively large distance by the carriers. Several alternatives have been proposed, but two have been studied more intensively than the other possibilities.

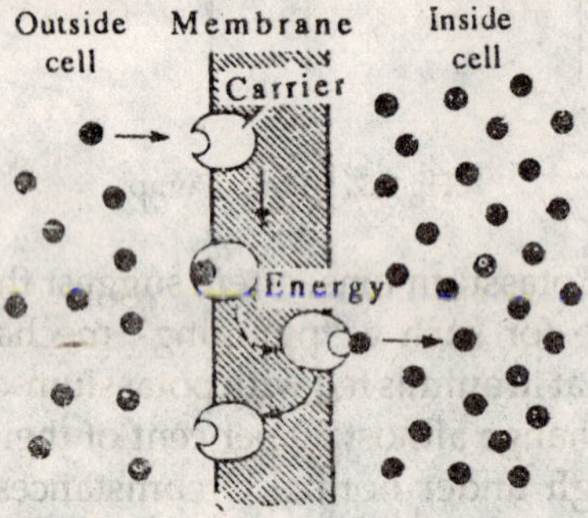

Fig. 2.8. Showing translocation across the Membrane

One alternative hypothesis postulates that the carrier binds with the hydrophilic molecule and that then the entire transport protein rotates across the membrane and delivers its bound metabolite to the other side. The second alternative proposes that the carrier is fixed in place within the membrane, and that the carrier molecule undergoes a conformational change that translocated the binding site across the membrane and the bound metabolite along with it at the same time. Once the metabolite has been translocated the binding site is freed and restored to its original conformation, ready to bind another hydrophilic molecule in another transport event. This second alternative has been referred to as the *fixed pore mechanism*. The first alternative is known as the *carrier mechanism*.

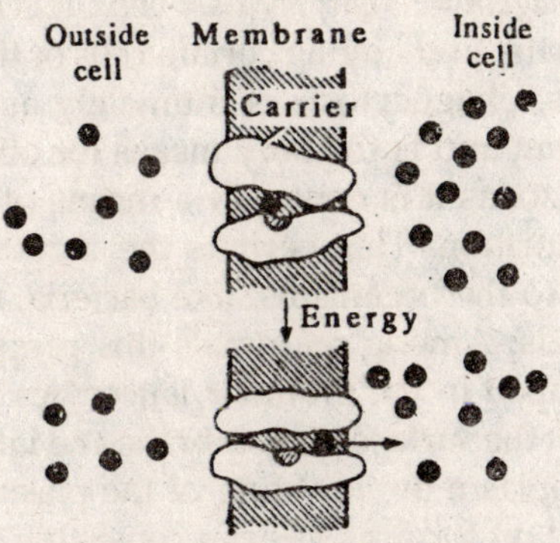

Fig. 2.9. Showing the fixed pore mechanism

Transport by Vesicle Formation : Most cell membranes can enclose materials in vesicles and bring the substances into the cell in this way, or package materials for discharge from the cell in a reverse process. The process is called *endocytosis* when materials are brought in, and *exocytosis* when vesicle discharge takes place. Endocytosis has features that are analogous to active transport.

For example, substances enter along an "uphill" concentration gradient, and energy is required to support the process. Endocytosis will stop if poisons that stops energy production in the cell are added, and the process can be stimulated by the addition to ATP to cells in suspension.

Various cell secretions are discharged from the cell by exocytosis. The mucus droplets of intestinal goblet cells, digestive enzyme precursors in granule package from pancreatic cells, and other cell secretions leave the cells in which they are produced by this general pathway. Although more difficult to see by light microscopy, numerous endocytotic infolded regions can be seen along the plasma membrane in suitable electron micrographs.

According to the nature of intake of food or foreign substances, the endocytosis may be classified into types:

(i) *Phagocytosis*. In some cases, cells may ingest rather larger, solid particles through plasma membrane. This activity is called *phagocytosis* (Gr. *Phagein* = to eat; Kytos = cell). It is found in large number of protozoans and among certain cells of the metazoans. Among metazoans, phagocytosis is intimately associated with amoeboid movement and is the only means for obtaining nutrition. Among metazoans it is generally a means of defence than serving the cell nutrition. This permits the ingestion of bodies which are foreign to the organisms, like bacteria, dust particles and various colloids. Among mammals this property is found very highly developed in the granular leucocytes. The particles become absorbed at the surface of membrane and later on they are taken into the cytoplasm by infolding of the plasma membrane which soon pitched off forming vesicles consisting of the particle envelope by a membrane. The vesicle so formed may then fuse and assume various sizes, or they may fragment.

Is the contact of transportant enough to stimulate the sequence of events culminating in the formation of vesicle? Certainly not. Whatever information available clearly indicate that the organism or substance to be phagocytized must be *cationic* in nature. There are, however, cases when the trasportant is not cationic in nature (for instance eating of bacterium by W.B.C.). In such cases it has been observed that the transportant first become coated by a phagocytosis-promoting substance (*Menkin*, 1956). The substance is called *opsonin*, which is cationic in charge.

Kinds of phagocytosis. According to the physical and chemical nature of foreign substance following types of phagocytosis have been recognised:

(a) *Ultraphagocytosis or colloidopexy*. The process in which plasma membrane ingests smaller colloidal particles is known as *colloidopexy* or *ultraphagocytosis*, e.g., leucocytes and the macrophagic cells of *mammals*.

(b) *Chromopexy*. When the ingestion of fluid material in bulk takes place by the cell through the plasma membrane, the process is known as *chromopexy*, e.g. some mesoplastic cells.

(ii) *Piocytosis*. When the ingestion of fluid material in bulk takes place by the cell through the plasma membrane, the process is known as *pinocytosis* (*Gr. pinein* = to drink). The process of pinocytosis was first of all observed by *Edward* in A moeba and by *Lewis* (1931) in the cultured cells.

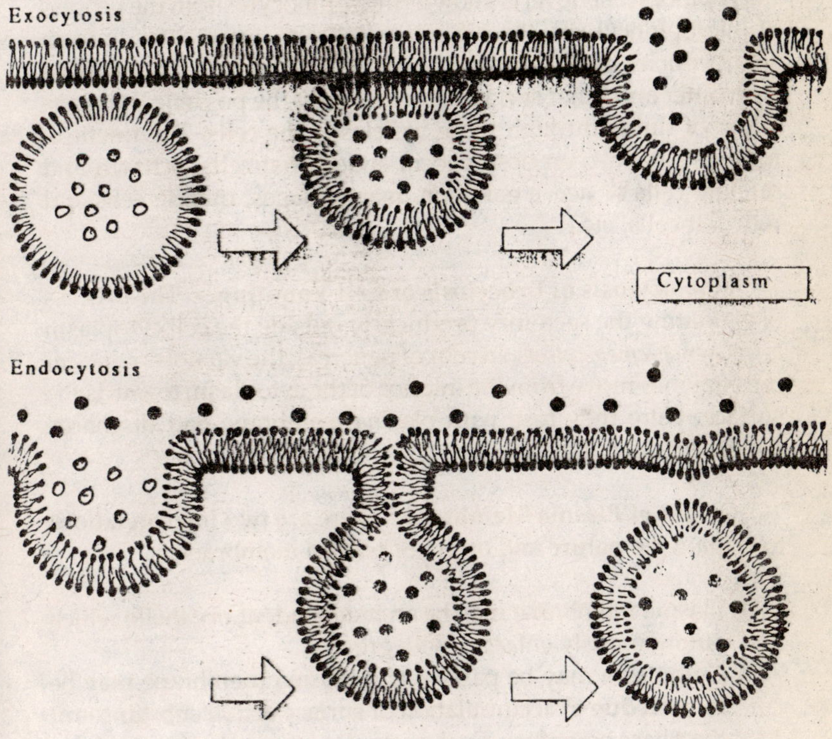

Fig. 2.10. Showing exocytosis and endocytosis

In the process of pinocytosis, the particle free globules of fluid are surrounded and ultimately engulfed by the clasping folds of the cytoplasm. The plasma membrane forms membranous vacuoles around the fluid globules. Such membrane-bound vacuoles are called *pinosomes* (*Lewis*, 1931). The pinosomes, later on, are transported to the interior of the cell where they are fused with the secretory granules or lysosomes. In the food vacuoles the digestion of food substances takes place and the digested food is diffused to the surrounding cytoplasm. The pinocytosis can be observed ordinary in the cells by light microscopy.

Micropinocytosis. Elecron microscopic observation have been made on the pinocytotic process at sub-cellular or sub-microscopic level in the cells. The pinocytosis which occurs at sub-micropinocytosis level is know as micropinocytosis. In the process of micropinocytosis, the plasma membrane invaginates to form small vesicles of 650Å diameter. These vesicles have openings on both outer and inner surfacs which suggest the possible transportation of fluids through these vesicles to the cells. The micropinocytosis have been observed in endothelial cells, Schawn and satellite cells of nerve ganglion, macrophages, muscle cells and reticular cells, etc.

Emeiocytosis or Exocytosis or Cell Vomiting : The process of exudating the secretory products to outside the cell cytoplasm is known as *emeiocytosis*. In cells of pancreas, the vacuoles containing enzymes move from the interior of the cytoplasm towards the surface. Here they fuse with plasma membrane and discharge their contents to the exterior.

Origin of Plasma Membrane : There are two interpretations to explain the nature and origin of plasma membrane:

(1) Plasma membrane may be an independent organelle which autonomously enlarges with growth.
(2) Cytoplasm may be passive and plasma membrane may be formed due to accumulation of surface active substances at the phase boundary. Such an explanation gets support from the observation that a new plasma membrane is formed wherever it is destroyed, resulting into new plasma surface. However, requisite quantities of lipoproteins must be present in the ground plasm, for the formation of plasma membrane.

A relationship between plasma membrane and other cell organelles has been postulated. In many cases, connections between plasmalemma and endoplasmic reticulum (ER) and also between plasmalemma and nuclear envelope have been shown. It has also been suggested that plasmalemma could give rise to endoplasmic reticulum. However, according to *Frey-Wyssling* and *Muhelethaler* (1955), published micrographs do not clearly settle this tissue. Therefore, it is doubtful whether or not there is a direct connection between plasmalemma and ER, but such a connection with Golgi membranes has been shown.

3

MITOCHONDRIA

Kolliker (1880) was the first who observed the granules (mitochondria) in muscle cell of insects. *Flemming* (1882) named the mitochondria as *fila*. *Altmann* in 1894 observed them and they were called *Altmann's granules bioplasts*. The term mitochondria was applied by *Benda* (1897-98) to these granules which were described as *cytomicrosomes* by *Velette St. George*. *Benda* stained mitochondria with alizarin and crystal violet. *Kingsbury* (1912) related them to cellular respiration and *Warburg* (1913) observed the presence of respiratory enzymes. In 1934 *Bensley* and *Horr* isolated mitochondria from liver cells and *Porter* and *Palade* described their electron microscopic structure.

Distribution. Ordinarily mitochondria are evenly distributed in the cytoplasm. They may, however, be localized in certain regions. In proximal convoluted tubules of the kidney they are found in the basal region of the cell, opposite the renal capillaries. In skeletal muscles they lie between the myofibrils. In insect flight muscle several large mitochondria are in contact with each fibril. In cardiac muscle the mitochondria are situated in clefts between the myofibrils, numerous lipid droplets are associated with the mitochondria. In many sperms the mitochondria fuse into one or two structures which lie in the middle piece of the tail, surrounding the axil filament. In columnar or prismatic cells they are oriented parallel to the long axis of the cell. In leucocytes they are radially arranged.

MORPHOLOGY

Shape. The shape is variable but is characteristic for a cell or tissue type, this too is dependable upon environment or physiological conditions. In general they are *filamentous* or *granular*. They may swell out at one end to become club-shaped or hollow out at one end to assume a shape of tennis racket. They may become vesicular by the appearance of central clear zone. Rod-shaped mitochondria are also observable.

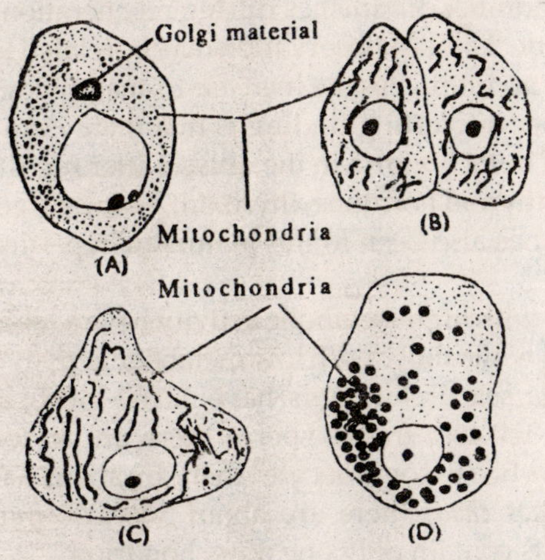

Fig. 3.1. Different sha pes and sizes of mitochondria

Size. The size of mitochondria also varies. In majority of the cells, width is relatively constant, about 0.5μ, but the length varies and, sometimes, reaches a maximum of 7μ. The size of cell also depends on the functional stage of the cell. Very thin mitochondria, about 0.2μ, or thick rods 2μ are also seen. The size and shape of the fixed mitochondria are determind by the osmotic pressure and pH of the fixative. In acid, pH mitochondria are fragmented and become vesicular. Mitochondria, in the rat-liver, are usually 3.3μ in length; in mammalian exocrine pancreas, they are about 10μ in length and in oocytes of Amphibia, they are approximately of the length of 20 to 40μ.

Number. Mitochondria are found in the cytoplasm of all aerobically respiring cells with the exception of bacteria in which the respiratory enzymes are located in the plasma membrane. The mitochondria content of a cell is difficult to determine, but in general, it varies with the cell type and functional stage. It is estimated that in liver mitochondria constitute 30 to 35 per cent of the total protein content of the cell and in kidney, 20 per cent. In lymphoid tissue the value is much lower. In mouse liver homogenates there are about 8.7 x 10^{10} mitochondria per gram of fresh tissue. A normal liver cell contains about 1000 to 1600 mitochondria, but this number diminishes during regeneration and also in cancerous tissue. This last observation may be related to decreased oxidation that accompanies the increase to anaeròbic glycolysis in cancer. Another interesting finding is that there is an increase in the number of mitochondria in the muscle after repeated administration of the thyroid hormone, thyroxin. An increased number of mitochondria has also been found in human hyperthyroidism.

Thus cells with high metabolic activity have a high number of mitochondria, while those with low metabolic activity have lower number. Large sea urchin eggs have 13000-14000, while renal tubules have 300-400. In the sperm there are as few as 20-24 mitochondira while in some oocytes there are about 300,000. In the protozoan *Chaos chaos* there are about 5000,000 mitochondria. Some algal cells contain only one mitochondrion.

STRUCTURE OF MITOCHONDRIA

A typical mitochondrion is sausage shaped with an average diameter of about 0.5μ. When it is properly fixed in osmimum containing fluid and studied under electron microscope it reveals that there is hardly any difference between plant and animal mitochondria. In both the cases the mitochondrion is bound by two membranes, the *outer membrane* and the *inner membrane.* The space between the two membranes is called the outer chamber or *inner-membrane* space. It is filled with the watery fluid, and is 40-70Å in width. The space bound by the inner chamber is called the *inner chamber* or *inner membrane space.* The inner membrane spaces is filled with a matrix which contains dense granules (300-500Å), ribosomes and mitochondrial DNA. The granules consist of insoluble inorganic salts and are believed to be the binding sites of divalent ios like Mg ++ and Ca++.

In some cases they apparently contain polymers of sugars. The side of the inner membrane facing the matrix side is called the *M-side,* while the side facing the outer chamber is called the *C-side.*

Two to six circular DNA molecules have been identified within mitochondria. These rings may either be in the open or in the twisted configuration. They may be present free in the matrix or may be attached to the membrane. The enzymes of the Krebs' cycle are located in the matrix.

The inner membrane is thrown up into a series of folds, called *cristae mitochondriales*, which project into the inner chamber. The cavity of the cristae is called the *intercristal space*, and is continuous with the *inter-membrane space*.

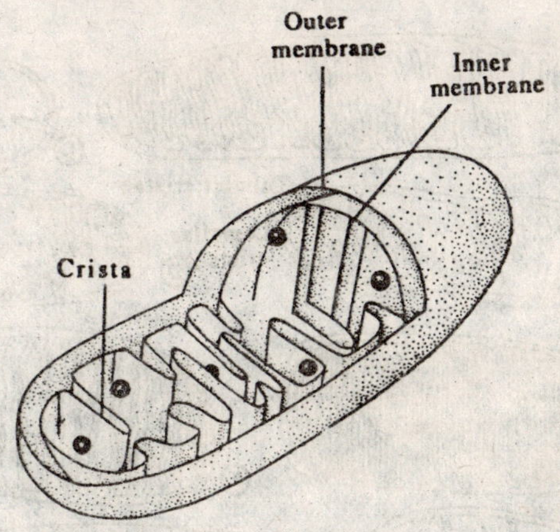

Fig. 3.2 Showing the structure of a mitochondria

Mitochondrial Cristae

The space and arrangement of crests is variable and may be of the following types:

(i) Parallel to the long axis of mitochondria as in the neurons and the striated muscle cells.
(ii) Concentrically arranged as in the matrix of certain spermatids.
(iii) Interlaced to form villi as in *Amoeba*.
(iv) Cristae in the form of vesicles which form a network of interconnected chambers as in the cells of parathyroid gland and W.B.C. of man.

(v) Arranged in a tubular fashion but perpendicular to mitochondrial axis as in the cells of adrenal gland.
(vi) Haphazardly distributed as in the cells of kidney of insects and hepatic cells.
(vii) Cristae extremely small and irregular as in the interstitial cells of *Opossum*.
(viii) Rarely the mitochondrial wall is smooth with no cristae. The number and size of cristae in a mitochondrion directly affects its efficiency. The greater and larger are the cristae, the faster is the speed of oxidation reaction.
(ix) Perpendicular to the long axis of mitochondria.

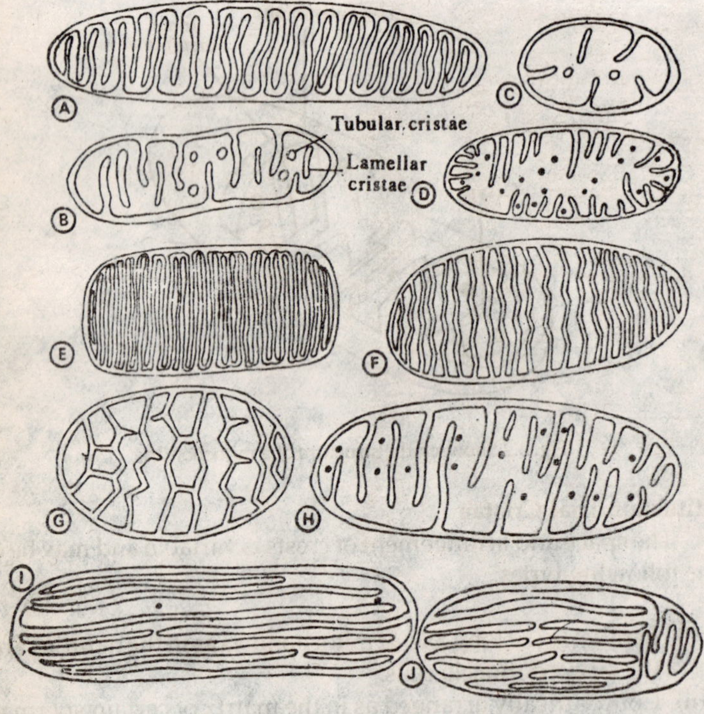

Fig. 3.3 Structural variations in mitochondrial cristae. A tubular cristae, B lamellar cristae C. cristae in salamander D. Plate like cristae E. parallel cristae F. cristal with sharp angulation G. Honey corubs cristae, H. usual cristae I. longitudinal cristae J. transverse and longitudinal cristae.

Mitochondrial particles

According to earlier descriptions (*Green* and *Perdue*, 1966) the outer surface of the outer membrane and the inner surface of the inner membrane were supposed to be covered with thousands of small particles. Those on the outer membrane were described as being stalkless and were called the *subunits of Parson*. There may be as many as 10,000 to 100,000 particles per mitochodrion. The stalked inner membrane particles were called the *subunits of Fernandez-Moran, elmentary particles, F_1 particles* or the *oxiosomes* or *ETP* or *electron transport particles*. These particles are about 85A° in diameter and are regularly spaced at intervals of 10 nm on the inner membrane. There may be as many as 10^4 to 10^5 elementary particles per mitochondrion.

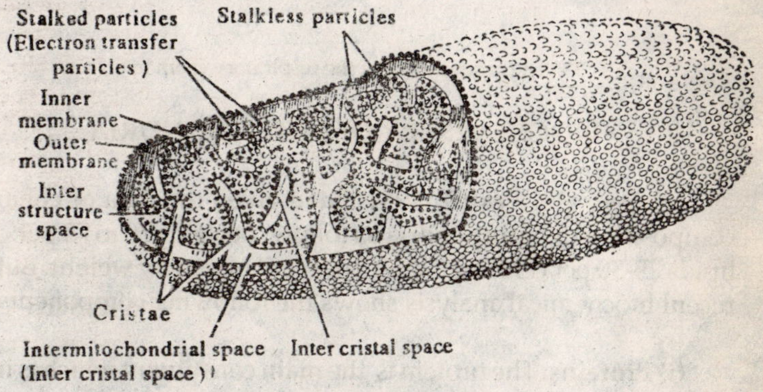

Fig. 3.4 Showing mitochondrial particles

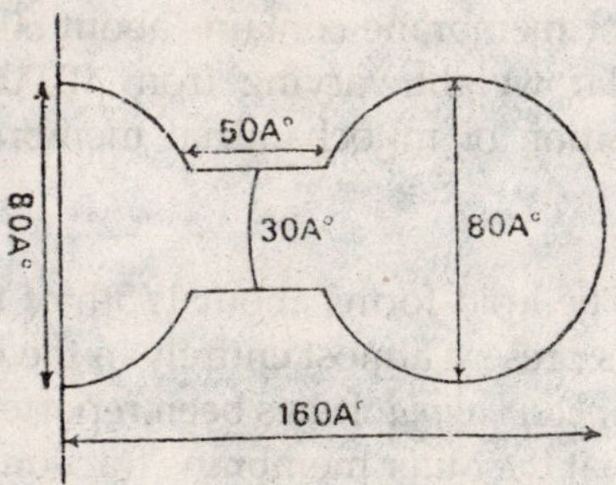

Fig. 3.5 Structure and measurements of the mitochondrion particles

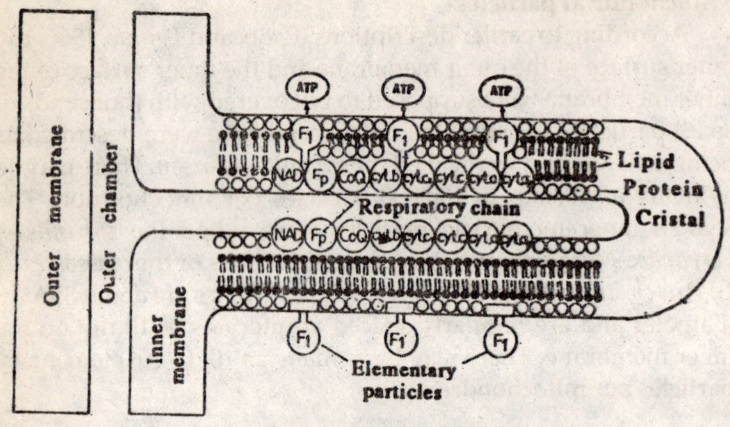

Fig. 3.6 The arrangement of the respiratory chain in cristae

BIOCHEMISTRY OF MITOCHONDRIA

Lindberg and *Ernster* (1954) have given the data of chemical composition of mitochondria as follow: proteins 70 to 75 per cent, lipids 25-30 per cent, and RNA 5 per cent of the dry weight. But the recent biochemical analysis shows the following components:

(i) Proteins. The protein is the main constituent which is insoluable in water. The outer limiting membrane of mitochondria contains less than 10 per cent of the total protein. There are about 14 different proteins having molecular weight from 12,000 to 22,000. The inner membrane contains about 60 per cent protein having molecular weight varying from 10,000 to 90,000. The protein composition of mitochandrial membranes is not fully known.

(ii) Lipid. The lipid forms about 1/5th of the weight of the membranes. It is present almost entirely in the form of the molecules known as *phospholipid*. It has been reported by *Meluick* and *Packer* in 1971 that the outer membrane fraction has a 40 per cent lipid contents as compared to 20 per cent in the inner membrane.

(iii) Enzymes. About 70 enzymes and 12 co-enzymes have

been recognized in the mitochandria. Enzymes lie in a non aqueurs membrane. region as solid arrays, with perhaps as many as 5000 to 20,000 such assemblages in a single liver or heart mitochondria.

Table 3.1 Localization of enzymes, obtained in fractionation studies

Mitochondrial fraction	*Enzymes located*
1. Outer membrane.	Monoamine oxidase "Rotenone-insensitive" NADH-cytochrome C reductase, Kynurenine hydroxylase, Fatty acid CoA ligase, Glycerolphosphate acyl transferase, Nucleoside diphosphokinase.
2. Inter membrane space.	Adenylate kinase, Nucleoside diphosphokinase, Respiratory chain enzymes.
3. Inner membrane.	Respiratory chain enzymes, B-Hydroxybutyrate, dehydrogenase, Ferrochelatase, Camitine palmityl-transferase, Fatty acid oxidation system, Xylitol dehydrogenase.
4. Matrix	Malate isocitrate and glutamate dehydrogenase, Fumarase, Aconitase, Citrate synthetase, Omithine-Carbomyl transferase, Fatty acid oxidation systems, Pyruvate carboxylase.

Mitochondrial DNA. Recently the DNA is also reported from mitochondria. The mitochondrial DNA is double stranded like the nuclear DNA. Each mitochondrion may contain one or more DNA molecules depending on its size. If, the mitochondrion is larger then that may have more DNA molecules, having a circular shape.

Mitochondrial DNA differs from nuclear DNA is several respects. The GC content is higher in mitochondrial DNA, and consequently the buoyant density is also higher. Another difference is the higher denaturation temperature of mitochondrial DNA and facility with which it denatures. The amount of genetic information carried by mitochondrial DNA is not sufficient to provide specification for all the proteins and enzymes present in this organoid. The most likely possibility is that mitochondrial DNA codes for some structural proteins.

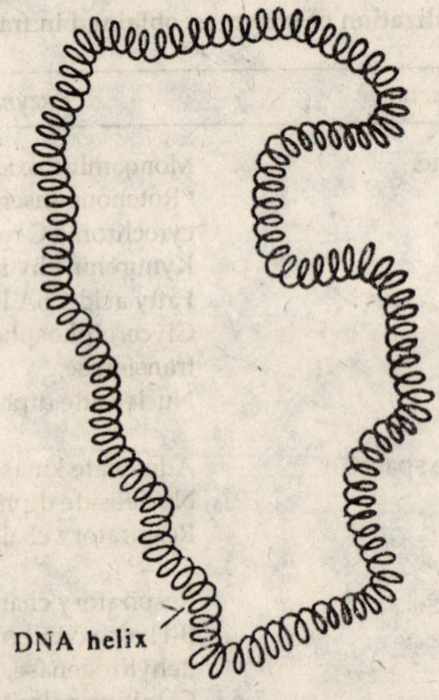

Fig. 3.7 Mitochandrial DNA

Yeast mitochondria have been shown to contain DNA polymerase (*Winters Berger*, 1966) and more recently *Kalf* '1968 has succeeded in isolating the enzymes from rat liver mitochondria. Mitochondrial DNA polymerase appears to be involved in DNA replication rather than repair (*Karol* and *Simpson* 1968) and possesses properties which are different from those of the nuclear enzymes. These include a differing requirement for metal ion (*Meyer* and *Simpson* 1968). Yeast mitochondrial DNA polymerase appears to be smaller than its nuclear counterpart, and is active at different stages of the cell cycle (*Iwashima* and *Rabinowitz*, 1969). Visual evidence showing what appears to be rat liver mitochondrial DNA in the process of replication has been presented by *Kirschner*, *Wolstenholme* and *Gross* (1968).

Mitochondrial DNA does not appear to have histones associated with it as has nuclear DNA of higher organisms. In this respect mitochondrial DNA resembles the bacterial DNA.

Mitochondrial RNA. *South* and *Mehlar* (1968) suggested that the amount of mt-RNA is about 10 to 20 times that of mt-DNA. All sorts of RNA have been identified in mitochondria. The present evidences point out conclusively that mitochondria contain complete set of t-RNA (*Wintersberger* and *Tuppy*, 1965), aminoacyl RNA synthetases (*Barnett, Braun* and *Epler*, 1967), as well as ribosomal RNA (*Rogers, Preston, Titchener* and *Linnane*, 1967). All these components differ from their respective counterparts in the groundplasm. The presence of m-RNA, transcribed from mitochondrial DNA is still uncertain. However, there are authorities who suggest its presence. Their ribosomal RNAs are coded for by mitochondrial DNA and are thus apparently synthesized within the mitochondria by a mitochondrial DNA-dependent RNA polymerase system (*Wintersberger*, 1964).

Mitochondrial Ribosomes. Mitochondria appear to contain ribosomes which are smaller in diameter than cytoplasmic ribosomes (*Swift*, 1965) and *Yeast* mitochondria contain RNA species of 35S and 16S (*Winter Berger* 1966) which would correspond to a 70S ribosome of bacterial type than rather the 80S ribosome of the cytoplasm. Ribosome like particles with sedimentation values of 81S and 55S have also been reported, and the extent of degradation suffered by the particles during isolation is not yet clear. Polysome like aggregation of ribosomes have been observed in sections of yeast mitochondria by *Vignais, Huet* and *Andre* in 1969. High molecular weight and RNA species associated with mitochondria which differ in sedimentation value from cytoplasmic ribosomal RNA have been reported in *Yeast, Neurospora* and *He-La cells*. Mitochondrial ribosom require a higher concentration of Mg^{++} ions to maintain their integrity than do cytoplasmic ribosomes.

Protein Synthesis. In general, mitochondria can code and synthesize protein, but the DNA present therein is insufficient to code for all the proteins. It is suggested that mitochondria can synthesize the proteins of structural nature (*cytochrome oxidase*), but much of the proteins if not all, of the soluble proteins of the matrix as well as the proteins of the outer membrane, and number of proteins located in the cristae (*Borst*, 1972) are under the control of nuclear DNA. Of the proteins coded by nuclear DNA, it is generally agreed that the m-RNA derived from nucleus are translated in the cytoplasm, and the resulting proteins are then transported into the mitochondria. How then protein enter the mitochondria? Two methods have been proposed:

(1) The precursors enter the mitochondrion and inside are changed into the end products, thereby affecting undirectional flow of material into the mitochondrion.
(2) There is the synthesis of lipoprotein vesicles which then merge and combine with the growing mitochondrion.

FUNCTIONS

1. Role of Mitochondria in Yolk Formation. There has been a good number of investigations, whose account reveals that, mitochondria help in the formation of yolk in a developing ovum. The first study in this field was made by *Loyez* (1911) and latest probably by *M.D.L. Srivastava* (1965), with the help of light microscope. The evidence adduced depends upon the topographical, and size relationship, and staining reactions of mitochondria and early proteid yolk.

In the modern cytology with the investigation of electron microscope a new era has started and the studies of yolk formation do not remain away from electron microscope. With the help of electron microscope *Farvard* and *Carasso* (1958) come to the conclusion that mitochondria was transformed into yolk granules in the egg of *Planorbis coneus*.

The main structural changes which they observed in the mitochondria are as follows.

(i) the cristae become disorganised in a few membranes, remaining concentric to the outer membrane before dropping completely,

(ii) In the matrix appeared a few minute granules which have scattered first, but become aggregated eventually in masses in regular pattern.

2. During Cell Division and Spermiogenesis. Early cytologists, *Benda, Dueberg* and *Meves* were of opinion that mitochondria also divide equally during the cytoplasmic division and perhaps play a part in inheritance.

Wilson (1928) commented that not the slightest proof has been produced of a fusion between the paternal and maternal chondrisomes. *Frederic* (1958) nas briefly summarized various changes in mitochondria during cell division. The first phase shows a decrease in the total volume of mitochondrial material; gradually ceases its movements, pronounced thinning, fragmentation into small spheres, loss of optical density and finally assimilation into the cytoplasm. In the second phase, when the cell divides into two, the modified mitochondria are separated passively, into the daughter cells. In the third phase, the modified mitochondria are reconstituted by addition of elements assimilated in the cytoplasm. Wilson found that in *Opisthacanthus*, during spermatogenesis, the number of mitochondria gradually reduces. *Pollister* (1930) describes in *Gerris* that mitochondria arranged themselves into a well defined ring, but without fusion. Modern microscopic studies provide firm conclusions regarding mitochondrial division during mitosis. *Pyne* (1952) noted in fowl adrenal cortex the mitochondria frequently appeared as pairs. This suggested that division, rather then fusion, was occurring. In the transformation of spermatids into spermatozoa many mitochondrial changes are observed. *Franzen* (1956) observed in those sperms, which are shed directly in water, that mitochondria are present in form generally of four or five spheres below the sperm head, and in the case of sperms discharged in viscous medium these spheres transform into two elongated ribbion like filamentous mitochondria. Sometimes these develop into *'nebenkern spheres'* which may elongate and twist around the axial filament to form the mitochondrial sheath. *Yasuzumi* (1958) found an electron opaque body within 'nebenkern' of spermatids of Drosophilla; it is described as 'indistinguishable from a lipid droplet.'

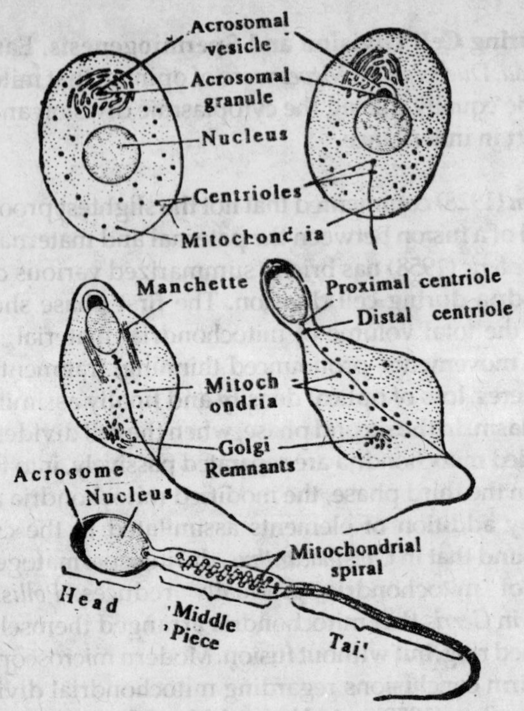

Fig. 3.8 Role of mitochondria during spermiogenesis.

3. Role of mitochondria in the production of energy. Mitochondria play a very important role in cellular respiration or the production of energy. Energy is produced inside the cell partly outside the mitochondria and mainly inside the mitochondria. The ATP molecules that are produced in the nonmitochondrial cytoplasm are generated by a process referred to as *anaerobic respiration*. Let us assume that the cell is going to break down one molecule of glucose and in the process extract all the possible energy from this molecule in the form of ATP. The breakdown of glucose starts in the nonmitochondrial cytoplasm and involves the splitting of glucose into two smaller molecules of *pyruvic acid* and the release of hydrogen atoms. In this process, there is a net production of two ATP molecules. At this point, the pyruvic acid may break down further to form either CO_2 and alcohol or two molecules of lactic acid, depending on the cell type. The process of *anaerobic* respiration is sometimes referred to as *glycolysis*. The breakdown of glucose by this pathway is not an efficient way to extract energy from the glucose. Indeed, the cell has an elaborate array of biochemical machinery that can take the two molecules of pyruvic acid as well as the hydrogen atoms released in the initial breakdown of glucose and generate 17 times as many ATP molecules as are produced by anaerobic respiration. This set of processes is collectively referred to as *aerobic respiration* and it occurs within the mitochondria.

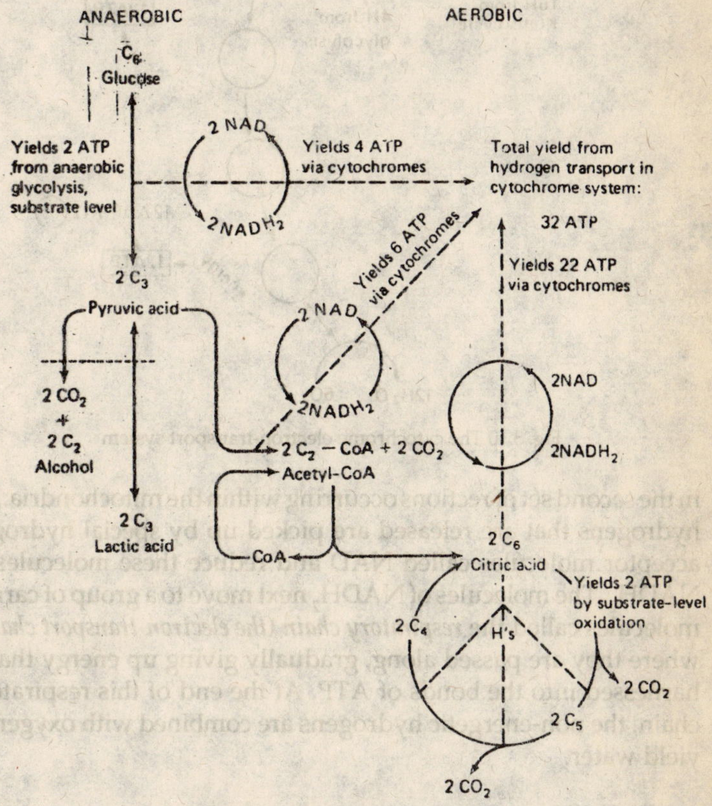

Fig. 3.9 Energy production showing both anaerobic and aerobic phases

There are two major groups of reactions involved in aerobic respiration. the first involves the hydrogens that were released earlier in the anaerobic process as well as those to be released later

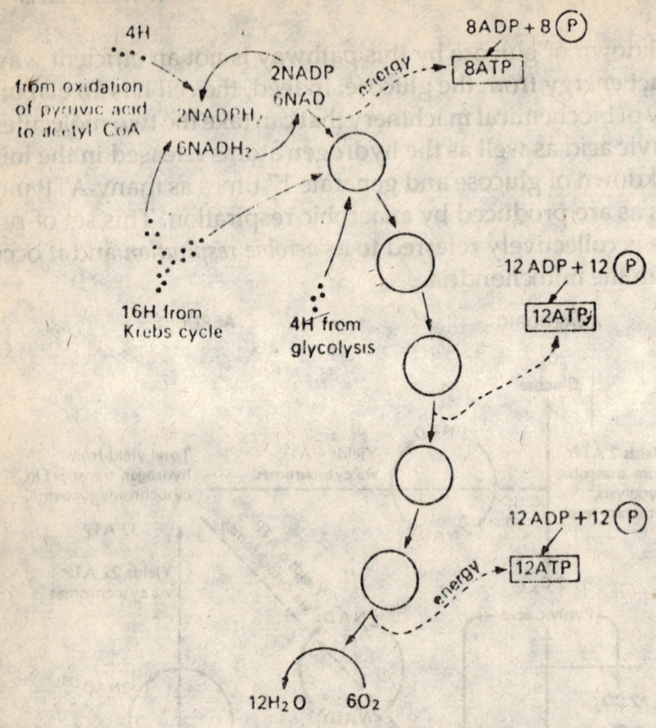

Fig. 3.10 The cytochrome electron-transport system

in the second set of rections occurring within the mitochondria. the hydrogens that are released are picked up by special hydrogen acceptor molecules called NAD and reduce these molecules to $NADH_2$. The molecules of $NADH_2$ next move to a group of carrier molecules called the *respiratory chain* (*the electron-transport chain*), where they are passed along, gradually giving up energy that is harnessed into the bonds of ATP. At the end of this respiratory chain, the non-energetic hydrogens are combined with oxygen to yield water.

The net result of this process is the production of three ATP molecules and H_2O for every two H^+.

The other major group of reactions involves the extraction of energy in the form of hydrogen from the pyruvic acid molecules. Instead of going on to form CO_2 and alcohol or lactic acid as in glycolysis, the pyruvic acids move into the mitochondria and react with an enzyme called coenzyme A to form two molecules of acetyl-CoA and CO_2. In the process of these reactions four hydrogens are released that are picked up by NAD (to form 2 $NADH_2$) and subsequently passed through the respiratory chain to yield ATPs.

The pyruvic acids are transported into the mitochondria and enter a cyclic group of reactions (called the *Krebs cycle*) that results in the generations of more hydrogens (and therefore more $NADH_2$ and more ATP via the respiratory chain). In addition, some ATP molecules are generated directly by the Krebs cycle. The end result is the production of 34 ATP molecules by the respiratory chain and the Krebs cycle—all of them just one molecule of glucose. One can certainly see how critical the mitochondria are for the generation of cellular energy. The breakdown of glucose by nonmitochondrial anaerobic respiration nets 2 ATPs, and by aerobic mitochondrial respiration, an addition 34 ATPs. The total number of ATPs produced in the breakdown of a single molecule of glucose can be as high as 36.

ORIGIN OF MITOCHONDRIA

Our understanding of the process whereby mitochondria are produced, is still very incomplete. *Lehninger* (1964) classified the various theories of possible routes of mitochondrial genesis into three main groups:

(1) Formation from other membranous structures in the cell,
(2) Growth and division of pre-existing mitochondria.
(3) *De novo* synthesis from submicroscopic precursors.

(1) Formation from other membranous structures in the cell. The formation of mitochondria by "pinching off" or budding from pre-existing cell structures has been suggested for a range of cell membranes including those of the plasmalęmma (*Robertson* 1959), endoplasmic reticulum, nuclear envelope, and Golgi complex (*Novikoff*, 1961). But the support for such evidence, in the absence of supporting biochemical data, can not be wholly conclusive. Part of the problem undoubtedly lies in our fragmentary knowledge of the structure and composition of, and differences between cell membranes in general. Indeed the similarities discussed in the literature between the mitochondrial membrane and the endoplasmic reticulum, could lend weight to the idea that probably mitochondria are formed when cytoplasm pushes into a cavity surrounded by an internal membrane, which then 'pinches off' and separates from the continuous system.

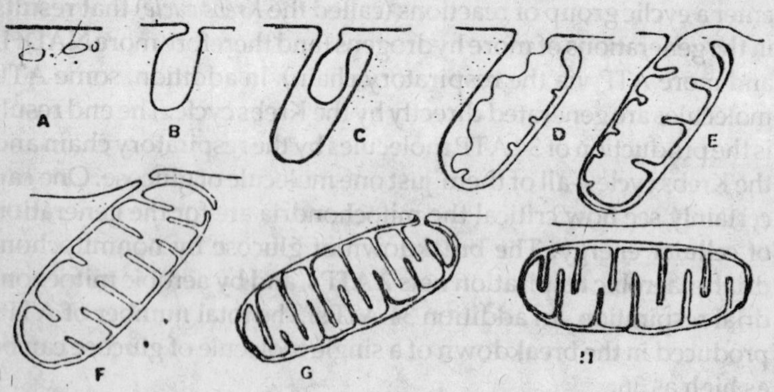

Fig. 3.11 A possible mechanism for the formation of mitochondria from the plasma membrane.

(2) Growth and division of pre-existing mitochondria. Electron microscopic evidence for mitochondrial division by fission, although plentiful is difficult to assess. The danger of producing artifacts is very real because of the harsh chemical and physical agents brought to bear on the test material during processing. Interpretation is not made easier by the ability of mitochondria to undergo extreme changes in shape in vivo which may or may not be associated with mitochondrial fission. There are numerous reports of mitochondria connected to each other by narrow bridges of membrane, especially in rapidly melopolizing tissue, and it is thought that such figures may represent mitochondria in an early stage of fission. By observing serial sections of rat liver *Stempak* (1967) was able to show that "dumb bell-shaped" mitochondria can be the sections of cup-shaped bodies. Such bodies have also been observed in rapidly growing tissues of fern and may represent the beginning stages of division.

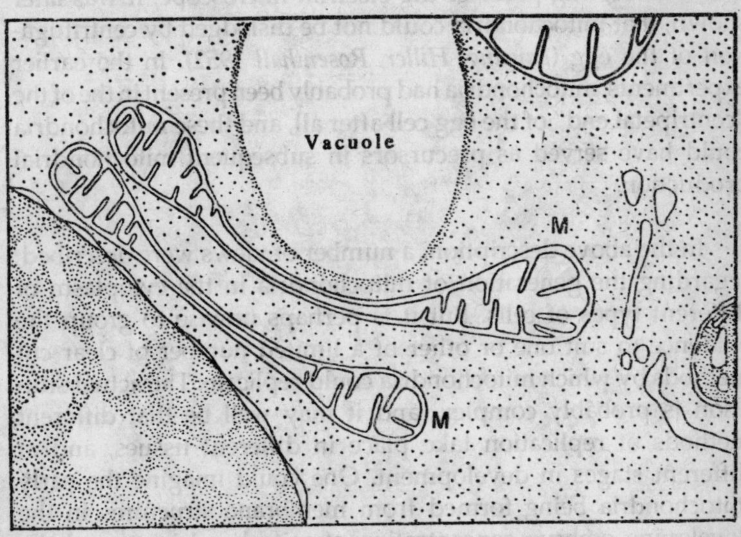

Fig. 3.12 Diagram showing the dividing mitochondria in developing callus tissue of fern

An early stage in mitochondrial division may involve the separation of mitochondrial contents into two or more compartments. The presence of mitochondria with internal "partitions" has been formed in several cell types (*Tandler* et. al., 1969) although the possibility that they are manifestations of mitochondrial fusion cannot easily be ruled out. *Lafontaine* and *Allard* (1964) have presented elections dividing the inner membrane complex into two masses, the whole being surrounded by continuous outer membrane. *Tandler et at* (1969) has demonstrated the partitions of mitochondria in liver which was recovering from riboflavin deficiency.

(3) De-novo synthesis. The possibility of *de-novo* synthesis of mitochondria arose with experiments in the early part of the century, when mitochondria containing larvae were seen to develop from sea urchin egg cytoplasm which had apparently been freed of mitochondria by centrifugation (*Novikoff* 1961). Using the greater resolving poser of the electron microscope, it was later shown, that mitochondria could not be dislodged by centrifugation of the egg (*Lansing, Hiller, Rosenthall* 1952). In the earlier experiments, mitochondria had probably been present in the of the "centripetal end" of the egg cell after all, and these mitochondria could have served as precursors in subsequent mitochondrial production.

In the above description, a number of views were described, regarding the generation of mitochondria in the cytoplasm of different types of cells. But it is perhaps unwise to group the evidence to suit one or other of a limited number of clear cut methods by which mitochondria could replicate. The actual situation is probably complex, and it may well be that different methods of replication take place in different tissues, and at different stages in development. One could imagine the early mitochondria being formed from membrane structures in the developing embryo concentration of mitochondria around the nuclear membrane have been noted in embryonic tissues from several phyla (*North* and *Pollak,* 1961) and formation of mitochondria from this membrane could involve the transfer of nuclear genetic information essential for subsequent mitochondrial growth and multiplication by division. the multiplication of mitochondria could then proceed by the incorporation of large pre-fabricated molecules and association of molecules, with division by fission, when the mitochondria reached a critical stage.

Prokaryotic Origin of Mitochondria. This fact that mitochondria can grown, divide and are capable of mutations support a long-held view that mitochondria originated with their host. Bacteria would have originated the mitochondria and blue green algae, the chloroplasts.There are numerous homologies between mitochondria and bacteria. In bacteria the electron transport system is localized in the plasma membrance which can be compared with the inner membrane of mitochondria. Some bacteria even have membranous projections extending from the plasma membrane (*Fitz-James,* 1960) which are comparable to mitochondrial crests since both contain the respiratory chain (*Salton* and *Chapman,* 1962). The inner membrance and matrix, it has been

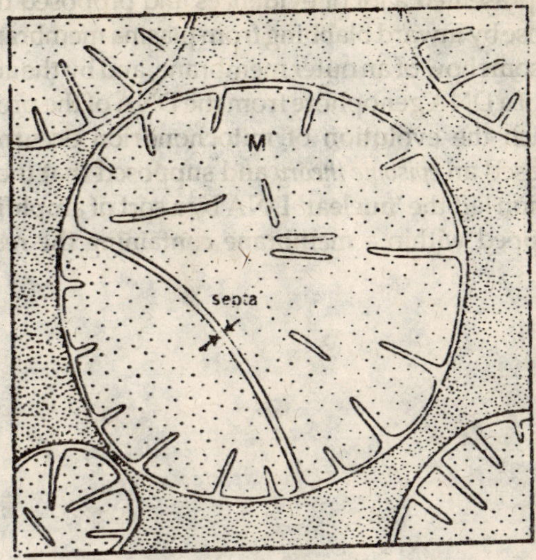

Fig. 3.13 A giant dividing mitochondria from the liver of a mouse

postulated may represent the original symbiont which may become enclosed within a membrane of cellular origin (ER). Further mitochondrial DNA is circular; it replicates and divides like that of bacteria. The ribosomes are also found which are, however, smaller than those of the bacteria. In mitochondria and bacteria, the protein synthesis is inhibited by chloramphenicol. From these similarities, one can easily conceive of mitochondria as being evolved from an ancient prokaryote (*Swift*. 1965), possessing all the attributes of an independent, probably aerobic organism. However, with the adaptation over a long period it became an essential and dependent symbiont, lost some of its identity to the cell, and conversely, the host cell lost some of its functions, deriving it now from the endosymbiont or mitochondrion. As a result, both became obligatory symbionts to each other.

This symbiont hypothesis for the origin of mitochondria and plastids has achieved wide popularity, but all biologists do not necessarily accept it. *Raff* and *Mahler* (1972) concluded that "while the symbiotic theory may be esthetically pleasing, it is not compelling." They presented a lot of evidences and proposed that mitochondria arose by inward blabbing from plasma membrane, by the acquisition somehow of an outer membrane, and by the additional acquisition of a DNA genophore from the DNA of the protoeukaryote in which the evolution of mitochondrion occurred. *Borst* (1972) proposed an *episome theory* and supposed that the DNA of mitochondrion left the 'nuclear' DNA by a sort of amplification to become mapped within a membrane containing the respiratory chain.

4

GOLGI COMPLEX

In 1898 by means of a silver staining method, *Golgi* discovered a reticular structure in the cytoplasm. The name *"Golgi apparatus"*, generally given to this structure, is confusing because it suggests a definite relationship with the physiological processes of the cell. Today it seems more appropriate to use the name *Golgi substance* or *Golgi complex*, to refer to this material that has special staining properties. Because its refractive index is similar to that of the matrix, the Golgi complex is difficult to observe in living cells. The use of the electron microscope has provided a distinct image of this component, and its submicroscopic structure has been revealed.

OCCURRENCE

The Golgi complex occurs in all cells except the prokaryotic cells (viz., mycoplasma, bacteria and blue green algae) and eukaryotic cells of certain fungi, sperm cells of bryophytes and pteridophytes, cells of mature sieve tubes of plants and mature sperm and red blood cells of animals. Their number per plant cell can vary from several hundred as a tissues of corn root and algal rhizoids (i.e., more than 25,000 in algal rhizoids, *Sievers*, 1965), to a single organelle in some algae. In animal cells, there usually occurs a single Golgi complex, however, developing oocytes of chordates may contain many Golgi bodies.

MORPHOLOGY

The morphology of the Golgi complex varies from cell to cell depending upon the type of cell in which they are found. Two forms of Golgi comples have been observed.

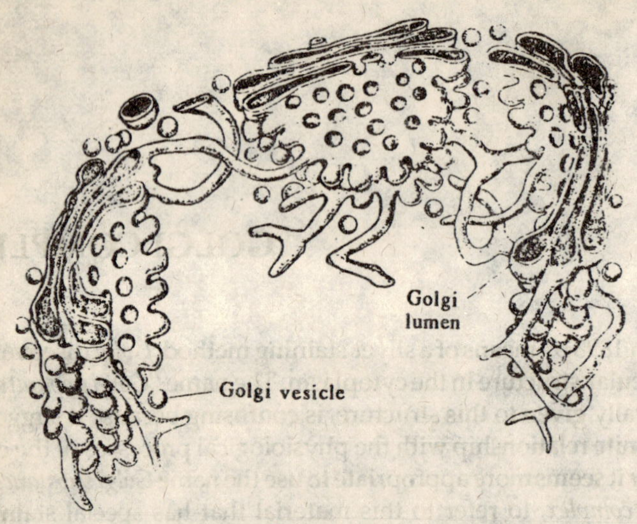

Fig. 4.1 Three dimensional representations of Golgi complex

1. Localized form. In polarised cells of vertebrates (which have base and apex), Golgi complex occurs singly and occupies a fixed position. It lies between the nucleus and secretory pole. This can be best seen in thyroid cells, in exocrine cells of pancreas and the mucous cells of intestine.

2. Diffused form. In some specialized cells of vertebrates (nerve cells and liver cells), in most plant cells and in the cells of invertebrates several units of Golgi complex are found scattered along with the elements of endoplasmic reticulum. Each unit is called a *dictyosome*. In liver cells there occur as many as 50 dictyosomes per cell and in certain plant cells their number may reach upto hundreds.

Shape. The shape of the Gogi complex is quite variable in different somatic cell types of animals. Even in the same cell there are variations in different functional stages. The shape is, however, constant with each cell type. It varies in form a compact mass to a disperse filamentous network.

Number. The number of Golgi stacks per cell varies enormously, depending on the cell type—from as few as one to the hundreds. There is a single large in some cells while in the case of *Paramoeba* there are two. In *Stereomyxa* (a species of *Amoeba*) there are many Golgi complexes. Nerve cells, liver cells and most plant cells also have multiple Golgi complexes, there being about 50 in liver cells. The Golgi complex can even account for a large fraction of the cell volume in some specialized cells. One example is the goblet cell of the intestinal epithelium, which secretes mucus into the gut; the glycoproteins in mucus are glycosylated principally in the Golgi complex.

Size. The size is likewise very variable. It is large in the nerve and gland cells and small in the muscles cells. In general the Golgi complex is well developed while the cell is in active state. When the cell grows old, the apparatus progressively diminishes in size and disappears.

Position. The position of the Golgi complex is relatively fixed for each cell type. In the cells of ectodermal origin, the Golgi complex is polarized from the time of the embryonic state between the nucleus and the periphery (*Cajal*, 1914). In the secretory exocrine cells that have in general a typical polarization the Golgi complex is found between the nucleus and the secretory pole. In the endocrine glands the polarity of this organoid is variable, except in the thyroid, where is oriented towards the centre of the follicle. In the younger cells and often in the older ones it lies most commonly at one side of the nucleus but in certain cases many completely surround it. In ganglionic cells of the mouse the position is perinuclear.

DETAILED STRUCTURE OF GOLGI COMPLEX

Dalton and *Felix* (1954) described the Golgi complex in the epididymis of the rat after taking the first electron micrographs. The following description of the Golgi complex is a composite one based on the work of several authors.

1. Cisternae : The cisternae or saccules are similar to the smooth surface ER, and appear in section as stacks of closely spaced membrane delimited sacs. The number of saccules varies from about 4 to 8 in most animal and plant cell types. In *Euglena*, the number may go upto 20. The membrane of the saccule is roughly 60 to 70Å in thickness which encloses a cavity about 150Å wide whose edges are often dilated. According to most authors, there are two well defined faces of the cisternae, i.e. convex and concave; the latter is generally referred to as the mature or forming or distal face and the convex side is assumed to be the immature or excit or proximal face. The cisternae lie in parallel array are separated from each other by a space of about 200 to 300 Å. What holds them together is not yet known but in few cells a thin layer of electron opaque, sometimes dense material is seen between the saccules which at certain regions are more prominent to which *Amos* and *Grimstone* (1968) applied the term nodes. *Mollenhauer et. al.*, (1973) explored in some detail intercisternal elements and plaques in certain plant Gogli complex.°

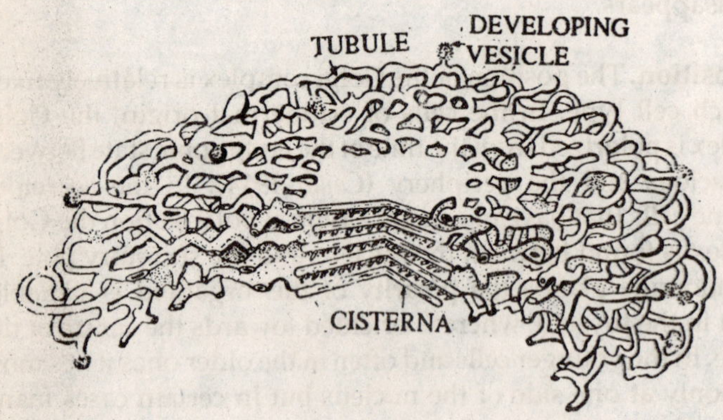

Fig. 4.2. Diagrammatic representation of the morophology of Golgi Complex

2. Tubules : From the peripheral area of cisternae arise a complex, anastomosing flat network of tubules of 300 to 500 Å diameter. *Clowes* and *Juniper* (1969) have compared this tublular network to disc of lace.

3. Vesicles : The vesicles are small droplet-like sacs which remain attached to tubules at the periphery of the cisternae. They are of following two types:

a. *Smooth vesicles* : The smooth vesicles are of 20 to 80mμ diameter. They contain secretory material (so often are called secretory vesicles) and are budded off from the ends of cisternal tubules within the net. Often more than one tubule connect to, and presumably fill, a single forming vesicle.

b. *Coated vesicles* : The coated vesicles are spherical protuberances, about 50 μ in diameter and with a rough surface. They are found at the periphery of the organelle, usually at the ends of single tubules, and are morphologically quite distinct from the secretory vesicles. Their function is unknown.

4. *Golgian vacuoles* : These are large rounded sacs present on the maturing face of Golgi. These are formed either by the expanded cisternae or by the fusion of secretory vesicles. The vacuoles are filled with some amorphous or granular substance.

CHEMICAL COMPOSITION

Regarding the chemical composition of Golgi complex, it has been demonstrated that the following substances are present:

1. Phospholipids. Phospholipids composition of Golgi membranes is intermediate between those of endoplasmic membranes and plasma membranes.

2. Proteins and Enzymes. Golgi complex from different plant and animal cells show great variations in the protein and enzyme contents. Some of the enzymes are ADPase, ATPase, CTPase, NADPHcytochrome-C-reductase, glycosyl transferases, galactosyl transferase, thiamine pyrophosphate etc.

3. Carbohydrates. Both plant and animal cells have some common carbohydrate components, like glucosarine, galactose, glucose, mannose, and fructose. Plant Golgi lack sialic acid, but it occurs in high concentration in rat liver. Some carbohydrates like xylase and arabinose are present in plant cells only.

4. Vitamin C. The function of vitamin C stored in the Golgi complex has been shown by *Tomitte.* According to him Golgi complex stores vitamin C and liberates it slowly into the cytoplasm in sufficient amount to prevent-oxidation of the cell products.

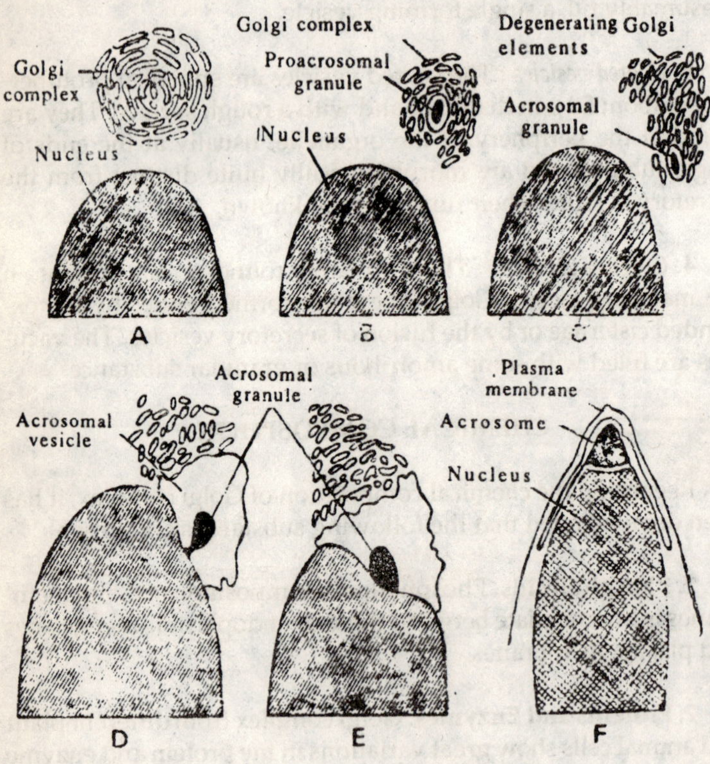

Fig. 4.3 Role of Golgi complex in the formation of acrosome

FUNCTIONS OF GOLGI COMPLEX

1. Formation of acrosome during spermiogenesis. During the maturation of sperm the Golgi complex plays a role in the formation of acrosome (*Burgos* and *Fawcett*, 1955).

In early stages, the Golgi appears as a spherical body, comprising cisternae arranged in parallel stacks and numerous small vesicles. The latter always pinched off from the cisternae. As development proceeds, the Golgi complex becomes irregular in shape and large vaculoles are formed by dilations of cisternal sacs. In the centre of these large vacuole or vacuoles is/are present a dense granule, the *proacrosomal granule.* This granule which is derived from Golgi complex continues to grow within the vacuole

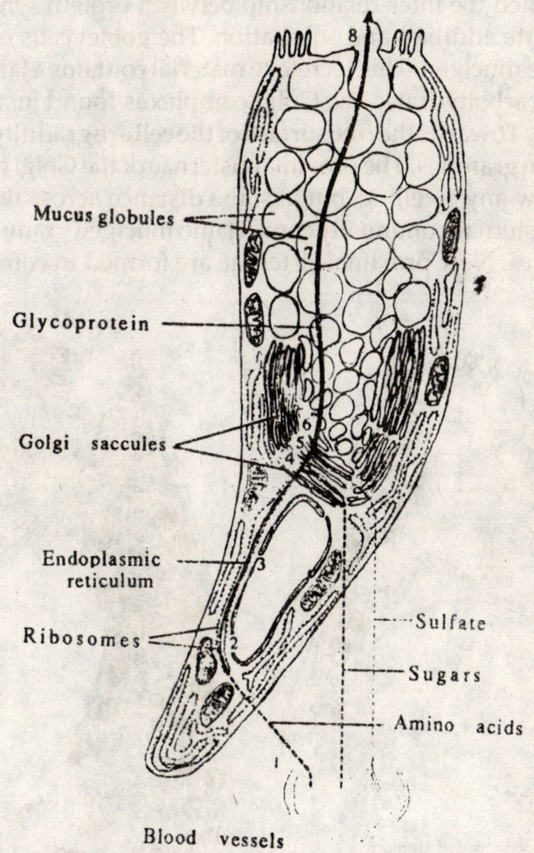

Fig. 4.4 Glycoprotein production through the intestinal goblet cell

by a process know as *accretion.* This vacuole and granule approaches the anterior pole of the nuclear membrane, constituting *acrosomal granule.* With the elongation of the spermatid, the *acrosomal vesicle* spreads over the nuclear surface and finally collapses with the nuclear membrane, forming the *cap material.* The acrosomal granule becomes the *acrosome* which lies at the apex of the nucleus and apparently comprises certain enzymes involved in the process of fertilization.

2. Synthesis and secretion of polysaccharides. Studies on goblet cells by autoradiography and electron microscopy have established the inter-relationship between protein synthesis, carbohydrate addition and sulphation. The goblet cells of the colon produce mucigen. This secretory material contains a large proportion of carbohydrate. The Golgi complex is found just above the nucleus. Towards the free surface of the cell are gradully enlarging mucigen granules. The proximal cisternae of the Golgi complex do not show any swelling, but at some distance across the stack the distal cisternae continually convert into mucigen granules every 2-4 minutes. New proximal cisternae are formed in compensation.

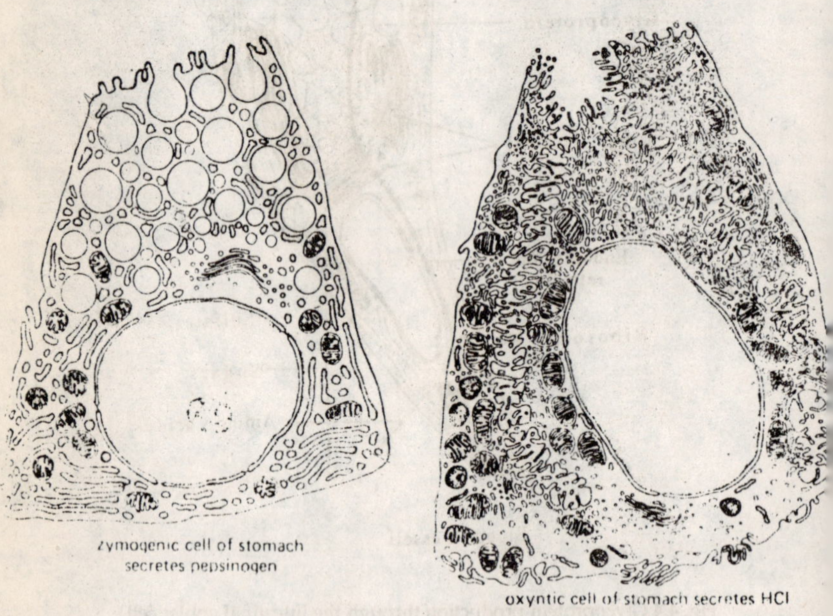

Fig. 4.5. Secretion in different cells

3. Role in secretion. Golgi complex is considered to play some role in the secretory functions of a cell. But the question is this that they are secreting or synthesizing some substances themselves or materials remain suspended in the nucleoplasm.

they are simply a store house in which the secrtory products which are secreted somewhere else in the cell, is simply stored and concentrated.

From the studies of *Palade et. al.* 1962 this secretory cycle is now well defined and includes four steps in case of pancreatic acinar cells and they are:

(i) The incorporation of aminoacids into protein at the surface of rough endoplasmic reticulum.
(ii) Transfer of these nascent secretory proteins into the cisternae of rough endoplasmic reticulum.
(iii) The intracellular transport of these proteins to the Golgi complex.
(iv) The migration or *zymogen granules* towards the apex of the cell where they discharged into lumens.

4. Role of Golgi body in oogenesis. *Srivastava* (1965) has given a brief review on the Golgi complex during oogenesis.

According to *Afzelius* (1956), the Golgi complex of a sea-urchin egg, as seen under electron microscope, consists of stacks of lamellae forming walls of flat pouches, which may occasionally be swollen. There is some indications of transverse divisions of these bodies. *Sotelo* (1959) and *Sotelo* and *Porter* (1959) have described the Golgi complex in rat-ovum as seen under the electron microscope and found juxtra nuclear localization of this organelle, in early oocytes. In the next stage, these resolve into fragments and in the third stage, these move towards the cortex. In all these cases, their structures remain to be of closely packed arrays of slender, double profiles (flattened sacs) and spherical vesicles. In the early oocytes the complex is compactly organized. In later stages, discrete bundles of profiles, surrounded by small vesicles are found scattered in the cortical zone. In the early oocytes, the Golgi complex and centrosome are closely associated.

5. Absorption of compounds. *Hirsch et al.*, have discovered that, when iron sugar is fed to an animal, iron becomes absorbed on Golgi complex (*Kedrowsky*). *Van Teel* has shown the Golgi systems also absorb compounds of copper and gold. *Kedrowsky*

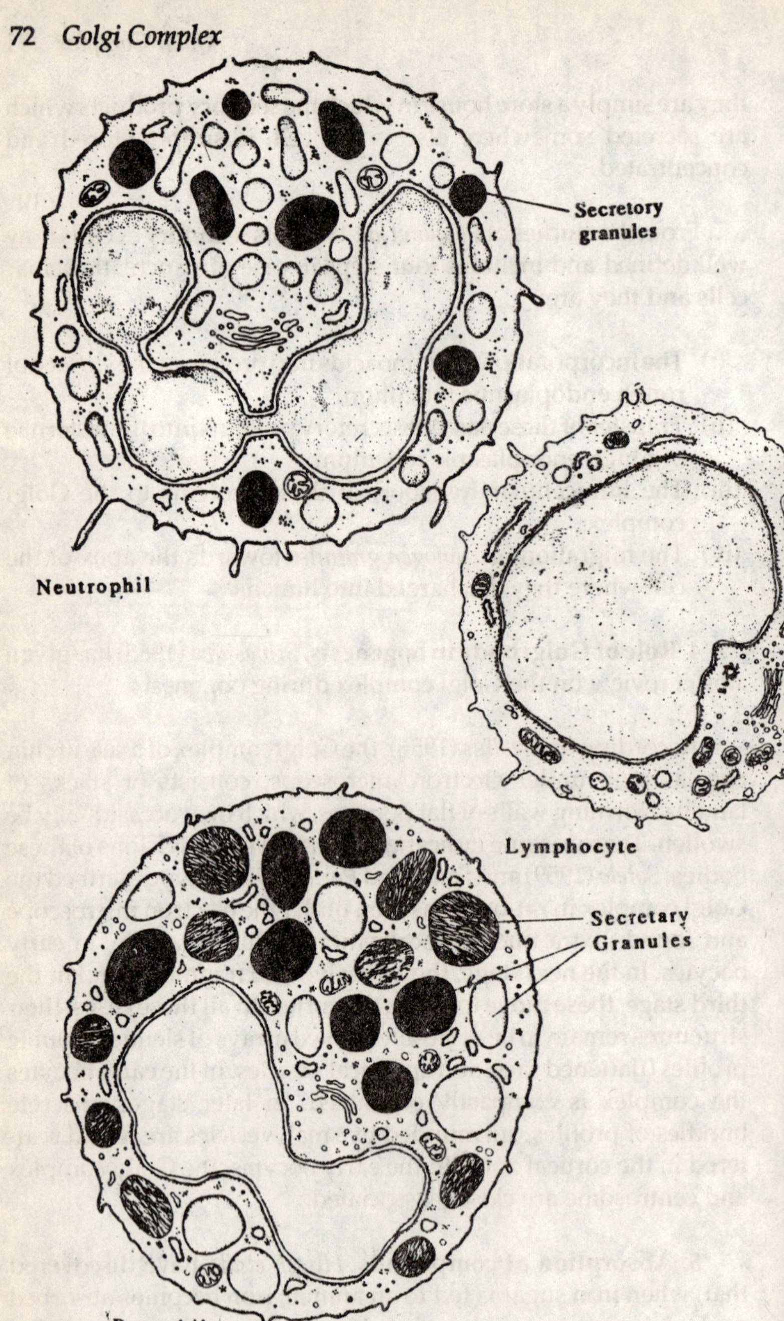

Fig. 4.6. Secretory granules in some leucocytes

has shown that Golgi complex of *Opalina* can absorb bismutose (compound of albumin and bismuth) and protargol (compound of albumin and silver). Thus, *Kirkman* and *Severing-haus* state that Golgi complex acts as a condensation membrane for the concentration of products into droplets or granules.

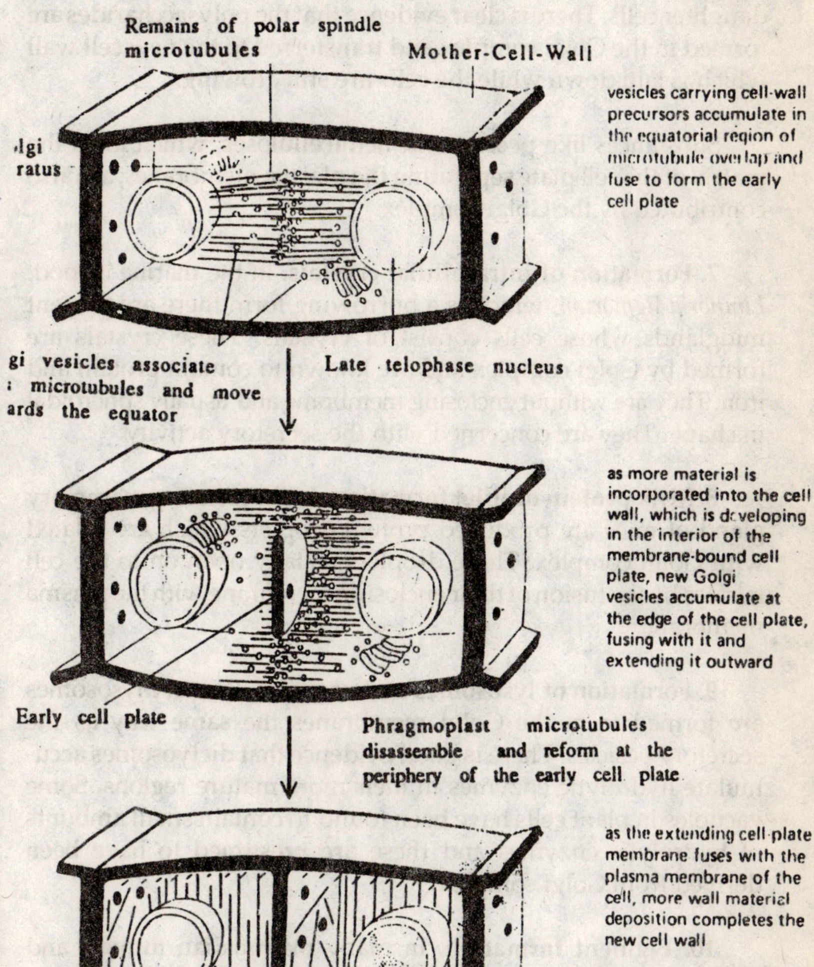

Fig. 4.7 Cell plate formation

6. Plant cell wall formation. The cell walls of plants are made up of fibrils which predominantly contain polysaccharides, along with some lipids and proteins. During cytokinesis a *cell plate* is formed between the two daughter nuclei, and has around it a membrane which later becomes the plasma membrane of the daughter cells. There is clear evidence that the polysaccharides are formed in the Golgi complex and transferred to the new cell wall which is laid down while the cells are still growing.

Substances like pectins and hemicelluloses, which form the matrix of the cell plate separating the plasma membranes, are also contributed by the Golgi complex.

7. Formation of intracellular crystals. In the marine isopod, *Limnoria ligmorum*, which is a burrowing form there are present midglands whose cells consist of crystals. These crystals are formed by Golgi complex and are known to contain protein and iron. They are without enclosing membrane and usually spheroidal in shape. They are concerned with the secretory activity.

8. Milk protein droplet formation. In the lactating mammary gland of mice are produced protein droplets which are related with Golgi complex. These droplets usually open on to the cell surface by the fusion of their enclosing membrane with the plasma membrane.

9. Formation of lysosomes and vacuoles. Primary lysosomes are formed from the Golgi membranes the same way as the secretory vesicles. There is good evidence that dictyosomes accumulate hydrolytic enzymes in their more mature regions. Some vacuoles in plant cells have been found to contain small amounts of hydrolytic enzymes and these are presumed to have been derived from Golgi complex.

10. Pigment formation. In many mammalian tumour and cancer cells the Golgi complex has been described as the site of origin of pigment granules (melanin).

11. Regulation of fluid balance. A homology has been suggested between the Golgi complex and the contractile vacuole of lower Metazoa and Protozoa. The contractile vacuole expel surplus water from the cell. In certain Protozoa the Golgi complex is also concerned with regulation of fluid balance.

ORIGIN OF GOLGI COMPLEX

Three different sources have been proposed from which new Golgi complex may arise:

1. From endoplasmic reticulum—*Eassner* and *Novikoff* (1962) and *Beams* and *Kessel* (1968) have proposed that Golgi cisternae arise from the ER. The rough endoplasmic reticulum after synthe-

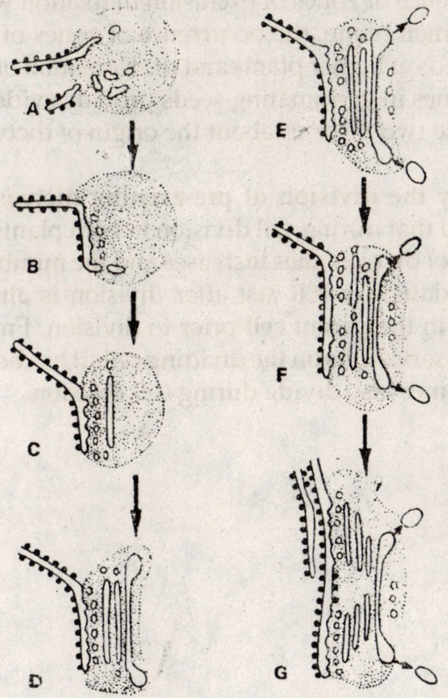

Fig. 4.8. Origin of dictyosome from endoplasmic reticulum from A to D and division of dictyosome—E,F,G.

sizing specific protein loses ribosomes and changes into smooth ER. Small transitory vesicles pinch off from smooth ER. These migrate to dictyosome. On reaching the forming face of dictyosome these fuse to form new cisternae and thus contribute to its growth. By the fusion of these vesicles new cisternae are formed continuously on the forming face and on the maturing face the old cisternae break down into secretory vesicles. Thus Golgi exhibit a phenomenon of 'membranous flow.'

2. From nuclear membrane. *Bouch* (1965) described the origin of Golgi from outer membrane of nuclear envelope in brown algae. Vesicles are pinched off from outer nuclear membrane which fuse to form cisternae on the forming face of dictyosome.

Presence of zones of exclusion in relation with smooth ER or nuclear membrane, the occurrence of zones of exclusion in dormant seeds of higher plants and the formation of dictyosome from these zones in germinating seeds provide evidence in support of the above two theories about the origin of dictyosome.

3. By the division of pre-existing dictyosome. It has been observed that during cell division in both plants and animals, the number of dictyosomes increases and the number of dictyosomes in each daughter cell just after division is almost equal to the number in the parent cell prior to division. From this and other direct observations on the dividing cells it has been presumed that dictyosomes also divide during cell division.

5

LYSOSOMES

The concept of the lysosome originated from the development of cell fractionation techniques by which different subcellular components are isolated. By 1949 a class of particles having centrifugal properties somewhat intermediate between those of mitochondria and microsomes was isolated by *de Duve* and found to have a high content of acid phosphatase and other hydrolytic enzymes. Because of their enzymatic properties they were named lysosomes (Gr., *Lysis* = disolution, *soma* = body). According to *Gohan* (1972) membrane bounded storage granules containing digestive enzymes are considered lysosomes of plant Alls. Hence *spherosomes, aleurone granules* and *vacuoles* of plant cells are supposed to have lysosome like functions.

OCCURRENCE

With the exception of mammalian R.B.C., the lysosomes have been reported practically from all the animal cells. The presence of lysosomal particles have also been suspected (and in some cases established) in protista (protozoan, slime-moulds, fungi, algae and prokaryotic protista). In plant cells, considering the evidences as a whole, there now seems little doubt about their presence. Further they have strong affinities with the lysosomes of animals and protista (*Pitt*, and *Galpin* 1973). In plants, further they should not be confused with spherosomes in function. According to *Pitt* lysosomes and spherosomes are two different organelles and the later are comparable to lipid droplets of animals. *Yatsu* and *Jack* (1972) have clearly shown that spherosomes are morphologically distinct organelles. *Gahm* (1973) reviewed the occurrence and histochemistry of plant lysosomes.

MORPHOLOGY

Shape and Size. The shape and size of lysosome is variable. Morphologically they can be compared with *Amoeba* and white blood cells (W.B.C.). Due to their changing habit they cannot be accurately identified as the basis of their shape. Normally lysosomes very in size from 0.4 to 0.8μ, but they may be as large as 5μ in mammalian kidney cells and are exceedingly large in phagocytosis.

Structure of Lysosomes : Like other cytòplamic complexes, lysosomes are like round tiny bags filled with dense material and digestive enzymes. They consist of two parts: (1) limiting membrane and (2) inner dense mass.

1. *Limiting membrane.* This membrane is single, unlike that of mitochondira and composed of lipoprotein. The chemical structure is homologous with the unit membrane of plasmalemma consisting of bimolecular layer as suggested by *Robertson.*

2. *Inner dense mass.* This enclosed mass may be solid or of very dense contents. Some lysosomes have a very dense outer zone and less dense inner zone. Some others have cavities of vacuoles within the granular material. Usually they are supposed to possess denser contents than mitochondira.

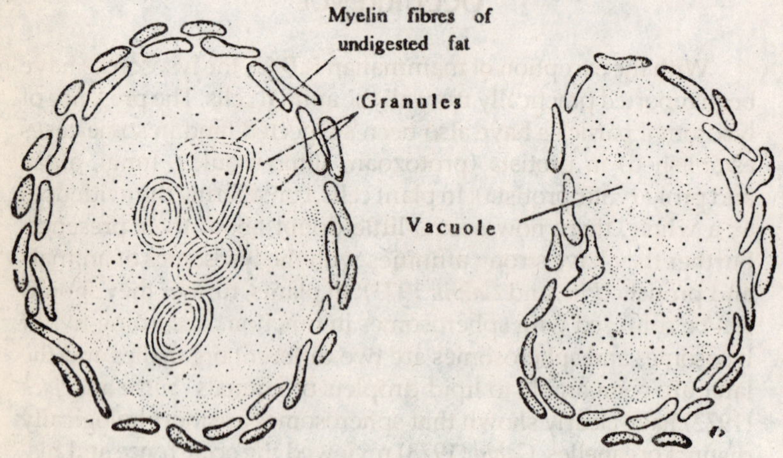

Fig. 5.1. Two types of Lysosomes from the kidney cells of rat

They show their polymorphic nature and their contents very with the stage of digestion, as they help in intracellular digestion.

Permeability of Lysosomal Membrane : The lysosomal membrane is impermeable to substances, of the enzymes contained in the lysosomes. Certain substances, called *labilizers*, cause instability of the lysosomal membrane, leading to release of enzymes from the lysosome. Other substances, called stabilizers, have a stabilizing action on the membrane. A list of some labilizers and stabilizers is give in Table 5.1.

Table 5.1 Lysosomal labilizers and stabilizers

Labilizers	*Stabilizers*
Vitamin A	Cholesterol
Vitamin B	Cortisone
Vitamin K	Cortisol
Vitamin E (high dose)	Vitamin E (low conc.)
Progesterone	Chloroquine
Testosterone	Phenothiazines
B-estradiol	Antihistamines
Ubiquinone	Heparin
Digistonin	
Polyene antibiotics	

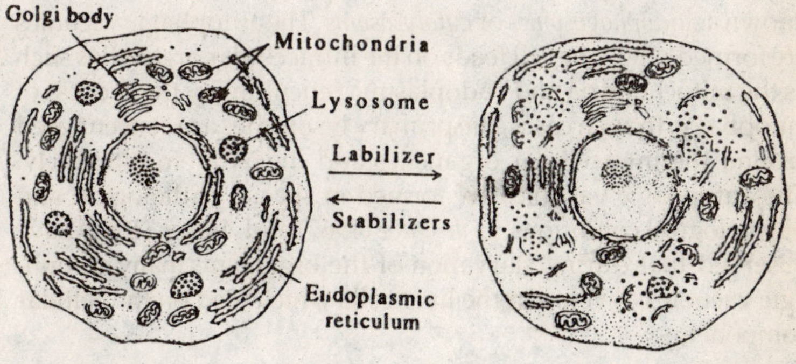

Fig. 5.2. Activities of the suicide bags in the cell

A labilizer might increase the permeability of the lysosomal membrane to small solutes like sucrose. The osmotic swelling which results might completely disrupt the membrane.

The limited permeability of lysosomal membrane explains why lysosomal hydrolases do not have a direct access to cellular components. This prevents uncontrolled digestion of the cell contents by the lysosomal enzymes.

Polymorphism: Lysosomes are polymorphic in nature. the polymorphic nature is due to variation in contents of lysosomes with different stages of digestion. Generally lysosomes can be traced in four forms given below:

(1) *Primary lysosomes.* These are also called the *true, pure* or *original lysosomes,* having a single unit membrane containing enzymes in the inactive forms.

(2) *Secondary lysosomes.* These are also called the *phagosomes* as they contain the engulfed material and enzymes. The fused mass is called the secondary lysosome. The enzyme present in such lysosomes gradually digests the engulfed material.

(3) *Residual or post lysosomes.* Lysosomal membrane characterized by the presence of undigested material like myelin figures is called residual body.

(4) *Autophagic vacuoles.* The autophagic vacuoles are also known as *autophogosomes* or *cytolysosoms*. The autophagic vacuoles are formed when the cell feeds on the intracellular organelles such as the mitochondria and endoplasmic reticulum by the process of autophagy. In such cases, the primary lysosomes are concentrated around the intracellular organelles and digest them ultimately. The autophagic vacuoles are formed in special pathological and physiological conditions. *C. de Duve* (1967) and *Allison* (1967) have observed that during starvation of the organisms many autophagic vacuoles develop in the liver cells which feed on the cellular components.

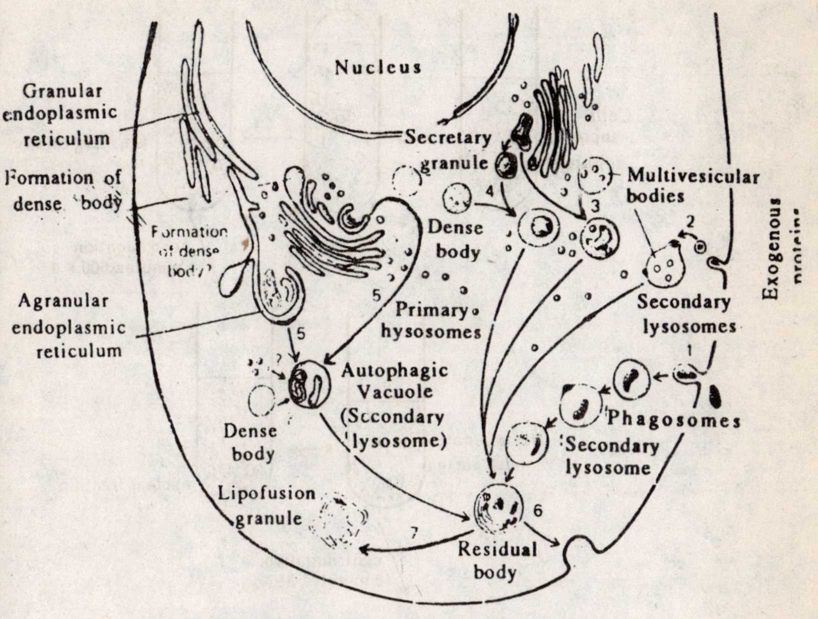

Fig. 5.3. Polymorphism of lysosomes

CHEMISTRY OF LYSOSOMES

Lysosomes contain variety of enzymes, upto the present time about 40 enzymes have been isolated in variety of tisue type. Some common enzymes, are B-galactosidase, B-glucuronidase, B-N-acetyl-glucosaminidase, x-glucosidase, x-mannosidase; cathepsin A (Acid protease), cathepsin B (Acid protease), aryl sulphatase A, aryl sulphatase B, acid ribonuclease, acid deoxyribonuclease, acid phosphatase, acid lipase, phospholipase A, phosphotidic acid phosphatase hyaluronidase, phosphoprotein phosphatase, amino peptidase A, dextranase, saccharase, lysozyme (muramidase), Mg++ activated ATPase, indoxylacetate, esterase and plasminogen activator. All these enzymes of the lysosomes are enclosed within the single lipoprotein membrane,. Most of these enzymes function more effeciently under slightly acidic medium, pH optima around 5.0, as such they are collectively called as acid bydrolases.

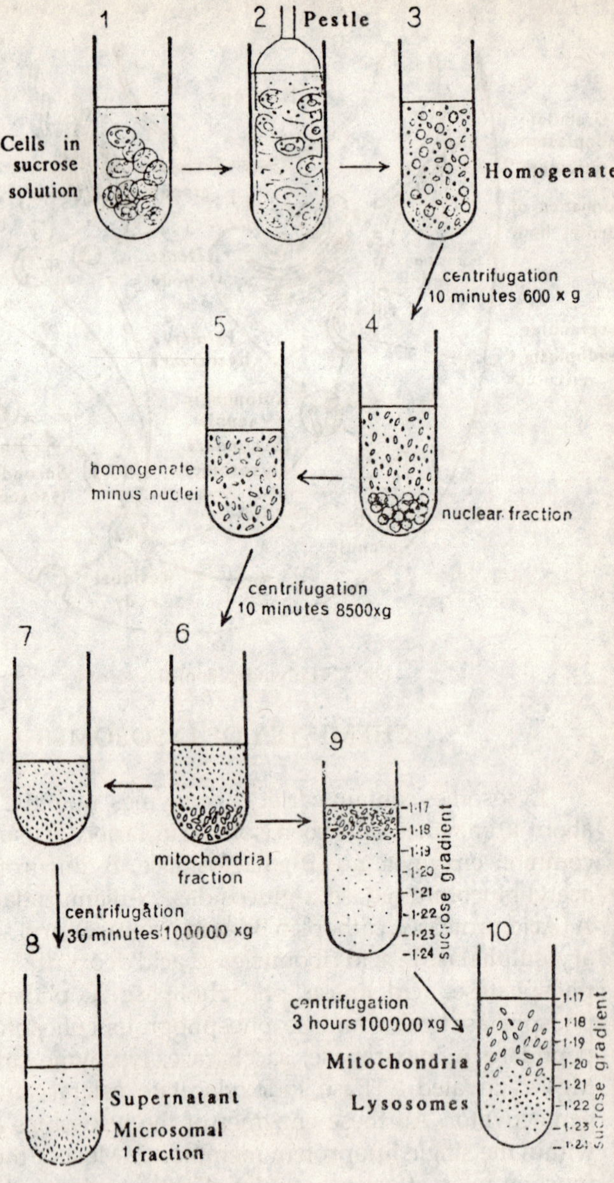

Fig. 5.4. Extraction of lysosomes by centrifugation

Table 5.2 Lysosomal enzymes, the substrate on which these work and the end products.

Enzymes	*Substrate*	*End produce*
1. **Nucleases**		
(i) Acid ribonuclease	Polynucleotides of RNA	Nitrogenous bases+ Phosphate+ribose sugar
(ii) Acid deoxyribonuclease	Nitrogenous base+ DNA	Phosphate+deoxyribose sugar
2. **Phosphatases**		
(i) Acid phosphatase	Phosphomonoesters	Monophosphates
(ii) Phosphodiesterase	Oligonucleotides, phosphodiesters	Monophosphates
3. **Proteases and Peptidases**		
(i) Cathepsins (A,B and peptides	Various proteins	Amino acids
(ii) Collagenase	Collagen	Amino acids
(iii) Peptidase	Peptides	Amino acids
4. **Glycoslidase**		
(i) B-galactosidase	B-galactosides	
(ii) x-glucosidase	Glycogens	
(iii) B-glucosidase	B-glycosides	
(iv) x-Mannosidase	x-mannosides	Monosaccharides
(v) B-glucuronidase mucopolysaccharides	Polysacharides and	
5. Sulphatases	Sulphate esters	Fragments of lipids
6 Lipases	Lipids	Fragments of lipids
7. Esterases	Fatty acids esters	Frageements thereof
8. Lysozyme	Mucopolysaccharides, bacterial cell alls	Frageements thereof
9. Sphingomyelinase	Sphingomyelin	Frageements thereof

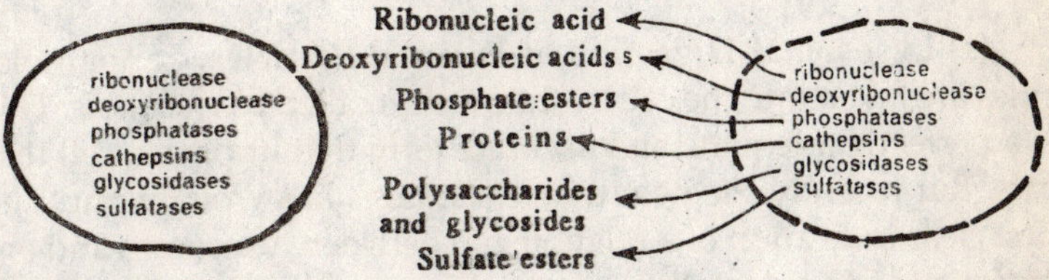

Fig.8.5. The enzymes of lysosomes and their substances.

Fig. 5.5. The enzymes of lysosomes and their substances

DIFFERENT NOMENCLATURE

The cytochemical definition of lysosomes based on the presence of a single unit membrane and a positive staining reaction for acid phosphatase and some related enzymes, may be considered for most pratical purposes equivalent to the biochemical definition. As our knowledge of the significance of lysosomes in cell physiology has progressed, it has become evident that the term lysosome covers a variety of different forms which can be distinguished on the basis of morphological and functional criteria. The following are the terms commonly used in the literature:

(i) **Autophagic Vacuoles.** It is a membrane lined vacuole containing morphologically recognizable cytoplasmic components.
(ii) **Cytolysome.** Same as Autophagic vacuoles.
(iii) **Cytosome.** Particles referred to cytosomes are usually lysosomes. Some workers include the unrelated microbodies under this term.
(iv) **Cytosegresome.** Same as Autophagic vacuoles.
(v) **Microbody.** A particle found in liver and kidney, bounded by a single unit membrane and containing a finely granulated material. According to *de Duve,* they are definitely not lysosomes.
(vi) **Multivesicular Bodies.** Structures lined by a single membrane and containing inner vesicles resembling Golgi complex and are considered to be lysosomes.
(vii) **Residual Bodies.** Membrane lined inclusions characterized by undigested residues comprises telo-lysosomes and hypothetical post-lysosomes.

FUNCTIONS

(1) Lysosomal Digestion of External Particles. Large molecules are taken into the cell by the process called *phagocytosis*. This is a perfectly adequate and accurate term that implies a cell that eats. But recently the new term *endocytosis* has won favour. The first clear indication of a relationship between lysosomes and engulfment of extracellar material was provided by *Stians* (1952,54,55). As shown in the figure, the cell engulfs the particles and then forms and invagination that becomes pinched off from the cell membrane to become an internal sac or body. It is referred to as a *phagosome*. A phagosome then moves towards the lysosome. Exposure of the material to the lysosomal hydrolases occurs through fusion of the phagosome with a lysosome. This results in the formation of a *secondary lysosome* or *digestive vacuole*. The lysosome involved in the process may be primary or secondary, depending on the relative sizes of the two partners. The process may appear to an observer as a lysosome discharging enzymes into a phagosome or as a phagosome shedding its contents into a lysosome, as may be the case in hepatic parenchymal cells; or simply as a mutual sharing of the contents of the two vacuoles, if they are of comparable sizes. Now the enzymes from the lysosome can come into contact with the molecules brought into the cell in the phagosome and digestion occurs. Once the molecules are digested, the digested products can diffuse out of the so called digestive vacuole into the cytoplasm of the cell leaving the residue in the digestive vacuole. The digestive vacuole now moves on to the cell membrane where the so called reverse phagocytosis or defecation occurs.

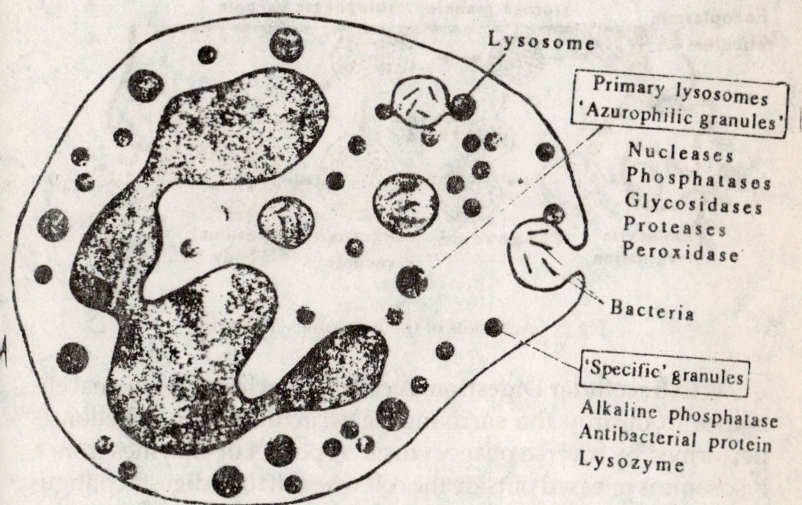

Fig. 5.6. A professional phagocyte

2. Digestion of Intracellular Substance. In certain cases portions of the cell, somehow, find their way inside the cell's own lysosomes and are broken down. This process is termed as *cellular autophagy*. How they get in, is not clear, and the role which autophagy plays in cell function can only be summarized. Proteins, fats and polysaccharides can all be synthesized, and stored in the cell. During the starvation of cell these stored food materials are digested by lysosomes to give energy. What stimulates autophagy to take place and how the large molecules get into the lysosome is not clear.

3. Cellular Digestion. When a cell dies, the lysosomal membrane ruptures. The liberated enzymes become free in the cell, which then quickly digest the entire cell. The hypothesis has been advanced that this is a built in mechanism for removing dead cells. In multicellular animals, many cells are constantly being formed, live for a short period of time, and then die. The self digestion may occur as a pathological mechanism just for example, if a cell is cut off from its oxygen supply or poisoned, the lysosomal membrane may rupture, thereby permitting the enzymes to dissolve the cell. Therefore, they are also considered as *suicide bag*s of the cells.

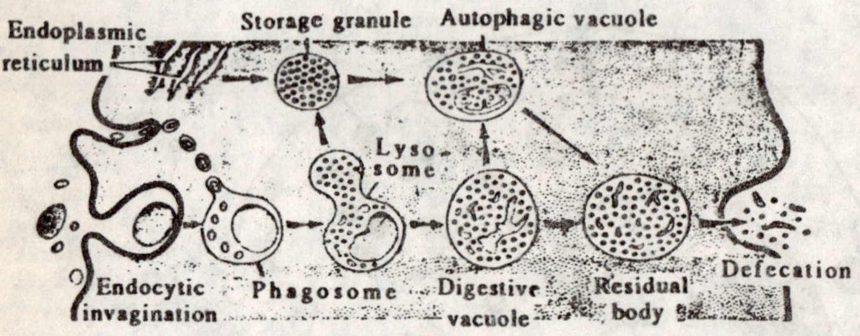

Fig. 5.7 Activities of the lysosomes in the cell

4. Extracellular Digestion. A cell can discharge lysosomal enzymes to destroy the surrounding structures. This function is performed by reverse phagocytosis. A pocket of enzymes from a lysosome is released outside the cell where it then digests contiguous structures. This is thought to explain, how sperms penetrate the protective coating of the ovum during fertilization. It may also explain how oesteoblast cells that destroy bones, function. This may also be the explanation for the well known ability of white blood cells to pass quickly out of the blood vessels and into the tissue spaces at the site of an infection.

5. Role in Secretion. In recent years evidences have started accumulating suggesting the role of lysosomes in the formation of secretory products in secretory cells. The phenomenon of lysosomes-mediated thyroid hormones secretion is the best known example of direct lysosomes involvement in secretory process. Lysosomes also play possible role in the regulation of hormone secretion. It is believed that mammotrophic hormones of the anterior pituitary is synthesized on the ribosomes of the RER and is packaged into secretory granules by passage through the Golgi.

The epithelial cells of the thyroid also contain lysosomes rich in lysosomal enzymes. The follicles of the thyroid gland contain high molecular weight protein thyroglobulin, which is stored as colloid in the lumen. The thyroid hormones thyroxine and tri-iodothyroxin are linked with this protein. The colloid containing thyroglobulin enters the epithelial cell by pinocytosis. The colloid droplets fuse with primary lysosomes to form secondary lysosomes or digestive vacuoles. The thyroid hormones are split from the thyroglobulin and released into the blood stream. Thus the thyroid hormones are released by hydrolysis of thyroglobulin.

6. Chromosome Breaks. Lysosomes contain the enzyme deoxyribonuclease (DNAse). This enzyme causes chromosomal breaks and their rearrangement. DNAase has two active sites and breaks down both the strands of DNA. The breaks have been produced experimentally in isolated chromosomes incubated in DNAase. These breaks lead to various syndromes.

7. Role in Development and Metamorphosis. Lysosomes are important in development. Good evidences have accumulated on the role of lysosomes in involutions of uterus and mammary glands immediately in postpartum. During metamorphosis, the process of resorption of the tadpole tail and regression of the various larval tissues, including the fat body and the salivary gland, are accompanied by increased lysosomal acid hydrolase activity (Weber).

8. Osteogenesis. During ossification conversion of cartilage into bone, the special osteoblast cells produce lytic substances which erode the matrix of the cartilage and help in the formation of bone.

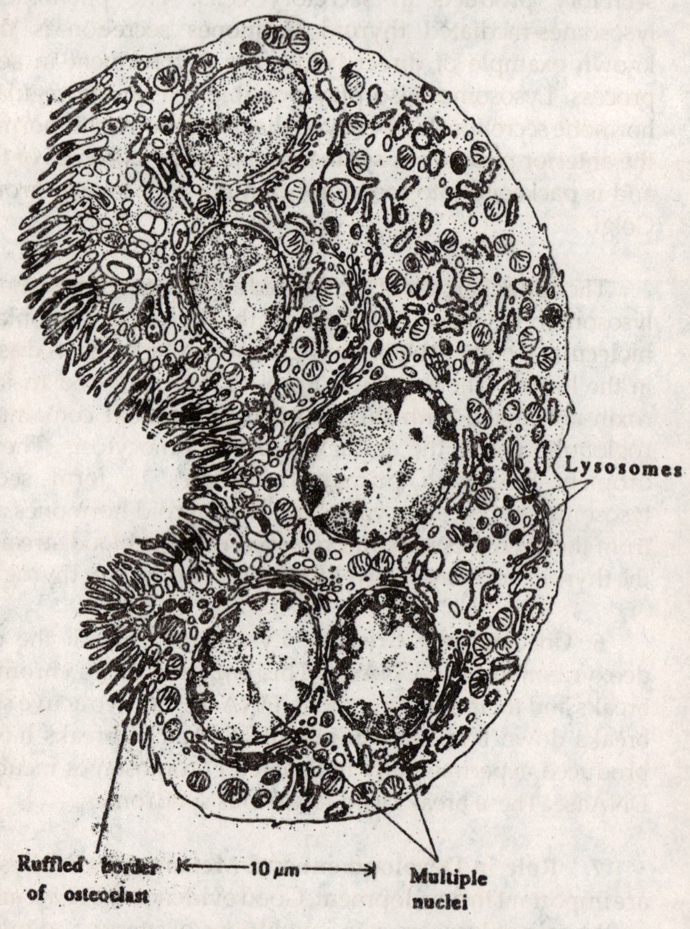

Fig. 5.8. Lysosomes in an osteoclast

9. Role of Lysosomes during Cell Division. During the cell division, the lysosomes of that particular dividing cell move towards the periphery instead of near the nucleus, as in usual cases they are seen. During the cytokinesis roughly equal number of them move towards opposite poles. Sometimes during cell-division certain repressors in cytoplasm inhibit call-division. Lysosomes secrete certain depressors which destroy the repressor and result in cell division (*Allison*, 1967).

10. Help in Protein Synthesis. *Novikoff* and *Essner* (1960) have suggested the possible role of lysosomes in protein synthesis. Recently, *Singh* 1972 has correlated lysosomal activity with the protein synthesis. In the liver and pancreas of some birds, lysosomes seem to be more active and developed showing possible relationship with cell metabolism.

11. Lysosomes and Cancer. Malignant cells are found to contain abnormal chromosomes. It is presumed that the chromosomal abnormality is caused by chromosomal breakage presumably produced by the lysosomal enzymes. The partial deletion of chromosome 21 in man is associated with the chronic myeloid leukemia (blood cancer).

12. Removal of Dead Cells. *Hirsch* and *Cohn* (1964) suggested that lysosomes help in the removal of dead cells in tissue. The lysosomal membrane ruptures in these cells, releasing the enzyme into body of cell, so that whole cell may be digested. This process of tissue degeneration (necrosis) is due to this lysosomal activity.

13. Fertilization. During fertilization the sperm release hydrolytic enzymes from the acrosomal vesicle. These enzymes help in the penetration of the sperm through the membranes of the egg. Fluorescence microscopy studies of acridine-stained spermatozoa of the guinea pig show that the acrosome vesicles contain several enzymes, including *hyaluronidase* and *proteases*, which are also found in lysosomes. In fact the acrosome vesicle has been looked upon as a *giant lysosome*. The acrosome vesicle enzymes also apparently activate the egg by breaking down its cortical granules.

14. Lysosomes and Disease. Inhalation of foreign particles like silica, asbestos etc. leads to inflammation and deposition of fibrous tissue in the lungs. The particles of silica or asbestos increase the permeability of lysosomal membranes and rupture of lysosomes. This leads to the lysis of lung cells resulting in their inflammation.

A metabolic disorder, the *gout,* is caused by the accumulation of sodium urate crystals in the joints. These are picked up by the phagocytes resulting in their lysosome rupture. This leads to acute inflammation and increased collagen synthesis. Pome's disease is another example which is caused due to absence of an lysosomal enzyme which hydrolize the glycogen. Thus liver cells are engorged with glycogen.

ORIGIN OF LYSOSOMES

They have multiple origin depending upon the tissue in which they are located or on their function in a specific cell.

(i) **Extracellular Origin.** Lysosomes may be the vacuoles absorbed into cell by the process, pinocytosis. The pinocytic vacuole may later become cytoplasmic particles and thereon enzymatic activity becomes developed.

(ii) **Origin from Golgi Complex.** There are evidences that lysosomes orginate from the Golgi complex and represent zymogen granules. Their similar function and structure with Golgi complex support this view. Recent studies have shown that accumulation of secretory products within Golgi vacuoles leads to the formation of lysosomes, and membranes surrounding the products are derived from Golgi membrane.

(iii) **Origin from ER.** *Novikoff* (1965) reported that the lysosomes originate directly from granular endoplasmic reticulum. by a process of blebbing.

6

ENDOPLASMIC RETICULUM

Endoplasmic reticulum was first of all observed in 1945 by *Porter*, *Claude* and *Fullam*. They noted the presence of a network of reticulum of strands associated with vesicle-like bodies in the cytoplasm of the cultural fibroplast or thinly-spread tissue culture cells. Further electron microscopy by *Porter* and *Thompson* (1947) has revealed that these strands of reticulum are vesicular bodies inter-connected, so as to form a complex network in the inner endoplasmic part of the cytoplasm. As this network is concentrated in the endoplasm of the cell more than in the ectoplasm, therefore, it is known as *endoplasmic reticulum* (ER), or *ergastoplasm* or *vaculolar system* of the cell. The endoplasmic reticulum is not visible in the cytoplasm of a living cell under the phase-contrast microscope but the observation by electron microscope on the fixed cell have revealed this structure.In 1952, studies with electron microscope further confirmed the presence of endoplasmic reticulum as reported by *Porter* and his colleagues. Recent studies have further confirmed and accepted the concept of a structural organization of cytoplasm. Recently, under the phase-contrast microscope, *Fawcett* and *Ito* (1958), and *Rose* and *Pomerat* (1960) have studied the structure and distribution of endoplasmic reticulum in the living tissue-culture cells.

OCCURRENCE

The endoplasmic reticulum occurs in all the eukaryotic cells except erythrocytes (R.B.Cs) of mammals. It is absent in prokaryotes. Its development varies considerably in various cell types. It is small and undifferentiated in eggs and in undifferentiated embryonic cells. Only a few vacuoles are present in the spermatocytes and muscle cells. However, it is highly organized in cells synthesizing proteins or in cells that are engaged in lipid metabolism.

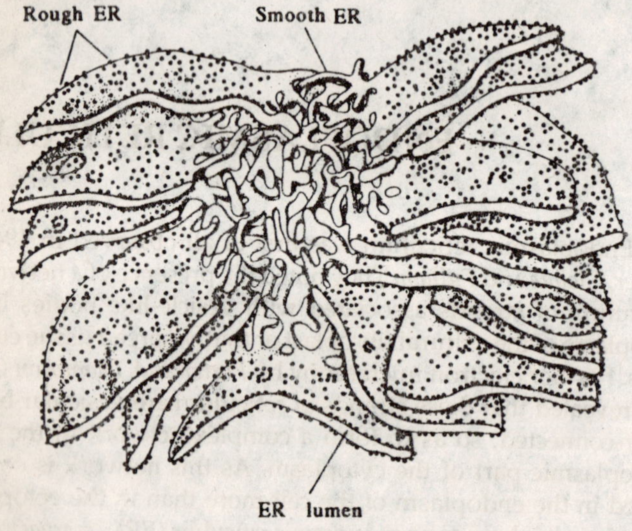

Fig. 6.1. Three dimensional view of rndoplasmic reticulum

MORPHOLOGY

The endoplasmic reticulum has been found in all kinds of mature cells except the mature mammalian erythrocytes, which is also devoid of a nucleus. Actually the first description of these structures seemed with electron microscope by *Porter, Claude,* and *Fullam* in 1945 in cultured cells. These are membrane bounded sacs in the form of double membranes (cisternae) by *Sjostrand* (1953) or the name *cisternae* was given by *Sjostrand* and the name *tubules* was given by *Kurosumi* (1954). Rounded and irregular *sacs* or *vesicles* were observed by *Weiss* (1953).

Morphologically the endoplasmic reticulum is composed of following three kinds of structure, viz., 1. cisternae, 2. vesicles and 3. tubules.

Cisternae or *lamellae*. They are long, flattened and usually unbranched tubules, which are arranged in parallel arrays. They are of uniform width throughout and their thickness varies from 40-50 μ. This pattern of reticulum is characteristic of basophilic regions of the cytoplasm and of those cells, which are active in protein synthesis. Lamellae or cisternae occur in the liver-cells, plasma-cells, pancreatic cells, brain-cells and in notochord cells etc.

Tubules. The tubules are small, smooth-walled, branched tubular spaces having a diameter of about 50-190 μ. These occur in cells that are busy in the synthesis of steroids like cholesterol, glycerides and hormones. These are haphazardly arranged in the cytoplasm of developing spermatids of guinea pig, muscles cells and other non-secretory cells.

Vesicles. The vesicles range in diameter from 25 to 500 μ and are for the most part rounded in shape. These are abundant in the cells engaged in the protein synthesis as in hepatic and pancreatic cells.

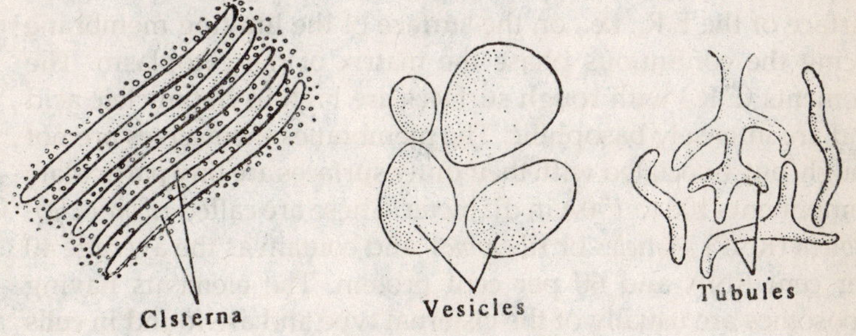

Fig. 6.2. Morphology of the endoplasmic reticulum

All these three patterns of endoplasmic reticulum may occur in the same cell or in different cells. Their arrangement also differs in different cell viz., in parallel rows in the liver-cells of mammals; haphazardly in pancreatic cells or in the form of a network of tubules in striated muscle-cells. In notochordal cells of *Ambyostoma* larva, the pattern of cisternae is of still another type.

Ultrastructure of Endoplasmic Reticulum : All the three structures of the endoplasmic reticulum are bounded by a thin membrane of 50 to 60 Å thick. Like the plasma membrane, nucleus, etc., its membrane is also formed of three layers—the outer and inner dense layers are composed of protein molecules, and the two middle thin and transparent layers are of phospholipids. The endoplasmic reticuluar membrane is continuous with the plasma membrane, nuclear membrane and membrane of Golgi complex. The lumen of the endoplasmic reticulum acts as a passage for the secretory products and *Palade* (1956) has observed the secretory granules in it.

TYPES OF ENDOPLASMIC RETICULUM

On the basis of presence or absence of ribosomes they are of two types :

(i) *Granular or Rough Walled Endoplasmic Reticulum*. When the particles or *ribosomes* are present on the wall of E.R., it is called rough walled E.R. These particles are always present at the outer surface of the E.R., i.e., on the surface of the limiting membrane facing the continuous phase the matrix of the cytoplasm. The elements (E.R.) with rough surfaces are high in ribonucleic acid and are intensely basophilic. The membranes themselves are not rough, but associated with their outer surfaces are tiny particulate components 100 to 150Å in diameter. These are called *ribonu-cleo-protein* (RNP) *particles* or *ribosomes* and contain as the average 40 per cent RNA and 60 per cent protein. The elements having ribosomes are usually of the cisternal type and are found in cells active in protein synthesis. Biochemical studies have indicated that the ribosomes are important in protein synthesis, even though the membranes are not always necessary for this activity. Other functions will be explained later.

The smooth surfaced E.R. is often continuous with the rough surfaced E.R. thereby making the absence or presence of ribosomes the only significant difference between the two. The continuity between smooth and rough E.R. has been repeated by demonstration. It has been suggested moreover that one grows from the other but which from which is uncertain. The ribosome can readily be dissociated from the endoplasmic reticulum membranes by treatment with deoxycholate.

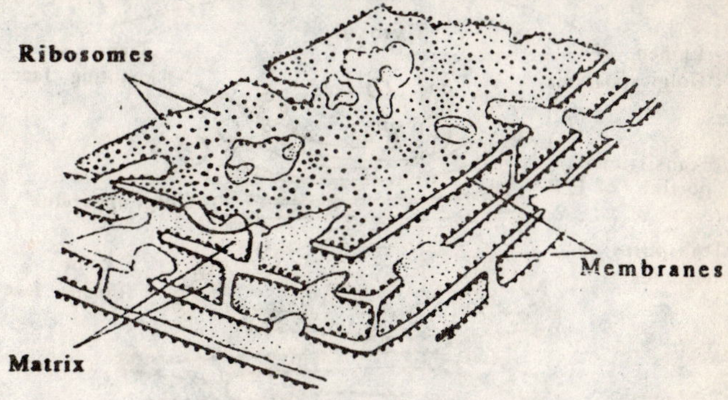

Fig. 6.3 Endoplasmic reticulum and ribosomes

(ii) *Smooth Walled Endoplasmic Reticulum.* The name smooth walled is given to that portion of endoplasmic reticulum that is devoid of ribosomes. Like the rough walled endoplasmic reticulum smooth form shows a characteristic morphology which is tubular rather then cisternae. These smooth walled endoplasmic reticulum is found in the cells that are active in the synthesis of steroid compounds such as cholesterol, glycerides, and the hormones (testosterone and progesterone). It is studied by Fawcett 1960 that they are also present in the pigmented epithelial cells of the retina which are involved in the metabolism of vitamin A in the production of visual pigment. Glycogen storing cells of the liver contain in the smooth, tubular elements of the endoplasmic reticulum.

Table 6.1. Differences between rough and smooth ER

	Smooth ER	*Rough ER*
1.	Well developed in steriod hormone secreting cells.	Well developed in protein-secreting cells.
2.	It tends to be tubular.	It tends to be cisternal.
3.	It is less stable and autolysis readily.	It is comparatively more stable. It may persist for some time after the death of the cell.
4.	If is devoid of ribosomes.	Ribosomes are found associated.

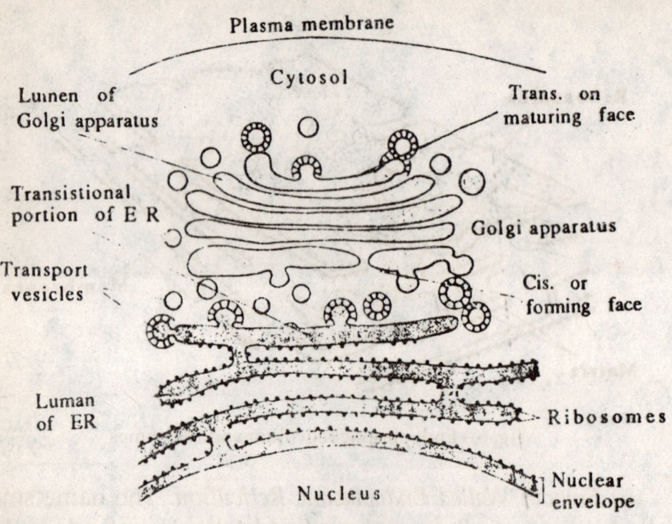

Fig. 6.4 Endoplasmic reticulum and other cell organelles.

MODIFICATIONS OF ENDOPLASMIC RETICULUM

(A) Sarcoplasmic Reticulum: Sarcoplasmic reticulum, found in the skeletal and cardiac muscles is a highly modified from of smooth ER. It was first reported by *Veratti* (1902) as delicate plexuses in skeletal muscles surrounding the myofibrils. Electron microscopy showed it to be composed of a network of membrane like tubules which run longitudinally in the interfibrillar sarcoplasmic space for the length of each sarcomere. At the level of H and I bands, these tubules merge with large cisternal structures. At the H band level this cisterna, called the central cisterna, forms a sieve-like structure round the myofibrils. At the level of I band, these tubules merge with the large terminal cisternae, from which transverse tubules extend peripherally to the sarcolemma and are continuous with and are deep invaginations of it. It is generally believed that sarcoplasmic reticulum plays a role not only in distributing energy-rich material needed for muscular contraction but also in providing the necessary action potential from the surface to the myofibrils within.

(B) Ergastoplasm : There are certain regions in the cytoplasm that stain with basic dyes. To these regions various names have been given like chromidial substance, basoplasm, ergastoplasm and so forth. The term *ergastoplasm* was given by *Garnier* in 1899 to those cytoplasmic filaments in the cells of exocrine glands which stained readily with basic stains. *Weiss* (1953) referred to the cisternal elements as ergastoplasmic sacs. In nerve cells, such areas are called *Nissil bodies*. Electron microscopic studies reveal it to be an accumulation or ribosomes situated on the parallel lamellae of ER stacks of accumulated freely in the groundplasm. Studies of *Caspersson* (1955), *Brachet* (1957) and others have demonstrated that the basophilic nature of ergastoplasm is due to the ribonucleic acid. Smooth E.R. areas of cytoplasm are never ergastoplasm.

ORIGIN OF ENDOPLASMIC RETICULUM

(i) *Multi Step Mechanism* : Although the origin of the new endoplasmic reticulum membrane has not been fully understood, The views are there. In fact, one of the possible function attributed to the endoplasmic reticulum is that of membrane biosynthesis. The protein components of endoplasmic reticulum and other membranes may be assembled by activity of the endoplasmic reticulum. There is certainly convincing evidence that Golgi membranes and many cytoplasmic vesicles can be derived from endoplasmic reticulum. Moreover, endoplasmic reticulum membranes appear to be continuously synthesized, having a relatively high rate of turn over. At the same time, the several elements of endoplasmic reticulum in the cell are asynchronous in this respect, they are not all replaced at the same time or with the same rate. It has also been suggested that membranes of the endoplasmic reticulum are formed not from pre-existing elements but from the ground substance of the cytoplasm. Thus the process by which a membrane is modified chemically and structurally is called membrane differentiation.

(ii) *From Nuclear Membrane* : The vacuoles are derived from the evagination of the outer membrane of the nuclear envelope, which separated from its inner partner, leaving cavities between. Shortly after the separation, small vesicles appear near the nuclear envelope, suggesting that parts of the envelope give rise to elements of

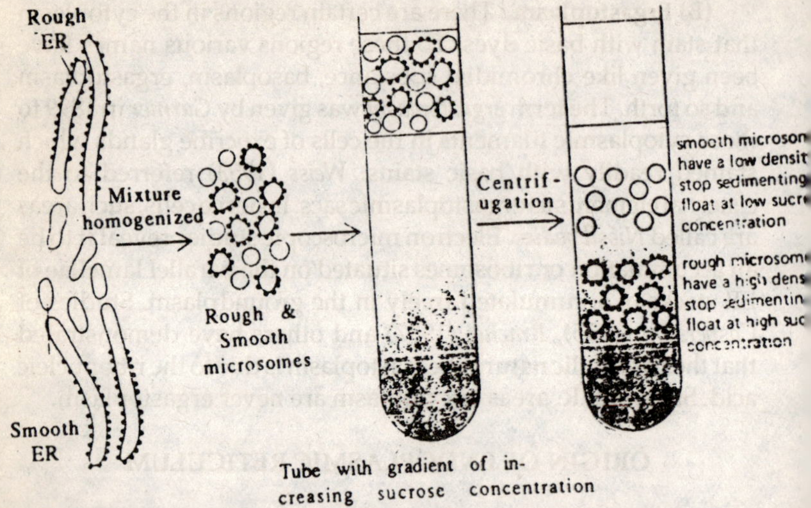

Fig. 6.5. Isolation procedure used to purify RWER & SWER

the endoplasmic reticulum. Thus the endoplasmic reticulum seems to have its origin in the nuclear envelope in undifferentiated cells.

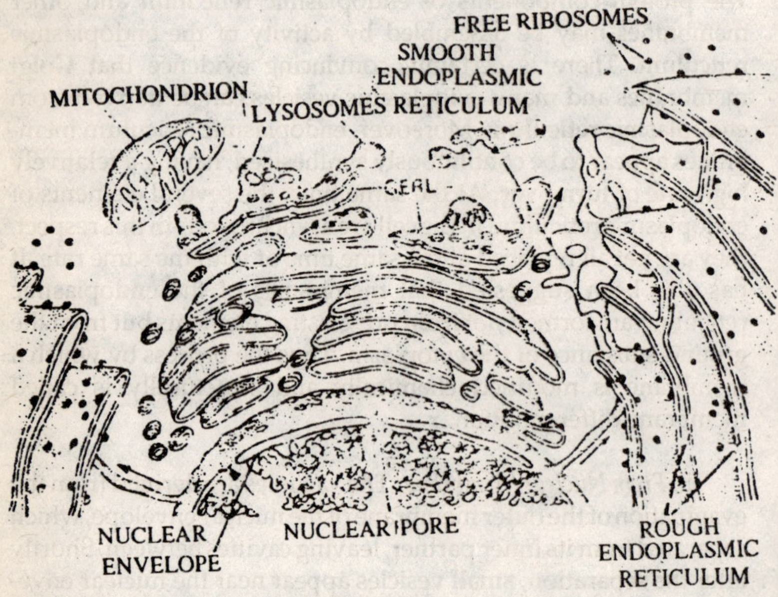

Fig. 6.6 Showing the origin of endoplasmic reticulum from nuclear envelope

ENZYMES OF THE ER MEMBRANES

The membranes of the endoplasmic reticulum are found to contain many kinds of enzymes which are needed for various important synthetic activities. The most important enzymes are the stearases, NADH-cyto-chrome C reductase, NADH diaphorase, glucose-6 -phosphotase-and-Mg++activiated AT Pase. Certain enzymes of the endoplasmic reticulum such as nucleotide diphosphate are involved in the biosynthesis of phospholipid, ascorbic acid, glucuronide, steroids and hexose metabolism. The enzymes of the endoplasmic reticulum perform the following important functions:

1. Synthesis of glycerides, e.g., triglycerides, phospholipids, glycolipids.
2. Metabolism of plasmalgens.
3. Synthesis of fatty acids.
4. Biosynthesis of the steroids, e.g., Cholesterol biosynthesis, steroid hydrogenation of unsaturated bonds.
5. $NADPH_2 + O_2$—requiring steroid transformations : Aromatization and hydroxylation.
6. $NADPH_2 + O_2$—requiring steroid transformations: Aromatic hydroxylations, side-chain oxidation, deamination, thio-ether oxidations, desulfuration.
7. L-ascorbic acid synthesis.
8. UDP-uronic acid metabolism.
8. UDP-glucose dephosphorylation.
10. Aryl-and steroid sulfatase.

FUNCTIONS

Many functional interpretations of endoplasmic reticulum are based on the polymorphic aspects of its components in a variety of cells and its different stages of activity. More reliable interpretations are based on the isolation studies just mentioned. The following functions are based on the same well known facts together with hypothesis.

(1) Mechanical Support : ER contributes to the mechanical support of the cytoplasm by dividing of fluid contents of the cell into compartments. This makes possible the existence of ionic gradients and electrical potentials along ER membranes. This concept has been specially applied to sarcoplasmic reticulum.

(2) Exchange of Ions and any other Fluid: These membranes of the endoplasmic reticulum may regulate the exchange between the inner compartment or cavity and the cytoplasmic matrix. The following statistic gives an impressive idea of the surface area available for exchange: 1 gm of liver contains about 8 to 12 square metre of endoplasmic reticulum. After isolation, microsomes expand or shrink according to the osmotic pressure of the fluid. Diffusion and active transports may take place across the membrane of the endoplasmic reticulum.

(3) Intracellular Circulation : The endoplasmic reticulum may act as a kind of circulatory system for intracellular circulation of various substances. Membrane flow may be an important mechanism for carrying particles, molecules and ions into and out of the cells by way of vascular system. The "pinocytosis", a "cellular drinking" also takes place by endoplasmic reticulum.

By this mechanism, particles attached to the surface of the cell or suspended in the fluid medium can be incorporated into the cytoplasm. The similar mechanism but working in a reverse direction can effect the transport of particle from the interior of the cytoplasm to the outer medium. The continuities observed in some cases between the endoplasmic reticulum and the nuclear envelope suggest that the membrane flow may also be active at this point. This flow would provide one of the several mechanisms for export of RNA and nucleoproteins from the nucleus to the cytoplasm.

(4) Protein Synthesis : Proteins may be synthesized to be utilized within the cell or these may have to be exported outside the cell to the site of their utility. It is the latter kind of proteins in whose synthesis, endoplasmic reticulum plays an important role. For instance, rough endoplasmic reticulum, which has attached ribosomes carries synthesis of secretory proteins on these ribosomes and export them. Synthesis of tropocollagen, serum proteins and secretory granules are some examples of secretory proteins. The protein molecules synthesized on attached ribosomes are discharged and penetrate into the cavity of ER, where they are stored or exported outside. During the transport of these products, three types of membranes ER-Golgi membrane-plasma membrane should interact and remain interconnected or disconnected due to fusion and fission repectively.

(5) Synthesis of Lipid : The cells in which active lipid metabolism takes place are found to contain large amount of the smooth type of endoplasmic reticulum. According to some workers as *Christensen* (1961) and *Claude* (1968) the smooth type of endoplasmic reticulum is related with the synthesis and metabolism of the lipids.

(6) Synthesis of Glycogen : The smooth endoplasmic reticulum of the glycogen storing cells of the liver and the cells of certain plants is found to be associated with the synthesis, storage and metabolism of the glycogen. But, *Porter* (1961) and *Peter* (1963) have suggested that smooth type of endoplasmic reticulum is related to glycogenolysis (digestion of glycogen) and not to glycogenesis (synthesis of the glycogen).

(7) Detoxification : Smooth ER is also involved in the detoxification of many endogenous and exogenous compounds. Prolonged administration of certain drugs (phenobarbitol) results in the increased activity of enzymes related to detoxification, as well as other enxymes, and a considerable hypertrophy of the SER (*Claude,* 1970). This is also applicable to administered steroid hormones.

(8) Synthesis of Cholesterol and Steroid Hormones : Cholesterol is an important precursor of steroid hormones. The major site of cholesterol synthesis is the ER. In liver cells the SER is believed to be concerned with both the synthesis and storage of cholesterol.

In the testis, ovary and the adrenal cortex the SER has a role in the synthesis of steroid hormones. The enzymes catalysing biosynthesis of androgens have been located in the SER. There is a strong correlation between the amounts of SEER in cells and the capacity to synthesize steroid hormones.

(9) Amphibian Development: There are evidences to suggest that the ER contributes in several ways to the development of the amphibian embryo.

(10) Cell Differentiation : Some specific instances of development have been studied in detail which more or less confirm the contention that the ER is important in the process of cell differentiation. Not only this much, ER also plays role in coordinating the differentiation.

(11) Formation of Microbodies : Closely related with the ER are microbodies, which are small granular bodies filled with an electron dense substance and limited by a single membrane. Microbodies are formed as dilations of the ER and frequently show connections with the ER cisternae. They are rich in the enzymes peroxidase (also called *peroxisomes*), catalase, and D-amino acid oxidase. In plant cells the enzymatic content is different and the bodies are called *glyoxysomes* because they, include enzymes of the glyoxylate cycle.

(12) Enzyme Activities and Cellular Metabolism : Numerous enzymes mainly those involved in the metabolism of steroid (cholesterol and glycerides), phospholipids and hormones (testosterone and progresterone) are associated with the membranes of smooth endoplasmic reticulum. These membranes provide an increased an inner surface for various metabolic reactions and they themselves take an active part in them by means of attached enzymes. This facilities free union of enzymes with their substrates.

(13) Role of Endoplasmic Reticulum in Intracellular Impulse Conduction : The existence of endoplasmic reticulum separating the cytoplasm into two compartments makes possible the existence of ionic gradients and electrical potentials across these intracellular membranes. This idea has been applied to the sarcoplasmic reticulum. A specialized from of smooth surface endoplasmic reticulum found in striated muscles which is now being considered as intracellular conducting system. On the basis of some evidences, it has been postulated that the sarcoplasmic reticulum transmits impulses from the surface membrane into deep regions of the muscles fibres.

(14) Formation of Plasmodestmata : Electron microscopic studies suggest that the endoplasmic reticulum in plants plays a special role in the interconnection of cells through the cytoplasmic strands called *plasmodesmata*.

(15) Role of E.R. during Cell Division : During cell division, some of the elements of reticulum contribute in the formation of the new nuclear membrane after karyogamy. The nuclear membrane breaks up into fragments in the early part of the division which finally disintegrate into small vesicles (*Moses* 1960). These vesicles moved towards the pole of the spindle as the metaphase starts, where they are indistinguishable from the elements of ER. From the polar ends of the cell, elements of ER as well as the fragmented vesicles migrate into the regions around the chromosomes, which are grouping at the poles. Most of these elements of ER join or fuse around each group of daughter chromosomes to form a new nuclear envelop.

(16) Transportation of Message from Genetic Material: ER provides passage for the genetic material to pass from the nucleus to the various organelles in the cytoplasm, thereby controlling the synthesis of proteins, fats and carbohydrates.

(17) ATP Synthesis : ER membranes are the sites of ATP synthesis in the cell. The ATP is used as a source of energy for all the intracellular metabolism and tranport of materials.

(18) Formation of Cell Organelle : Most of cell organelles like Golgi complex, mitochondria, lysosomes, nuclear membrane and cell plate etc. are usually developed from endoplasmic reticulum.

7

RIBOSOMES

Ribosomes are the basophilic granules present in the cytoplasm of the cell. Since this material had an affinity for basic stains similar to that of chromatin granules of the nucleus, so it was for a time called *chromidial* or *chromophil substance*. The ribosomes were first noted in plant cells by *Robinson* and *Brown* in 1953 while studying bean roots with the electron microscope and shortly afterward *Palade* (1955) observed them in animal cells. He isolated the ribosomes and detected the RNA in them. That is why it was also called *RNP* or *ribonucleo protein particles* or *Palade granules*. *Claude* named them as *microsome* but the name *ribosomes* was designed by *Robert* in 1958.

Occurrence. They are universally distributed throughout the animal kingdom and plant kingdom. In prokaryotes too, they are found. The only cell types devoid of ribosomes is the mammalian RBC. The density of ribosomes per unit area being rather constant for any given type, it is high in the cells which are active in protein synthesis and low in cells where protein synthesis is low.

Distribution. In prokaryotic cells the ribosomes often occur freely in the cytoplasm. In eukaryotic cells the ribosomes either occur freely in the cytoplasm or remain attached to the outer surface of the membrane of endoplasmic reticulum. When they are not attached to the ER they are called free ribosomes. Free ribosomes serve as sites for the synthesis of proteins that are required to maintain the enzyme constitution of the cytoplasmic matrix.

Number and Concentration of Ribosomes. In all cells that contain endoplasmic reticulum, a good number of ribosomes can be observed. For example, at the base of gland cells, in plasma and liver cells, in all rapidly growing plant and animal cells and in bacteria, quantity of RNA can be related with the concentration of ribosome. In reticulocytes of rabbit nearly 100 ribosomes are found per 3 μ, which corresponds to 1 x 105 particles per reticulocyte and about 0.5 per cent of total volume of the cell. In growing *E. coli* (bacteria), ribosomes account for 25 to 30 per cent of the cells mass, or about 20,000 to 30,000 per cell. However, if the rate of protein synthesis is slowed down by unfavourable nutritional conditions, the number of ribosomes can drop considerably in protein synthesizing cells and in bacteria.

Structure of Ribosomes : Ribosomes are remarkable for their uniformity in size and composition through the wide range of cells in which they have been studied. Ribosomes of higher plants and animals are oblate, spheroids and their diameter is approximately 250Å. However, the ribosomes of bacteria are somewhat smaller because they contain less amount of proteins than the higher animal ribosomes. However, in quantity of RNA per particle, bacterial ribosomes resemble all the other presently studied ribosomes.

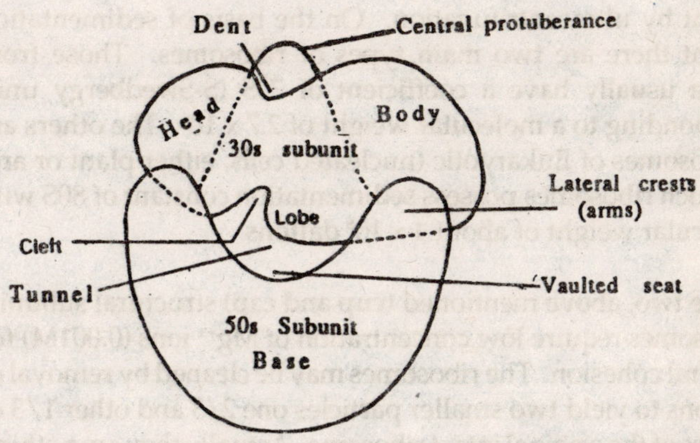

Fig. 7.1 70S ribosome of *E. coli* (Stoffler and Wittmann's model)

In the electron microscope studies negative staining reveals a cleft that divides the ribosomes into a larger sub-unit and a smaller sub-unit. In *E. coli* the larger particle is somewhat 'Cup' shaped or dome shaped (140 to 160 Å) and smaller one forms a 'Cap' (90 to 110 Å) that is applied to the flat surface of the other (*Huxley* and

Zubey, 1960). In higher animals and plants it was shown that the ribosomes are attached to endoplasmic reticulum by the large subunits.

The fine structure of the ribosome is very complex and not yet fully elucidated. Since the ribosomes are highly porous and hydrated, the RNA and protein are probably intertwined within the two subunits. In sections, stained with uranyl ions (RNA selective stain), each ribosome appears as a star shaped body with four to six arms implanted on a dense axis. The isolated 50S subunit of *Bacillus subtilis* appears as a compact particle of 160 to 180 Å having a pentagonal face, in the centre of which is a round area to 40 to 60 Å (Nanninga, 1967). An electron transparent core, which in negative stained ribosomes correspond to an electron opaque region, has been described in the large subunits. The 40S subunit is not regular and tends to be sub-divided into two portions that are inter-connected by a strand 30 to 60 Å thick.

Ribosomal Subunit. Another property which is common to all ribosomes is their subunit structure and their sedimentation constant by ultracentrifugation. On the basis of sedimentation constant there are two main types of ribosomes. Those from bacteria usually have a coefficient of 70S (S-Swedbergy unit) corresponding to a molecular weight of 2.7×10^6. The others are the ribosomes of Eukaryotic (nucleated cells, either plant or animal), such ribosomes possess sedimentation constant of 80S with a molecular weight of about 4×10^6 daltons.

The two, above mentioned (cup and cap) structural subunits of ribosomes require low concentration of Mg^{++} ions (0.001M) for structural cohesion. The ribosomes may be cleaned by removal of Mg^{++} ions to yield two smaller particles one 2/3 and other 1/3 of the mass of the original intact ribosome. Actually they are nothing but same subunits which are observed with the help of electron microscope. These subunits are referred to by their sedimentation constants. The one unit of ribosome possesses a sedimentation constant of 80S or 70S as mentioned earlier, while the 2/3 subunit has a sedimentation constant of 60S or 50S and the 1/3 subunit 40S or 30S respectively. Both the subunits are bound together through magnesium ions which interact with the phosphodiester groups of

RNA. The fully magnesium saturated particle contains Mg^{++} ion per three phosphodiester groups. Removal of calculated 1/3 of these magnesium ions result in cleavage of the 80S to form 60S and 40S (subunits). Removal of further Mg^{++} results in the case of pea and yeast ribosomes at least in further cleavage liberating what are apparently 1/6 subunits. This further cleavage, in contrast to that to 2/3 and 1/3 subunits is, however, irreversible in the sense that restoration of magnesium ions, does not result in the restoration of 80S particles. If the Mg^{++} concentration increases ten folds, two ribosomes combine and form a "dimer' with twice the molecular weight of the individual ribosome. The 'dimer' can be convered back into two ribosomes by lowering the Mg^{++} concentration.

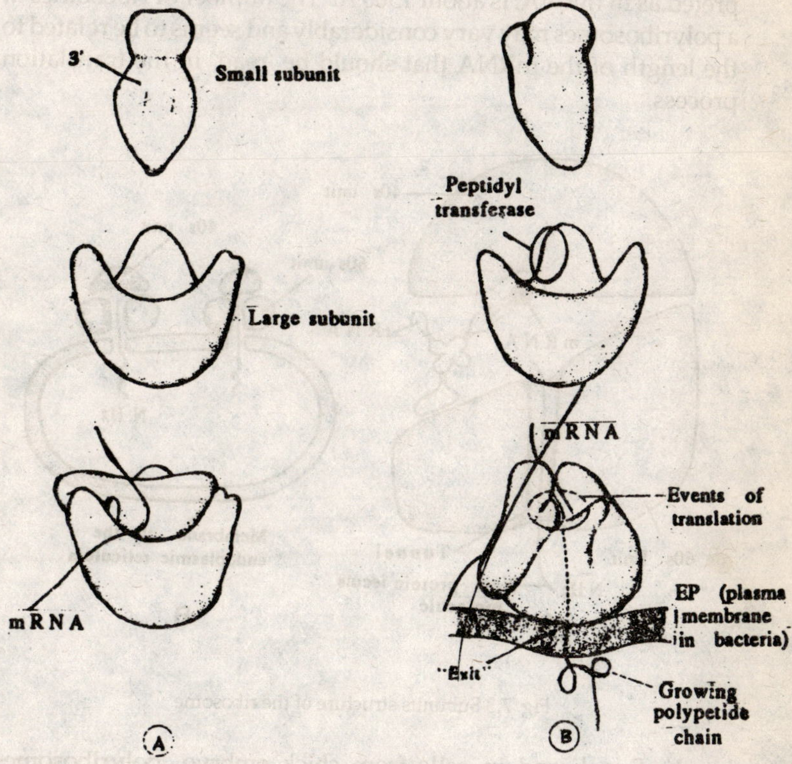

Fig. 7.2 Two proposed models of ribosome structure in prokaryotes

The early electron microscopic observations of cell sections revealed that ribosomes were frequently associated in groups occasionally forming recurrent pattern. It was not until 1962 that the function of these poly-ribosomes, or polysomes, in protein synthesis was discovered (*Warner* and *Rich*, 1962). After treating reticulocytes with C^{14} labelled amino acids and using gentle methods for disruption, it was found that in addition to the typical sedimentation constant of single ribosome (80S) some larger units were present. The sedimentation constant of these particles vary from 108S to 170S or even more; this corresponded to a polyribosome of five units (a pentamer). It was confirmed by electron microscopy that about 75 per cent of the ribosomes which show 170S peak, were presented as pentameres. A thin filament, interpreted as in mRNA, is about 1500 Å. The number of ribosomes in a polyribosomes may vary considerably and seems to be related to the length of the mRNA that should be 'read' in the translation process.

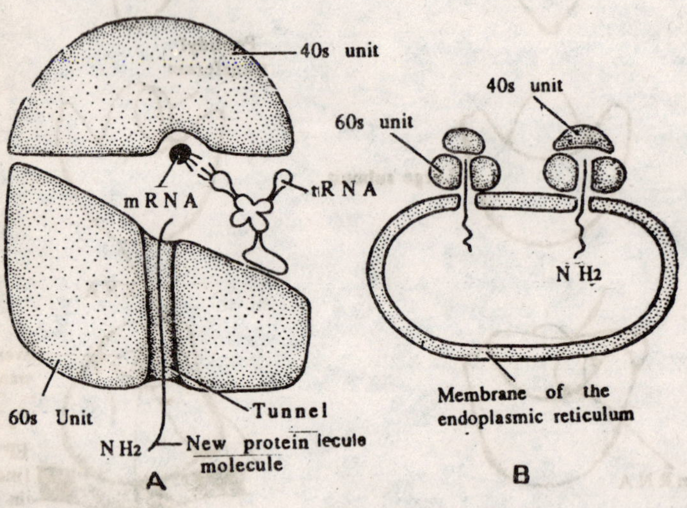

Fig. 7.3 Subunits structure of the ribosome

In *E. coli* and in cells from chick embryo, polyribosomes composed of about 50 units have been observed (*Rich* 1967). Polyribosomes may be free in the cytoplasm or bound to the membranes of the endoplasmic reticulum. For free polyribosomes, a helical configuration has been postulated with the small subunits arranged around the central axis and the large subunits disposed at the periphery. In sections of various cells polyribosomes have been observed in a helical array (*Weiss* and *Grover*, 1968). It is assumed that in the polysome the mRNA is situated in between the two subunits of the ribosome.

TYPES OF RIBOSOMES

The ribosomes are of two basic types, 70S and 80S ribosomes. The S refers to Svedberg units. Actually it is the sedimentation coefficient which shows how fast a cell organelle sediments in an ultra centrifuge. Sedimentation coefficients are not additive. 80S ribosomes are found in eukaryotes (organisms whose cells have true nuclei bounded by nuclear envelopes), e.g. algae, fungi, higher plants and animals. The 80S ribosome of animals consists of a large 60S subunit and a small 40S subunit (Table 7.1).

70S ribosomes are relatively smaller and are found in prokaryotes (organisms whose DNA is not bounded by a nuclear envelope), e.g. bacteria. The 70S ribosome consists of a large 50S subunit and a small 30S subunit.

Ribosomes found in mitochondria and chloroplasts of eukaryotes are closer to prokaryote ribosomes rather than the 80S eukaryote ribosomes. Vertebrate mitochondria, for example, contain 55S ribosomes, each with a large 40S subunit and a small 30S subunit. The sedimentation coefficients 80S, 70S and 55S are rounded off values. Actual S values in different organisms may be

Table 7.1 Characteristics of different ribosome types.

Ribosome type	*Found in*	*Large subunit*		*Small subunit*	
		Size	*RNAs*	*Size*	*RNAs*
80S	Eukaryotes (animals)	60S	28-29S+5S +5.8S	40S	18S
80S	Eukaryotes (plants)	60S	25S+5S +5.8S	40S	16-18S
70S	Prokaryotes	50S	23S+5S	30S	16S
55S	Mitochondria	40S	16-17S+5S	30S	12-13S

CHEMICAL COMPOSITION

The main constituents of ribosomes are RNA and proteins. The lipids are entirely absent or present in traces. The ribosomes of *E. coli* possess nearly 60-65 per cent of RNA and 35-40% protein of their weight. Table 7.3 is showing approximate quantity of RNA and protein in different types of ribosomes.

Table 7.2 Differences between 70S and 80S ribosomes.

Presence	*In prokaryotes (bacteria)*	*In eukaryotes (algae, fungi higher plants and animals).*
Sedimentation Coefficient	64S-72S (average 69S)	79-85S in fungi, 80S in mammals.
Size	Relatively smaller	Relatively larger.
Molecular wt.	3×10^6	$4\text{-}5 \times 10^6$
Subunits	Small 30S and large 50S	Small 40S and large 60S
RNA	3 molecules of RNA: 16S RNA in 30S subunit, 23S and 5S RNA in 50S subunit.	4 molecules of RNA: 16S-18S RNA in 40S subunit; 25-29S, 5.8S and 5S RNA in 60S subunit.

cont.....

MW of RNA	16S RNA-550,000 23S RNA-1,100,000 5S RNA-40,000 5S RNA-39,000	18S RNA-70,000 28S RNA-1,700,000 5.8S RNA-51,000
No. of proteins	21(S1-S21) in small subunit 34(S1-L34) in large subunit Total in prokaryotes: 50-60 proteins.	33 in small subunit 49 in large subunit. Total in eukaryotes: 70-80 proteins
Average MW of protein	18,000	21,000
No. of amino acids	8,000	16,000
RNA-Protein ratio	2:1	1:1

TABLE 7.3 Showing the chemical composition of ribosomes

Ribosomes	*Sedimentation constant*	*Subunits*	*S.U. of % RNA*	*RNA in complete Ribosomes*	*% Protein in complete ribosomes*
Liver.	80S	60S	28S	45%	55%
Yeast	80S				
Neurospora	80S	40S	18S		
Mitochondira	70S	50S	23S		
E.Coli	70S			65%	35%
Chloroplasts	70S	30S	16S		

Ribosomal RNA differs in size and base contents from tRNA and from other RNA classes of most cells. Two types of RNAs are found in all ribosomes. They are the integral component, and cannot be removed easily. RNA of rat liver particles contain chiefly the common bases adenine, guanine, cytosine, and uracil with small amount of pseudo-uridine, the usual bases which occur in the soluble RNA are found in particles RNA only in very small amount.

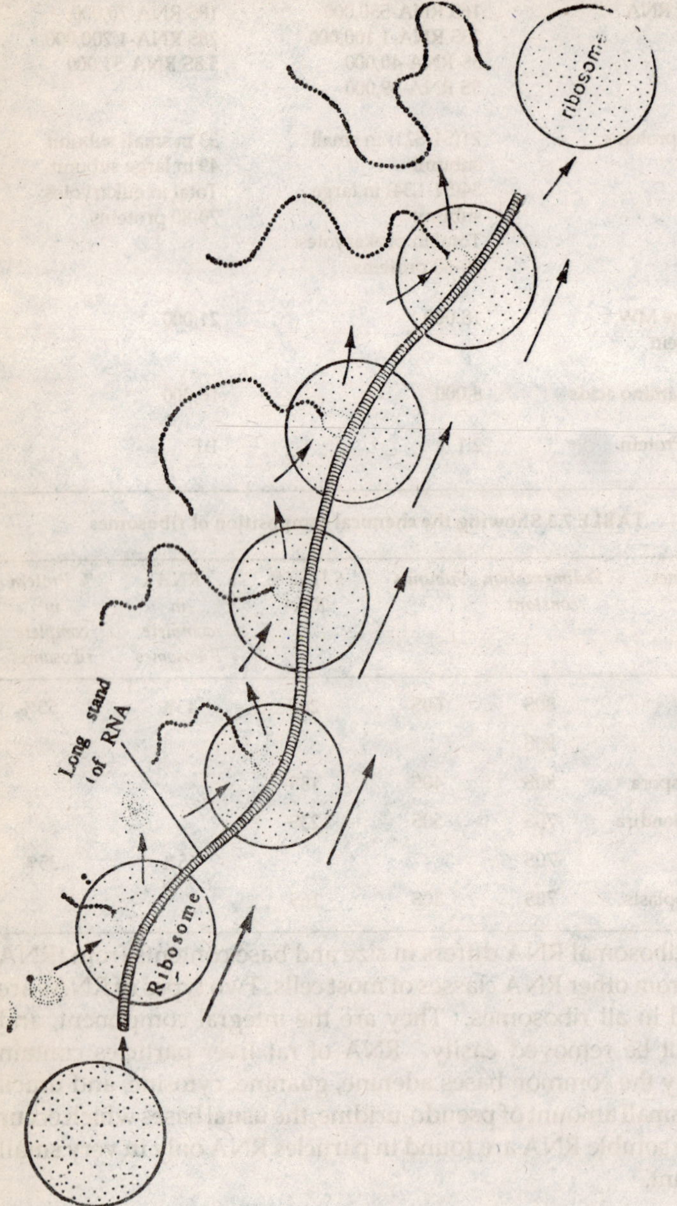

Fig. 7.4 A polysome

Ribosomal RNA

The 70S ribosomes contain three types of rRNA, viz., 23S rRNA, 16S rRNA and 5S RNA. The 23S and 5S rRNA occur in the larger 50S ribosomal subunit, while the 16S rRNA occurs in the smaller 40 S ribosomal subunit. The 23S rRNA consists of 3200 nucleotides, 16S rRNA contains 1600 nucleotides and 5S rRNA includes 120 nucleotides in it (*Brownlee*, 1968, *Fellner*, 1972).

The 80S ribosomes also contain three types of rRNA, viz., 28S rRNA, 18S rRNA and 5S rRNA. The 28S and 5S rRNa occur in the larger 60S ribosomal unit while the 18S rRNA occurs in the smaller 40S ribosomal subunit.

The 28S rRNA has the molecular weight 1.6 x 106 daltons and its molecule is double stranded and having nitrogen bases in pairs. The 18S rRNA has the molecular weight 0.6 x 10 6 daltons. The molecules of 5S rRNA has a clover leaf shape and a length equal to 120 nucleotides (*Forget* and *Weissmann*, 1968).

Other Constituents. The metal contents of ribosomes are also a difficult question. There is little doubt that magnesium is the chief ion physiologically, since it is present in high concentration in rat liver ribosomes. It is the most active in maintaining the 80S structure (*Hamilton* and *Petermann*, 1959) as it is essential for amino acid incorporation in vitro (*Rendi* and *Hultin*, 1960). The other metals which are present in the ribosomes are chromium, manganese, nickel, iron and calcium (*Walker* and *Valle* 1958 and *Tso* 1958).

FUNCTIONS

It is a well known fact that the ribosomes are factories of manufacturing of protein in a cell but actually one ribosome cannot take part in the protein synthesis. It was known from 1962 when a report was published which showed that active units are not individual ribosome, but a group of these units, which is called as polyribosome. A detailed role of polyribosome was published in *Scientific American* Dec. 1963 by *Grick* and *Hall*. There is much evidence that ribosomes are alike and are at least interchangable.

In case of hemoglobin with a chain of 150 amino acids the most usual number of ribosomes which were linked together was 5. There may be large number of ribosomes and upto 40 ribosomes have been described. So the name polysome can also be applied at the place of polyribosome.

Protein cosists of linear chain of amino acids. The chain may be short or long, in both the cases it is called polypeptide chain. Polypeptide can be folded in a specific manner often combine to form a complex protein.

The ribosomes in a polysome are separated by gap of 50-150A°. Positive staing by Uracil-acetate reveals that the ribosomes are connected by a thin thread 10-15A° in diameter, which is about the thickness of a single strand of RNA. From the size of the gap between ribosomes, the total measurement of the gap containing five ribosomes, is about 1500A°, the five ribosomes have inter ribosomal gap of 50-150A° each.

8

PLASTIDS

The plastids are characteristic large cytoplasmic bodies of the cell intimately related to the metabolic processes and impart colour to the tissues. They are found mostly in plants with possible exception of the very lowest group of plants. However, plastids are also found in few animals, especially the protozoans flagellated. They are not found in bacteria, certain large, myxomycetes and fungi. On the basis of presence of the plastids, the living world has been distinguished into plant and animal kingdoms. Old literature indicates that *Pringshetn* was the first to investigate the plastids. The term plastid was used in 1885 by *A.F. W. Schimper* to include the cell organelles which are primarily involved in the formation and storage of soluble and insoluble carbohydrates. *A Meyer* in 1883, *F. Schmitz* in 1884 and *A.F. W. Schimper* in 1885 made detailed cytological studies of these cell organelles and showed that green plastids now known as chloroplasts could not be formed from cytoplasm, but only from existing chloroplasts. The plastids very in size, number, shape and chemical organization with the particular tissue and organism concerned. In contrast to the smaller cytoplasmic granules such as the mitochondria. important physical and chemical diferences in the plastids can be easily recognized, such as changes in size or shape, the presence or absence of the chloroplastic chlorophyll, carotenoids and starch. Mature plastids can be shown to arise from more or less undifferentiated plastid primordia which occur in the meristematic cells, or those of the developing embryo.

The plastids are self-duplicating bodies and their life history, especially of the chloroplast, may be divided into three phases. In the first phase self duplication and enzymatic activities with some concern to RNA takes place. The second phase is mainly concerned with differentiation to form the enzymes required for photosynthesis. In the third phase the activities of the enzymes that predominates are those concerned with photosynthesis.

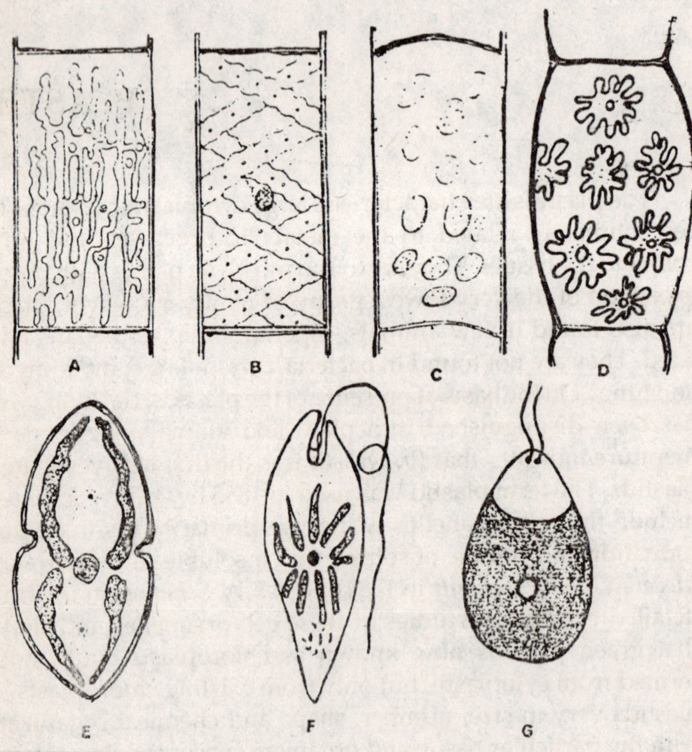

Fig. 8.1. Various types of chloroplasts. A-Oedogonium, B-Spirogyra, C-Phyloiella, D-Rhodochlorton, E-Euastrun, F-Euglena, G-Chlamydomons.

VARIOUS TYPES OF PLASTIDS

Plastids may be divided into two general groups; the *chromoplasts* (coloured plastids); and the *leucoplasts* (colourless plastids). The chromoplasts may be further divided into two subgroups; those that are photosynthetically active and those that are not.

(A) Photosynthetically active Chromoplasts : The photosynthetically active chromoplasts are chloroplasts, pheoplasts, rhodoplasts, blue-green chromoplasts and chromatophores of photosynthetic bacteria.

(1) *Chloroplasts.* These are green plastids of green algae and higher plants and contain chlorophyll A and B in the ratio of 2.3:1. These have different appearance and varying sizes.

(2) *Pheoplasts (Brown or yellow plastids).* This type of plastid is commonly present in the brown algae, diatomos and dinoflagellates. In these pheoplasts, brown carotenoids mask the chlorophyll.

As reported by *Strain* (1951) the yellow or brown colour of the pheoplasts appears to result from the physical state or condition of the pigment from their geometrical arrangement in the plastids. Brown algae contain fucoxanthin which can absorb light and transfer energy to chlorophyll.

(3) *Rhodoplasts.* Various members of Rhodophyceae contain red coloured plastids. The red colour is due to a pigment phycobilin and protein phycoerythrin (*Strain* 1949). The colour of plastids may be the result of light absorption. There may be phycocyanin too in traces. *Haxo, Blink* and *Young* (1952) found that light is absorbed by phycobilin and is transmitted to chlorophyll *a*.

(4) *Blue-green Chromatophore.* Two accessory protein phycocyanin and phycoerythrin impart blue-green colour to algae. These pigments and chlorophyll *a* alongwith carotenoid form lamellar structure, the *chromatophore.*

Wilson and *Morrison* (1967) mention that all the organisms capable of performing photosynthesis do not necessarily contain plastid structures; for example, blue-green algae and photosynthetic bacteria. In blue-greens, the light sensitive pigments are chlorophyll and phycobilin pigments. These pigments are associated with a system of membranes and lamellae in the cytoplasm of the cell. In photosynthetic bacteria also wide diversity of structures are associated with the photosynthesis. These structures are as follows:

(1) Lamellae in some purple bacteria; for example, *Rhodomicrobium*, (2) Vesicular membrane-bound structures, known as chromatophores found in non-sulphuric and purple sulphur bacteria; for example, *Rhodospirillium*, *Chromatium*, and (3) Ribosome like granules found in green sulfur bacterium, *Chlorobiumthio sultatophilum*. All these photosynthetic bacteria possess a pigment system consisting of a specialized form of chlorophyll, known as bacteriochlorophyll and various carotenoid pigments.

(B) Chromoplasts without Photosynthetic activity : These types of chromoplasts contain carotnoids only. They are red to yellow in colour and are much more variable in shape. They impart specific colour to various plant tissues, fruits and flowers. The new colour that arise often due to the formation of special carotenoids, for example the *leucopene* of tomato fruits, *prolycopene* of berries, and *capsanthin* of red pepper. Xanthophyll is also present in adequate proportions. Coloured carotenoids are also important constituents of the coloured parts of plant. These may be found in fungi and bacteria. Acidic carotenoids of fungi are similar to astaxanthin. *Haxo* (1949) isolated a mixture of carotenoids from the *Neurospora crassa* which includes lycopene, carotene, and spiriloxanthines as the main components. the growth of carotenoid becomes double in presence of light.

These chromoplasts are supposed to develop from the leucoplasts that contain starch. As the carotene increase in concentration the starch disappears. The older chromoplasts appear thin plates as needles with typical crystalline appearance. They are direfringen and dichroic (*Frey Wyssling*, 1935).

Leucoplasts. The non-coloured plastids are called leucoplasts. They do not contain pigments and the membranous structures are absent. They are found mainly in the embryonic and sexual cells. They are also found in merestemetic cells and in those regions of the plants which do not receive light. They serve mainly for the storage of starch, oils and proteins. Plastids. located in cotyledons and the primordium of stem are first colourless but eventually become filled with pigments and become coloured plastids. Leucoplasts are further categorized into following three types.

(1) *Amyloplasts.* These are mature plastids with predominant starch contents and generally found in storage tubers, cotyldons and endosperm. Starch is characteristic of the coloured and the colourless plastids of green algae and the higher plants. the deposition of other carbohydrates may not necessarily be with the plastids. For example, in red algae starch is formed at the surface of the plastids. In *Euglena,* Paramylum grains are considered to be produced outside the plastids. The starch grains may be of two types: assimilative starch and reserve starch. The former is characteristic of actively photosynthesizing chloroplasts and the latter is most familiar in storage organs. The starch grains are made of a series of concentric layers successively deposited about a centre, the *hilum.* As starch continues to be deposited, the walls of the amyloplast become greatly distended. *Frey Wyssling* (1953) observed that the formation of a new concentric layer begins as a dense region of high refractive index, then it becomes a dense layer due to more hydration. Chemically starch contains two components: mainly α-amylose (which stain red with iodine) and minorly B-amylose (only 20-30 per cent forming helical chain structure and stains blue with iodine), *Hassid* (1954).

(2) *Elaioplasts.* The plastids storing oils are known as elaioplasts. In most monocotyledons, the chloroplasts after losing their chlophyll start storing oil in epidermal cells of Orchidaceae and Liliaceae. The disorganised plastids fuse to form oil droplets. In brown algae the reserve storage is oil and this oil appears to be formed in the pheoplasts (*Sharp,* 1934).

(3) *Aleuroneplasts.* These are the plastids that contains much protein and often termed as the *proteinoplasts.* Protein crystals and granules are produced in the seeds of numerous plants especially in those seeds that also from large amount of oil, e.g. the Brazi Neof and seeds of *Ricinus. Mottier* (1921)referred that protein and oil formation involves the activity of permanent plastic primordia. Protein crystals may develop independently in the cytoplasm without any aid of the aleuroneplasts, as for example in cells poor in starch in peripheral layers of potato. Protein crystals in epidermal cells may also represent virus material or may be the result of virus action (*Granide*).

Amyloplasts are the most important of all the different types of leucoplasts. The amyloplasts resemble proplastids and differ from them only in size. They contain fewer lamellae, but in presence of light they can build up a thylacoid structure found in chloroplasts. However, chloroplasts can also synthesize starch and store in the stormal region. The starch in chloroplasts disappears quickly and is, therefore, known as transitory starch. The starch present in leucoplasts on the other hand can be stored for longer periods and is, therefore, known as reserve starch.

The starch development begins with the formation of a particle in the stroma. This particle has several bubuli and thylcoids and is surrounded by additional rings of starch. It grows till the amyloplasts is filled with starch. As a result, the tubuli are pressed against the wall and ulimately starch granule exceeds the size of amyloplast. The wall of the plastid ruptures and finally withers away so that only the starch granules can be seen.

CHLOROPLASTS

Chloroplasts are the plastids that are most common and of greatest logical importance, since by *photosynthesis* they produce most of the chemical energy used by living organisms. Without chloroplasts there would be no animals, because animals feed on the foodstuff produced by plants.

Distribution and Orientation : Chloroplasts are sometimes distributed homogeneously within the cytoplasm, but are frequently packed near the nucleus, or close to the cell wall. The distribution and orientation of the chloroplasts within the cells may vary with the amount of light energy. Chloroplasts apparently multiply by division—elongation of the plastid and constriction of the central portion. They have a higher density than the cytoplasm and migrate to the centrifugal pole of the cell when submitted to the action of centrifugal force.

Table 8.1 Showing occurrence, functions and pigments of various plastids.

Kinds of Plastids	*Occurrence*	*Functions*	*Pigment*
I Chromoplasts			
A. *Photosynthetically active chromoplasts.*			
1. Chloroplats	Higher plants and green algae	Photosynthesis	Chlorophyll-a and chlorophyll-b
2. Pheoplasts	Brown algae, diatoms and dinoflagellates	Light absorption	Fucoxanthin
3. Rhodoplasts	Red algae (Rhodophyceac)	Light absorption	Phycoerythrin
4. Blue-green	Blue-green algae	Photosynthesis	Phycocyanin Phycoerythrin Chlorophyll-a and Carotenoids
5. Chromoplasts of Photosynthetic bacteria	Purple and non-purple sulfur bacteria	Absorption of infra red portion of light	Bacteriochlorophyll
B. *Chromoplasts devoid of photosynthetic activity*			
6. Carotenoids	Tomato, red peppar, flower parts, fungi, ornamental bacteria and fruits.		Lycopene and Capsanthin
II. Leucoplasts			
7. Amyloplasts	Storage tubers, cotyledons and endosper	Starch-storage	None
8. Elaioplasts	Epidermal cells of Orchidaceae and Liliaceae	Oil-storage	None
9. Aleuronplasts	Epidermal cells of *Helleborus* and seeds of *Ricinus* and Brazil nut	Protein-storage	None

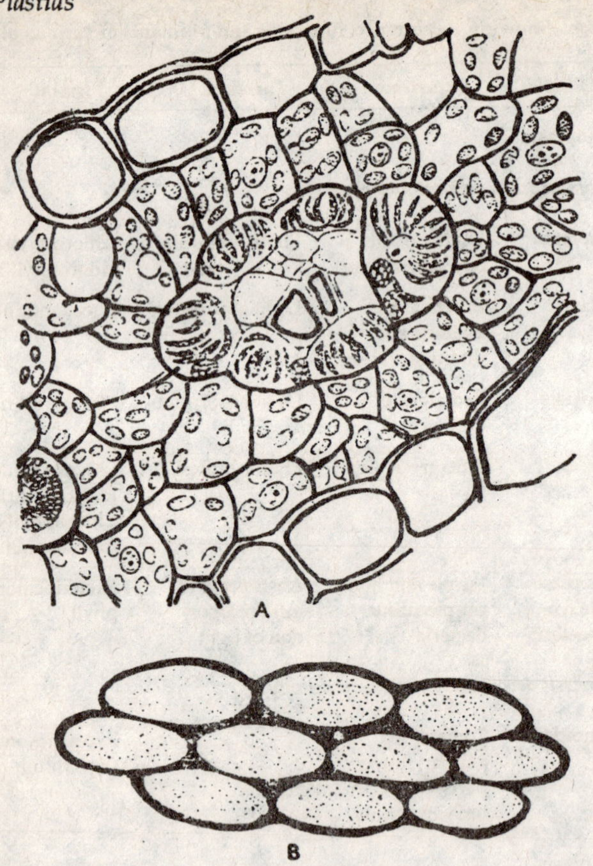

Fig. 8.2 Plastides in the nature leaf A-Ellipsoidal starch containing plastids in a sing layered parenchyma, B-Ellipsoidal plastid, showing the arrangement of starch grains.

MORPHOLOGY

Shape. Higher plant chloroplasts are generally biconvex or planoconvex. However, in different plants cells, chloroplast may have various shapes, viz., *filamentous, saucer-shaped, spheroid, ovoid* or *discoid shaped*. They are vesicular and have a colourless centre. Some chloroplasts are *club shaped*, having their middle zone and bulging ends filled with chlorphyll. Algae often possess a single huge chlroplast that appears as a network, a *spiral band*, or *stellate plate*.

Size. The size of chloroplasts varies from species to species but in constant for a given cell type. The average size of chloroplasts in higher plants measure 4-6μ in diameter and 1-3μ in thickness. The chloroplasts of polyploid plant cells are larger than those in the corresponding diploid cells. In general, chloroplasts of plants grown in the shade are larger and contain more chlorophyll than of those plants grown in sunlight.

Number. The number of chloroplasts is relatively constant in the different plants. In higher plants there are 20 to 40 chloroplasts per cell. It has been calculated that the leaf of *Ricinus communis* contains about 400,000 chloroplasts per square millimetre of surface area. When the number of chloroplasts is insufficient, it is increased by division; when excessive, it is reduced by degeneration.

Conformational changes and ion movements.

Chloroplasts undergo striking conformational changes which are dependent on the action of light. In the dark they undergo swelling and separation of the membranes of the thylakoid. This phenomenon is reversible; in the presence of light the membranes again return to close apposition. It was mentioned in Chapter 9 that mitochondria eject H^+ ions during the electron transport and that the interior becomes more alkaline. In the case of chloroplasts the opposite reactions occur; under the action of light H^+ ions are absorbed, and the interior becomes acidified. At the same time K^+ and Mg^{++} are ejected into the medium. In the dark, H^+ is ejected and K^+ and Mg^{++} are reabsorbed by the chloroplasts. Thus, the chloroplast membrane has a vectorial organization that is the reverse of the mitochondrial membrane. In physical terms it is understood that dark reactions, being of a thermochemical nature, do not need an ordered structural arrangement (i.e. they are carried out by soluble enzymes). On the contrary, photophosphorylation requires the separation of positive and negative charges into specific pathways of electron flow.

CHEMICAL COMPOSITION

Chloroplasts of spinach leaf cells contain about 56% protein, 32% lipid and 8% chlorophyll. The lipids include xanthophylls, carotenoids, triglycerides, steroids, waxes and phospholipids. Chloroplasts of higher plants contain approximately 35-55% proteins, 20-30% lipids, 9% chlorophyll, 4-5% carotenoids and 2-3% nucleic acids. In cytoplasm the protein-lipid ratio is generally 90:1. In plastids this ratio is about 40:30. Thus the grana have a high concentration of lipid. The nucleic acid DNA and RNA have been demonstrated in the chloroplasts of higher plants.

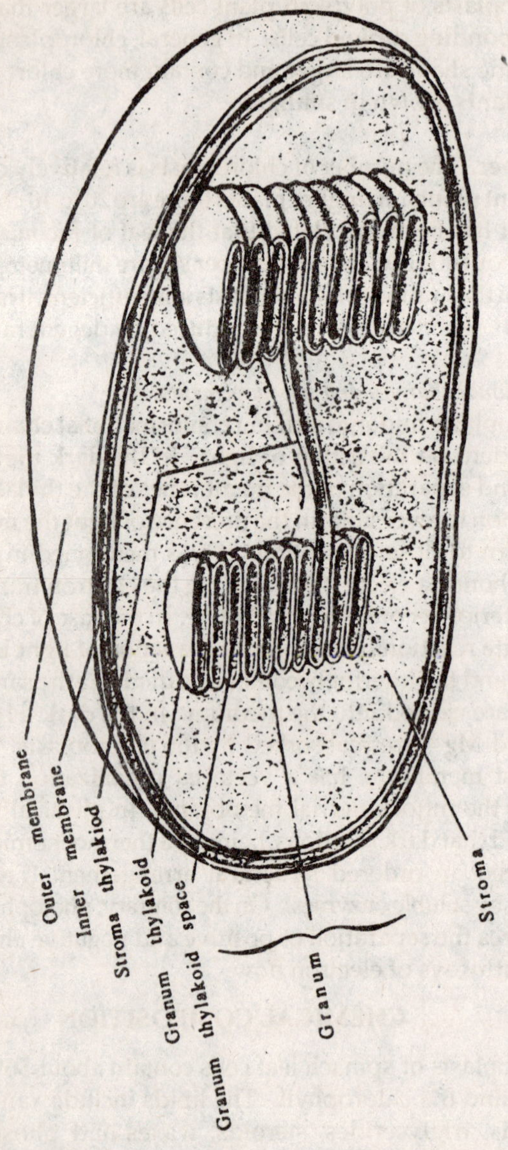

Fig. 8.3 Sub microscopic Structure of mature chloroplast

Chlorophyll has a tetrapyrrole structure and consists of a hydrophilic head and a hydrophobic tail. The head is made up of a magnesium atom surrounded by four pyrrolic nuclei (tetra-pyrrole structure). The long tail consists of a phytol china. Green plants have two types of chlorophyll, *chlorophyll a* and *chlorophyll b*. In *chlorophyll b* one of the methyl (-CH_3) groups of chlorophyll a is replaced by a formyl (-CHO) group.

Structure. Chloroplasts are dynamic organelles whose structure changes in response to changes in environment. A mature chloroplast has following parts:

(1) Limiting membrane
(2) Stroma
(3) Grana

(1) Limiting Membrane. Each mature chloroplast is covered by a double membrane as in mitochondira, each unit is about 40 to 60 A° in thickness. The limiting membrane functions as a semipermeable membrane as well as a boundary.

(2) Stroma. The inner space which is formed by a limiting membrane is filled with a proteinaceous matrix called the stroma. A number of starch grains and sometimes osmiophilic droplets are embedded in the stroma. When the plastid becomes inactive or ages, the number of osmiophilic droplets may increase.

(3) Grana or lamellar system. These are flat bodies shaped like platelets or discs, which in a lateral view appear as dense bands perpendicular to the limiting membrane of plastid. A number of grana are embedded in the stroma or matrix of plastid. The size of the grana varies between 0.3-1.7μ depending on the species. Each granum consists of a stack of double membrane or lamellae. The lamellar membranes are composed of lipids and proteins. Protein contents are about 45% while lipids contents are 55% in amount. Each lamella is 30-35 Å thick and the space between two such lamellae is of 65-70°. The lamellae can be placed under two groups:

(i) Stroma lamellae
(ii) Grana lamellae

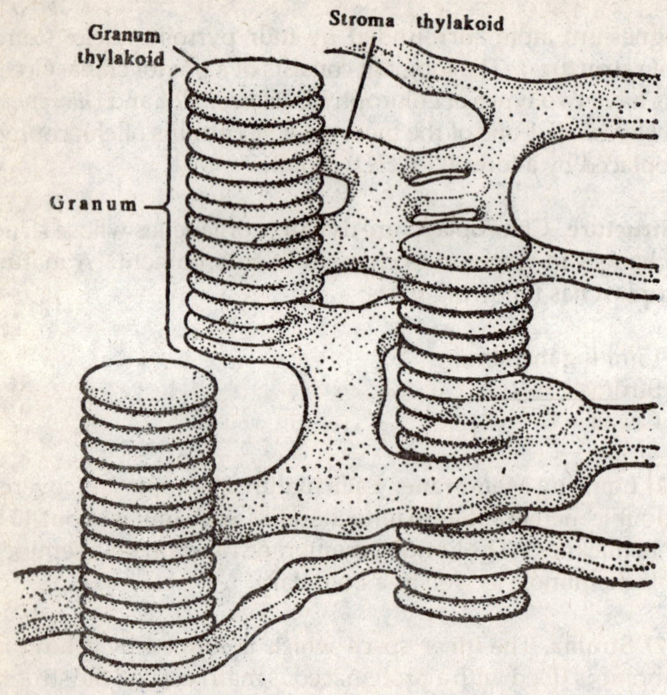

Fig. 8.4. Diagram showing the three dimensional arrangement and inner relationships of grana.

Those lamellae, extending through the entire length of the plastids are called the stroma lamellae. These are not directly connected with the cell wall. The grana lamellae are always densely packed. Anyway, the system of lamellae represents a closed unit, and thus both stroma and grana lamellae are closely related to one another, i.e., each granum lamella represents a local adhesion of two or more stroma lamellae. Both stroma and grana lamellae may stay coupled for a long distance and then separate again from each other. Another term *thylakoid* (*Greek*; sac like) has been used for the double membranous lamellae already explained. The stroma lamellae are larger thylakoids while the smaller, stacked thylakoids are the grana lamellae. One more term has been added by Weier and others, which is *fret* to describe stroma lamellae as a flattened tubular channel connecting adjacent grana.

Recent studies have provided evidence that the membranes within the chloroplasts form a continuum and the cavities of the thylakoids (locuili) communicate via fret work connection.

The total number of grana in plastids of certain plants have been calculated. There is a considerable variation in the number of grana in a single plastid, depending upon the species. In *Euglena* only one granum is present in one plastid while in Spinach, where about 40-60 grana are present in each plastid.

In *Chlamydomonas*, the plastid envelope is sometimes continuous with elements of the endoplasmic reticulum. In *Ochromonas* as well as in *Chlamydomonas*, connection with other cytoplasmic membranes with single plastid have also been traced.

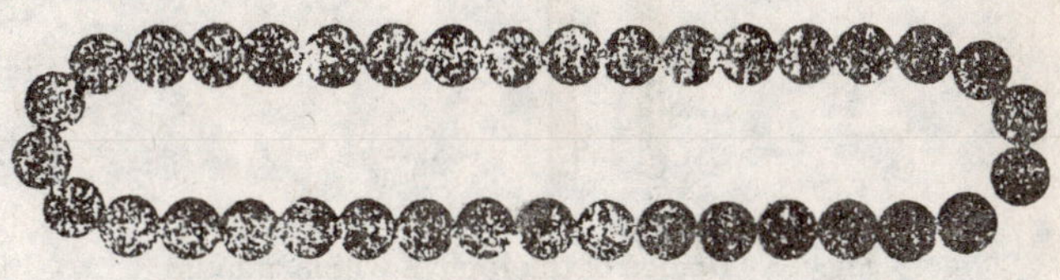

Fig. 8.5. Grana membranes consisting of a string of the particles

QUANTOSOME CONCEPT

The membranes of thylakoids are composed of many paracrystalline spheroid particles known as the quantosomes (*Park* and *Pon*, 1963). The quantosomes are about 160Å by 180Å and about 100Å thick. *Sauer* and *Calvin* (1962) have shown that 3 to 6 quantosomes may aggregate together to form a large particle of 500 x 100Å. *Park* and *Beggins* (1964) have reported that each quantosome is composed of four subunits. According to *Howelland Moundrianakis* (1967) these quantosomes are the smallest units capable of carrying out the photochemical reaction and each of them contains about 200 chlorophyll molecules.

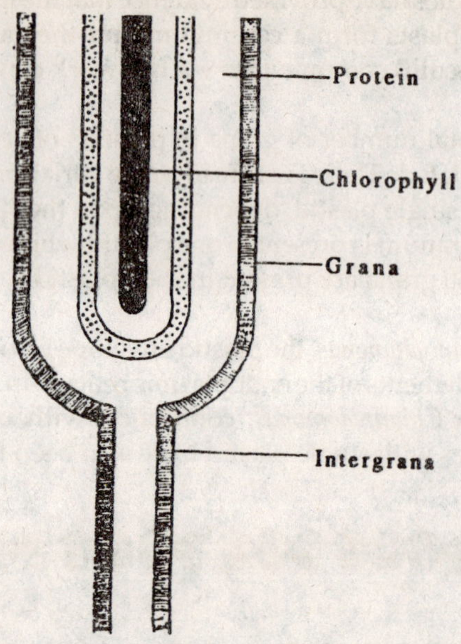

Fig. 8.6. Location of chlorophyll within granum

According to the size, nature and arrangement of quantosomes in the membrane of thylakoids and stromal *lamellae, Branton* and *Park* (1967) have recognised three types of membranes which are as follows:

1. Membrane with quantosomes.
2. Membrane with smaller particles (110Å).
3. Membrane with rough surface and with a few or no particles.

The chloroplasts, thus, act as elaborate biochemical machines and transform the energy at the molecular level.

FUNCTIONS

Photosynthesis : Photosynthesis involves two major sets of reactions, each set consisting of many steps. One set, the *light reactions*, transform ("transduce") energy acquired through the absorption of light into usable chemical forms, namely ATP and the reduced form (NADPH) of the coenzyme NADP. This is accomplished via oxidation-reduction sequences that include the removal of electrons from water, releasing oxygen and protons (H^+). These protons and others transferred across the thylakoid membranes during the oxidation-reduction reactions contribute to an ATP-producing proton gradient like the one described for mitochondria in the last chapter.

The other reactions in photosynthesis, the dark reactions, occur both in the light and in the dark. They use the ATP and NADPH to build carbohydrates from CO_2. The most common pathway by which this is done is the "carbon reduction cycle" (the *Calvin cycle*), which starts with the reaction of CO_2 with the 5-carbon sugar ribulose 1,5 - diphosphate. This generates two 3-carbon molecules that undergo the cycle schematized. This initial CO_2 fixation is catalyzed by the enzyme rubulose 1,5-diphosphate ("bisphosphate") carboxylase, often called RuDP carboxylase or carboxydismutase.

The Light Reactions. The green colour of chlorophyll is due to its selective absorption of light with wavelengths of 650 to 700 nm. (Light of these wave-lengths appears to the eye as red; when red light is removed from white light, as by absorption, what is left appears green). Chlorophyll also absorbs light at shorter wavelengths (400 to 475 nm, corresponding to the violet-blue region of the spectrum). Two major chlorophyll types are present in eukaryotic plastids: Chlorophyll a shows absorption maxima (peak absorption) at about 670 nm and at about 490 nm, Chlorophyll b absorbs maximally at about 650 to 470 nm. Wavelength is an indicator of the energy carried by packets (photons) of light. The shorter the wavelength, the greater the energy. the absorption maxima of the chlorophylls and other photosynthetic pigments indicate the portions of the spectrum of sunlight that can be captured for energizing photosynthesis. When a chlorophyll molecule absorbs a photon, an electron of the chlorophyll's porphyrin ring acquires the photon's energy and thereby is excited. This is the basis of the chloroplast's ability to transduce light energy to chemical energy. The excited electron can enter a series of electron transport reactions involving iron-containing proteins (ferrodexins, cytochromes), a copper-containing protein (plastocyanin), lipid-soluble molecules (plastoquinones) resembling

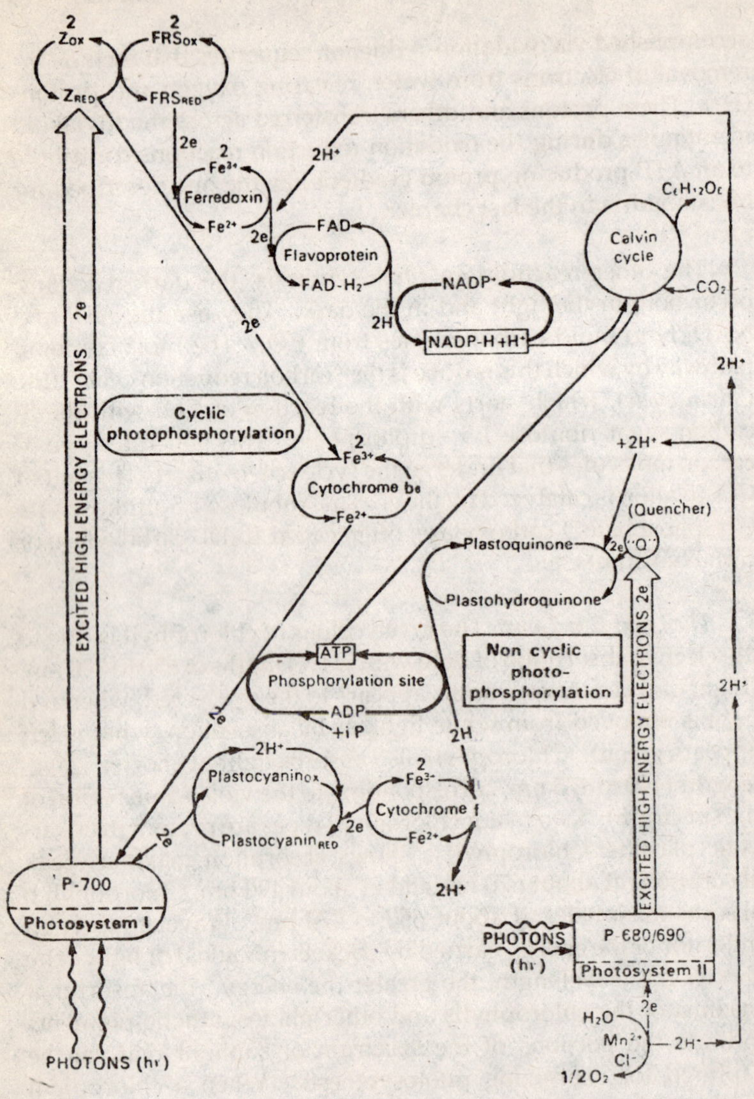

Fig. 8.7. Figure showing legal and dark reaction

coenzyme Q and other participants, some yet to be identified. Two distinguishable "photochemical units", *photosystems*, cooperate in photosynthesis. This cooperation as currently envisaged by a majority of investigators. The functional heart of each unit is a reaction centre (action centre) that carries out the essential processes by which energy derived from light is made available to the electron transport sequences and other phenomena of the light reactions. Each photosystem is characterized by a particular form of pigment molecule associated with the reaction centre; the pigments almost certainly are chlorophylls. In photosystem I (PSI), the reaction centre pigment absorbs light maximally at 700 nm and hence is called P700. Excited electrons from P700 pass from the PSI reaction center to the electron transport sequence that reduced NADP. The electrons "lost" from P700 in this process are replaced through electron transport from photosystem II (PSII); the cyclic pathway diagrammed in Figure represents an alternative replenishment mechanism, which some investigators believe is actually the predominant one, at least under some physiological circumstances. The reaction centre pigment PSII, P680, absorbs light preferentially at 680 nm. The PSII reaction centre transfers electrons from this pigment to an electron transport chain that links PSII to PSI. The "loss" electrons from P680 is made up by the removal of electrons from water molecules; it is this PSII-mediated oxidation ("splitting") of water that generates O_2.

In net effect the two photosystem collaborate via electrons transport to transfer electrons from water to NADPH. Accompanying this transfer is the establishment of an electrochemical H^+ gradient across the thylakoid membranes: The thylakoid interior is maintained at low PH relative to the stroma. The H^+ ions feed in the "splitting" of water also contribute to this gradient. The proton gradient is used to generate ATP (photosynthetic phosphorylation). As with mitochondria, vesicles formed from fragmented thylakoids are capable of both electron transport and phosphorylation but can no longer phosphorylate if broken open or otherwise treated to disrupt the permeability barrier inherent in the membrane. Moreover, chloroplast vesicles can produce ATP for a brief period if simply soaked for a time in a medium of low PH, until their interior equilibrates with the medium, and then transferred into a medium of high pH, establishing a transient H^+ gradient across the vesicles' membranes. Experiments of his sort were crucial in verifying the plausibility, in general of chemiosmotic mechanisms for production of ATP.

ORIGIN OF THE PLASTIDS

Plastids are generated only by other prexisting plastids or proplastid body. They are self reproducing cell organelles like the chromosomes and the centrioles. The proplastid may be regarded as the "stem" plastid, giving rise to metabolically active leucoplasts or chloroplasts which may later develop into other types of chromoplasts through a kind of degeneration. Plastids are transmitted directly to daughter cells during division, providing a genetic continuity in plastid lineage. Although the origin of intials that develop into proplastids is not entirely clear, some observations in fern suggest the nuclear envelope as a possible source.

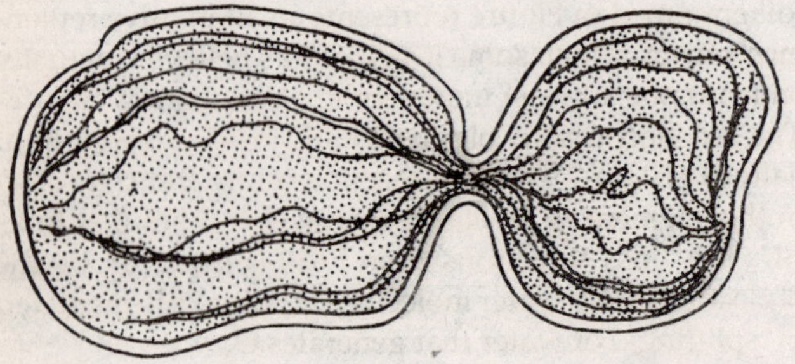

Fig. 8.8. Young chloroplast of germinating corn embryo showing equal division

In lower plants. In algae and lower plants, the plastids are quite large and often of different shapes and the process of their division is easy to follow. Here the division begins with an infolding of the inner membrane of the limiting chloroplast envelope. Later on the outer membrane invaginates until the plastid is divided into two. The daughter plastids thus formed, may or may not be equal in size.

In higher or *superior plants.* In higher plants the process of formation of plastids is more complicated. The process can be effected even by sunlight, as the formation of plastids in sunlight and in dark show vast differences in either case.

In Sunlight. During the development the proplastids increase in size. Protoplastids are limited by a double membrane. In the presence of light the inner limiting boundary invaginates at several places, producing small vesicle like structures. These vesicles later on pinch off as free units, which then aggregate in several arrangements to form the lemellae of the mature plastid.

In Dark. If the proplastids are left in dark, the process of formation upto vesicle stage is the same, as in presence of light. But the arrangement of vesicle is different. In dark the clusters of vesicles of discs constitute the lamellar system or a series of concentric rings are developed.

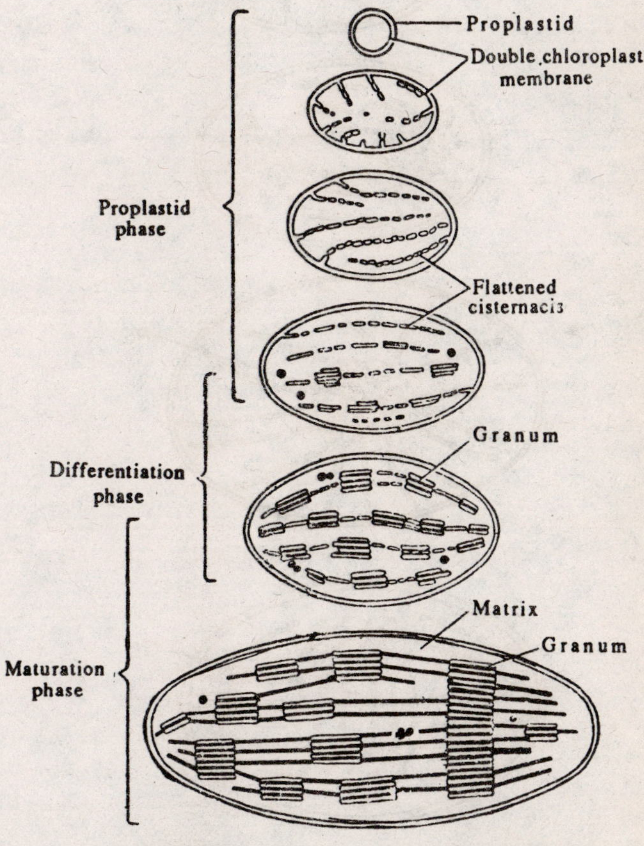

Fig. 8.9. Development of a chloroplast in sunlight

Formation of Leucoplasts, Chromoplasts and Chloroplasts from Proplastids. The non-lamellated proplastids can also transform themselves into leucoplasts. These, in turn, can develop into

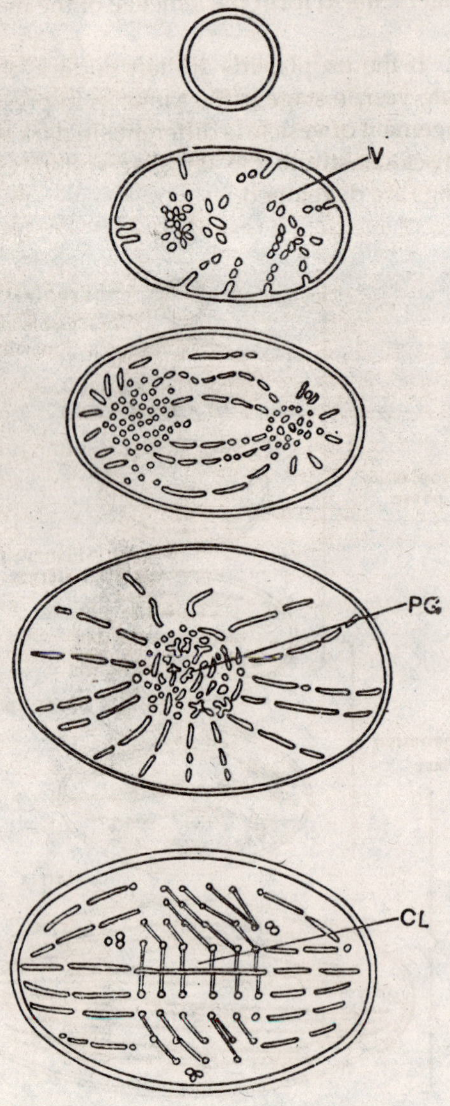

Fig. 8.10 Development of a chloroplast in dark

immature lamellar plastids or, by a reversible process, into starch containing amyloplasts. The still mature proplastids then grow to become either mature chloroplasts or other chromoplasts or even, by storing proteins, aleurone plastids. Mature chloroplasts can become chlorophyll free chromoplasts or, by absorption of many lipids elaioplasts.

Nuclear Origin : A large number of intials around the nucleus have been observed under special conditions, where the cell organelles are breaking down. This suggested that the initials originated due to evagination of the double nuclear membrane and gave rise to mitochondira and proplastids.

Symbiotic Origin : Resemblance has been observed between mitochondria and bacteria on the one hand and chloroplast and blue-green algae on the other hand. They are not only some what similar in shape and structure but also in function. All possess DNA, much smaller than nuclear DNA and circular, not organised in chromosomes; they ribosomes are all about the same size, smaller then the cytoplasmic matrix ribosomes of animal and plant cells. In bacteria the respiratory chain is localised in the membrane comparable to inner membrane of mitochondria. Further comparable to cristae of mitochondria, in foldings of plasma membrane (mesosomes) have been reported in certain bacteria. In mitochondria and bacteria both, the protein synthesis is inhibited by chloramphenicol, whereas the extracellular protein synthesis of higher cells is not effected. These similarities have led some to consider the mitochondria and chloroplasts of today as generally modified descendants of an ancestral free living bacteria and blue green-algae respectively (autotrophic micor-organisms) which at one time came together with the ancestral eukaryotic cell (heterotrophic host cell) to form a symbiotic relationship. This hypothesis is no doubt highly attractive, but still is the evident that the electon-transport system in chloroplasts and the enzymes required for making the photosynthetic pigments are controlled by the nuclear genes (*Kirk* 1960).

9

NUCLEUS

The most prominent particulate feature of a cell when viewed under the microscope is the nucleus. Originally it was detected by *Leeuwenhock* in 1700 as refractile bodies in the centre of blood corpuscles of salmon blood. These structures, which must have been nuclei, were seen with the simple lenses which were found by him in his spare time. *Fontana* in 1781 observed similar oval bodies inside the skin cells of an eel, and the full description was given by the Scottish botanist *Robert Brown* in 1835. It is an almost universal structure of cells at sometime during their life cycle, although such cells as the sieve tubes of vascular plants and the red blood cells of mammalian vertebrate may lose their nuclei by the time they are fully differentiated. The nucleus is not homogeneous, but contains thread like structures which were discovered some years later that these structures could be obtained with aniline dyes for which reason they become known as *chromosomes* (*Gr-Chroma*=colour and *Soma*=body). *Sutton* in 1903, first suggested that hereditary factors or genes are carried on chromosomes. And in 1871 for the first time it was isolated by *Miescher*, its morphological anlysis was much less advanced than that of the cytoplasm. *Kossel* was able to demonstrate the presence of nucleic acid, and for this he was awarded the Nobel Prize in 1910.

Cell without nuclei have very limited futures. The only common animal cell type without a nucleus, the mammalian red blood cell, lives only a few months; aside from its role in oxygen transport, it is extremely restricted in its metabolic activities. Egg cells from which nuclei have been experimentally removed may divide for a while, but the products of division never differentiate into specialized cell types, and eventually they die. Fragments without a nucleus, cut from such large unicellular organisms as amoeba or the algal, *Acetabularia*, survive temporarily, but ultimately they die unless nuclei from other cells are transplated into them.

The nucleus is essential to long-term continuation of metabolism and to the ability of cells to alter significantly their structure and function (as in differentiation). In large part, this reflects the primary role of the nucleus in producing the RNA required for protein synthesis. When cells change, their new functions and structures require new proteins. Even cells that are constant in metabolism and structure show continual replacement (turnover) of macromolecules and probably of organelles, including portions of the cytoplasmic protein-synthesizing machinery.

SIGNIFICANCE OF NUCLEUS

Hammerling's Experiment : *J. Hammerling,* a German biologist, experimentally proved the significance of nucleus. If a fragment containing the nucleus is cut from an Acetabularia of one species, characterized by a given morphology, the fragment will regenerate a whole cell of that species. This regenerative ability permits experiments of the type illustrated in Figure 9.1 in which nuclei of one species are combined with cytoplasma from different species. *Hammerling* conducted certain experiments using two species of a green alga, *Acetabularia.* The two species, namely *A. crenulata* and *A. mediterranea* used in this experiment differ in the shape of their caps. While in *A. crenulata* the cap has loose rays, in *A. mediterranea* an umbrella-like cap is found. The nucleus in both the species is situated in rhizoid at the bottom of stalk. If cap is cut off, it will develop again and its shape will be that of the original type. However, if after removing the caps, stalk of one species is grafted on rhizoid (containing the nucleus) of the other species, shape of cap will be determined by nucleus and not by stalk. If the nucleus belongs to *A. crenulata,* shape of cap will be of the crenulata type. If the nucleus comes from *A. mediterranea,* cap will be of mediterranea type. When both nuclei are present, shape of cap will be intermediate. The conclusion drawn from such experiments is that the nucleus produces material that enters the cytoplasm and participates in the control of cell growth and cell morphology. The crucial finding is that the morphology of the regenerated cells eventually becomes like that of the species from which the nucleus is taken. In the hybrid fragments with the nucleus from one species and most of the cytoplasm from the other species, old cytoplasmic material persists for a while and may influence cell form. Eventually, however, this is depleted and replaced by newly produced material from the nucleus.

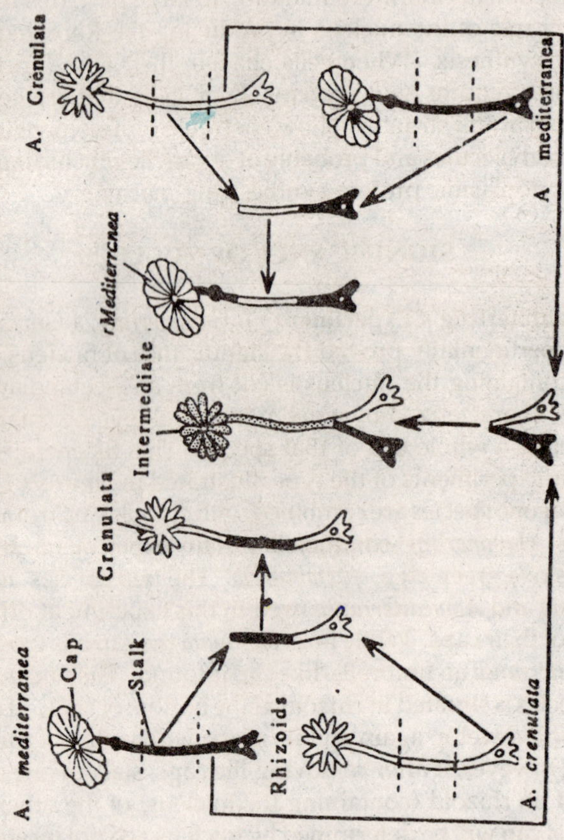

Fig. 9.1 Hammerling's experiment in Acetabularia

MORPHOLOGY

Shape. In general the nucleus tends to be spherical, but may be fusiform, ellipsoidal, flattened, depending on cell shape and function. In young cells it is more often spherical and centrally located, but in differentiated ones it may be displaced and irregular in shape. The nucleus may be *elongated* as in columnar epithelium and muscle cells. In certain cases it becomes *irregular* and has often been observed in particular cases to undergo slow amoeboid changes of form in the living cells, e.g., cartiliage cells, leucocytes or in animal ova. Nuclei (Nucleus-singular) of irregular or amoeboid form are frequent in cells characterized by very active metabolism, in which case the nuclei are often not only of large size, but show a marked further increase of surface by the formation of lobes, sacculations, or even in extreme cases of complex branches ramifying through the cell. An extreme example of this is offered by the spinning glands of certain insect larvae (Lepidoptera and Trichoptera), in which the nucleus, originally spheroidial, finally assumes labyrinthine appearance with convolutions occupying a large area in the cell.

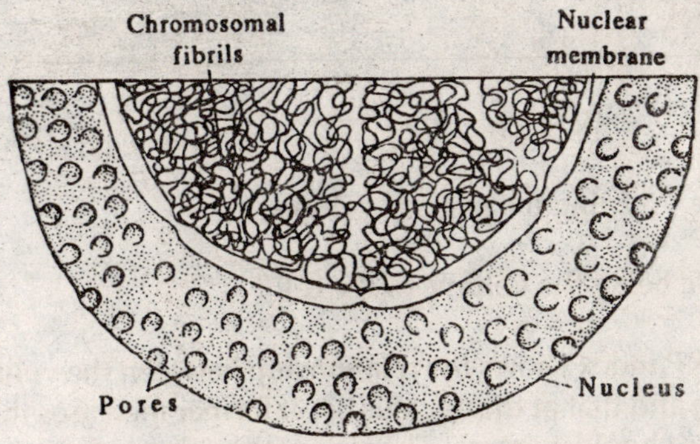

Fig. 9.2 Nucleus with the chromosomal fibrils and nuclear pores

In certain types of cells the surface of the nucleus may also be increased by its breaking up into more or less separate vesicles or *Karyomerites*, thus forming "Polymorphic" nuclei or nuclear nest. Vesicular or spherical shaped nuclei generally occur in the tissue cells of most multicellular animals and plants. Massive nuclei occur typically in the male germ cell of animals generally and of many lower plants (in coenocytic plants like *Vaucharia* etc.).

Position. The position of the nucleus is determined by many causes, such as surface tension, the position of the vacuole, the relative density of the cytoplasm in different portion of cell. In embryonic cells it almost always occupies the geometric centre. In non-vacuolated cells of plants even it occupies the centre of the cytoplasmic mass. In adipose cells, in eggs rich in yolk the nucleus is forced toward the periphery by the accumulation of the paraplasm. In glandular cells it is located in the basal position, the granules occupying the apical cytoplasm. The position of the nucleus is also related to the function of the cell.

Size. In 1895 *Boveri* showed that the size of the nuclei in merogeic echinoderm larvae is dependent upon the number of chromosomes each contains. *Gates* 1909, however, adduced evidence to show that this rule is by no means universal. The size of the nucleus is variable, but in general it bears some relation to that of the cytoplasm. This may be expressed numerically in the so called nucleoplasmic index (NP) by *O. Hertwig* (1906).

$$NP = \frac{Vn}{Vc - Vn}$$

where Vn being the nuclear volume

and Vc being the volume of the cell

This NP index shows the relationship between the volume of cytoplasm and that of the nucleus i.e., if former increases then the second also should increase. The ratio of the volume of the nucleus to that of the cytoplasm in a cell is called the '"nucleoplasmic ratio" or "Karyoplasmic ratio".

Number. The number of nuclei present in any mass of protoplasm depends largely upon the bulk of the mass since within limits a certain ratio of nuclear surface to cytoplasmic volume must be maintained for the proper action of the whole system. Generally all the cells are uninucleate or *mononucleate* i.e., one nucleus in one cell. But in certain cases *binucleate* conditions occur as in *Paramoecium caudatum,* here one nucleus is smaller which is micronucleus while the larger one is called the macro — or meganucleus. In few others the poly - or multinucleate condition exists as in Opalina, striated muscles and certain syphonal algae etc.

The nucleus consists of four components : (1) Nuclear envelope (2) Nuclear sap (3) Nucleolus and (4) Chromatin network.

(1) Nuclear Envelope : The nuclear envelope has only recently enjoyed much investigation. As viewed with the standard phase contrast microscope, it appears as little more than a dark line, this line separating the nuclear contents from the cytoplasm. In most cells, it is observed to break down and reform as the cell enters and completes division. However, in some algae, protozoans, and fungi, it does not break down during division. Observation with the light microscope shows that the nuclear envelope serves as a barrier between the nucleus and the cytoplasm. The way in which the nuclear envelope regulates the flow of material is just beginning to be studied.

Ultra structural studies reveal that the nuclear envelope is actually comaposed of two membranes separated by a *perinuclear space* 110 to 400 Å wide. The inner membrane appears to be in contact with the nuclear chromatin, which can be seen condensed along its surface, the outer membrane is contiguous with the cytoplasmic endoplasmic reticulum and is often observed with ribosomes bound to its surface. The association of the outer membrane with the ER results in a continuity between the nucleus and the cytoplasm. However, this continuity is not complete because of the presence of the inner nuclear membrane, which still serves as a structural barrier. The occurrence of direct channels between the nucleus and the cytoplasm in the form of nucleopores does provide for a complete continuity between the two major cell compartments. The pores are circular or oval regions of 5 μ to 1000 Å in diameter and appear to have a specific substructure consisting of annuli.

The pores are often plugged with material that appears to be in the process of moving either from the nucleus to the cytoplasm or vice versa. The mechanism of control over the movement of material through the pores are not well known. In addition to the direct movement of material through the nuclear pores, there appear to be specific transport mechanisms associated with the non pore regions of the nuclear membrane.

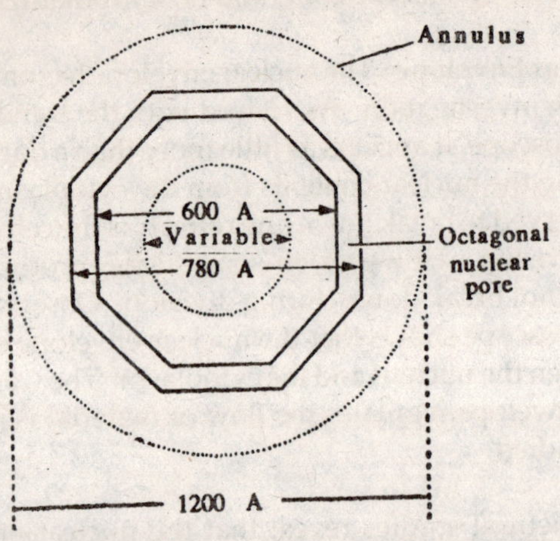

Fig. 9.3. Diagram of nuclear pore structure

Pore Complex: At certain points the nuclear envelope is interrupted by structures called pores. around the margins of these nuclear pores both membranes are in continuity. At their nuclear side the pores are generally aligned with channels of nucleoplasm situated between more condensed lumps of chromatin. The number of pores varies from 40 to 145 per square micrometre in nuclei of various plants and animals. At their highest density the pores are packed in hexagonal array with centre-to-centre pore distances of about 150 nm.

In nuclei of Mammalia it has been calculated that nuclear pores account for 10 per cent of the surface area; membranes constitute the remaining surface area. The pores are enclosed by circular structures called *annuli*. The pores and annuli, together, are designated the *pore co   lex*. Negative staining techniques have demonstrated that the nuclear pores are octagonal in shape and are about 60 nm in diameter. The annular material is a kind of amorphous cylinder that extends through the pore into either side of the pore margin. It has an outer diameter of about 120 nm, which exceeds that of the pore. The central hole of the annulus varies from from 30 to 50 nm. This material is digested by trypsin and remains untouched when exposed to ribonuclease and deoxyribonuclease. These findings suggest that the annular material is protein in nature. The pore complex is apparently a rather rigid structure present in a fixed number according to cell type. In certain physiological stages, however, they may change in number. For example they are reduced in number in maturing erythroblasts and in spermatids.

In amoebae there is a layer of electrodense material with a honeycomb structure at the inner surface of the nuclear envelope. This component is made of prisms that are attached at one end to the nuclear envelope at the site of each pore. In other cells, a layer of fibrous material known as fibrous lamina, has also been observed on the nuclear side of the envelope.

(2) Nuclear Sap. An unstained or light acidiophilic mass, the "Karyolymph" or "Nuclear Sap" fills completely the nuclear space where the other components are found. It was *Caude* who in 1943 precipitated out the nuclear sap by histological fixative and stained with acid dyes. In eggs and in larger cells (e.g., *Acetabularia*), the nuclear sap is clearly visible. According to *Stich* (1951, 58) it gives positive cytochemical test for RNA, protein including-SH groups and glycoproteins.

Many metabolic pathways have also been demonstrated in nuclear sap, similar to cytoplasm. These include glycoysis, hexose monophosphate shunt, citric acid cycle, etc. The hexose monophosphate shunt is important since it supplies the nucleus with pentose. Further, in the nucleus NAD is synthesized which is the coenzyme of numerous dehydrogenases. Characteristic enzymes of the nucleus are DNA and RNA-polymerases.

PERMEABILITY OF THE NUCLEAR ENVELOPE

Several experiments suggest that the pore complexes may be temporary or permanent openings in the nuclear envelope. By injecting colloidal gold particles, varying in size from 2.5 to 17 nm, into the cytoplasm of amoebae, it was found that those with diameters upto 8.5 nm rapids entered the nucleus. Particles with diameters of 8.9 to 10.6 nm penetrated more slowly, and the larger ones did not enter at all. These results indicate that the openings are smaller than the pore size would indicate.

Evidence has been obtained with these techniques, suggesting that the pores are pathways for the exchange of macromolecules. The annuli may regulate the exchange in relation to the size and possibly to the chemical nature of the penetrating substance. It is important to consider that the permeability of the nuclear envelope is not fixed, but varies in different cell types and within a given cell—at least during the division cycle. Such differences are attributable to changes in the nature of annular material (*Feldher*, 1971).

The presence of pores in the nuclear envelope should be correlated with some of the electrochemical properties of this structure, which can be investigated with fine microelectrodes. Two types of nuclear envelopes have been recognized with this technique. When giant cells from the salivary gland of *Drosophila* are penetrated with a microelectrode, there is an abrupt change in potential at the plasma membrane (-12 m V); then, as the microelectrode enters the nucleus, there is another drop in negative potential at the nuclear membrane (-13 mV). These results suggest that the nuclear envelope may be a diffusion barrier for ions as small as K+, Na+, or Cl^-. In the nuclear envelope present in oocytes, however, there is no detectable potential, thus indicating a free interchange of ions between the nucleus and the cytoplasm.

There are several morphological observations that suggest there is passage of ribonucleoproteins and other macromolecules across the nuclear pores. The relationship of the pores with channels in the nucleoplasm was mentioned earlier. Dense material extending through the nuclear pores has been observed in oocytes of Amphibia. Some of the material may correspond to ribosomal subunits, other to messenger RNA. The mechanism by which the passage of these substances is achieved is unknown. Cytochemical studies, however, have revealed the presence of an ATPase in the pores which may provide the necessary energy for the transfer of macromolecules.

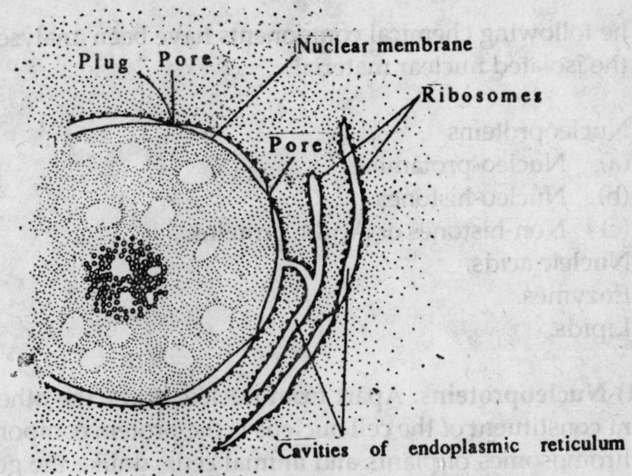

Fig. 9.4 Formation of nuclear envelope from E.R.

ORIGIN OF NUCLEAR MEMBRANE

The nuclear membrane is considered as a specialized cytoplasmic structure originating from the cytoplasmic membrane system. During telophase, it is formed by the accumulation of vesicles of endoplasmic reticulum around the chromosome group, which later on fuse to form a complete membrane.

There are basically two theories as to how the nuclear envelope reconstitutes after telophase, either the pair of lamellae is synthesized *de novo* at the sites where chromosomes and cytoplasm are in contact with each other. (*Jones*, 1960) or parts of the already present endoplasmic reticulum adjoin the telophase nucleus and merge to form the nuclear envelope. In locust spermatocytes, for instance, the 0.5μ vesicles which are formed at the surface of the chromosomes, are indistinguishable from the vesicles of the endoplasmic reticulum (*Bahr*, 1959, 61). They gradually arrange themselves so as to lie parallel to the surface of the nucleus and then merge to form a continuous nuclear envelope.

CHEMICAL COMPOSITION OF NUCLEUS

The following chemical components have been analysed out from the isolated nuclear material.

(1) Nucleoproteins
  (a) Nucleo-protamine
  (b) Nucleo-histones
  (c) Non-histones or Acidic proteins.
(2) Nucleic acids.
(3) Enzymes.
(4) Lipids.

(1) Nucleoproteins. Apart from nucleic acids, the other important constituent of the cell nucleus is the protein components. The chromosomes of plants and animal cells, unlike the genetic material of bacteria, consists of DNA associated with proteins. In giant polytene chromosomes protein has been found in the banded and interbanded regions of gene activity. Protein is associated with the extended loop of lampbrush chromosomes. Nucleoli contain high proportions of protein and there are of course protein present in the nuclear sap or nucleoplasm, and, in association with lipids, in the nuclear membranes.

The protein part of the nucleus is certainly very complex and has several components. Of these the best known are two strongly basic and simple proteins: the protamines and the histones. In addition to these there are Acidic proteins, the so-called nonhistone proteins and enzymes present.

(a) Protamine or Nucleo-protamine. It was *Miescher* who discovered the protamine in Salmon sperm. These are simple basic proteins having a very low molecular weight. These are very rich in basic amino acid arginine and are found in spermatozoa of some fishes and are tightly bounded to DNA by salt linkage. As the protamines are smaller than histones, which means that the chromosomes and nuclei can be packed into a smaller space, allowing greater mobility of the sperm. In general they consist of about 28 arginine polypeptides, with a total length of 100 A°, and contain 19 arginines and 8 or 9 non-basic amino acids. During development there is a progressive replacement of the histones by protamine. This may be due to the higher affinity of protamine for DNA.

(b) Nucleo-histones. Histones were discovered in the goose erythrocytes by *Kossel* and soon thereafter were found in the thymus gland by *Lilientfeld.* Histones have also been found in certain plant cell nuclei, notably wheat and cedar nut embryo by *Mirsky.*

The nucleoproteins are also basic proteins having a molecular weight about 12000. In addition to about 13% *arginine, histones* contain other basic residues including *lysine* and *histidine.* Several histones of different compositions have been isolated, and three main types have been characterized :

(i) Very lysine rich
(ii) Arginine rich
(iii) And slightly lysine rich

These are heterogenous and consists of several components. Histones are found in all nuclei of higher organisms, although they have been little studied in plants. Those found in plants, however, resemble the histones found in vertebrates.

The main function of histone ascribed is that of acting as a chromosomal 'glue' binding together the genetic units of DNA. It is also known that DNA—histones complexes are more resistant to denaturation by heat that DNA alone, and that proteins (mainly histones) in the nucleo-proteins complex can partially protect DNA from radiation damage. Evidence now indicates, however, that the really important role played by histones lies in representing the genetic activity of cells. It was suggested by *Stedman* and *Stedman* in 1950 that histones interact with DNA in a specific way preventing it from acting as a template for RNA synthesis and thus preventing the transfer of genetic information to the cytoplasm.

(c) Non-histones or Acidic Proteins. Chemical analysis of isolated nuclei and chromatin threads led to the demonstration of another type of protein which is generally called non-histone protein. This protein contains tryptophane and has acidic properties. Another non-histone fraction has been identified from isolated chromatin threads. The insoluble residue appears under the microscope as spiral threads which maintains the characteristics of the interphase chromosomes. From a chemical stand-point it is very interesting that these residual chromosomes contain more ribonucleic acid (RNA) than DNA.

The considerable amount of non-histone proteins present in a metabolically active cell contrast markedly with the composition of the spermatozon, which is much less active.

(2) Nucleic Acids. Nucleic acids, which are of two types : Ribonucleic acid (RNA) and Deoxyribonucleic acid (DNA) have been observed in the nuclear region of the cell. (For the detailed account please see the relevant chapter.

(3) Nuclear Enzymes. A number of enzymes have been found in the isolated germinal vesicles of frog oocytes by *Brachet* and *Dupsiva*. Their actual concentration is difficult to ascertain because of high permeability of the nuclear membrane and enzymes are also liable to leak out of the isolated germinal vesicles during their isolation. According to recent studies the nuclear enzymes fall into two classes. Some have a general distribution whereas others are found preferentially in certain tissues. In the first group, only some enzymes related to the nucleoside metabolism, such as adenosine diaminase, nucleoside phosphorylase and guanase are found in high concentration. Other enzymes as esterases are present in varying concentration. Still others, such as alkaline phosphates, nucleotide phosphatases and B-glucoronidase are either present in low concentration or lacking entirely. Of the special enzymes, catalase and arginase appear to be concentrated in some nuclei but are lacking in others.

(4) Nuclear Lipids. The lipid content of the nucleus has been investigated in isolated nuclei. Recently it has been reported that the lipo-protein complex nuclei from ox spleen and chicken erythrocytes is approximately 10% lipid, these give positive tests for phospholipids and cholesterol.

(3) Nucleolus. The nucleus contains a large, spherical and acidophilic dense granule known as the nucleolus. The nucleoli were discovered by *Fontona* in 1781. It was well established in 19th century that the size of the nucleous is related with the synthetic activity of the cell. Therefore, the cells with little or no synthetic activities, e.g., sperm cells, blastomeres, muscle cell, etc., are found to contain smaller or no nucleoli, while the oocytes, neurons and secretory cells which synthesize the proteins or other substances contain comparatively large size nucleoli. The number of the nucleoli in the nucleus depends on the species and the number of the chromosomes. The number of the nucleoli in the cells may be one, two or four. The position of the nucleolus in the nucleus is eccentric.

FINE STRUCTURE OF NUCLEOLUS

Regarding the fine structure of the nucleoli, it has been reported by *Estable* and *Sotelo* (1955) that they are formed of two parts — a filamentous *nucleolonema* and *a pars amorpha*. The nucleolonema is said to divide and to be equally distributed into the daughter nuclei during mitosis, and is regarded as a permanent structure which persists throughout mitosis in association with the chromosome. It is believed that the filamentous part of the nucleoli contains DNA while the parts amorpha is partially made up of RNA. Pars amorpha undergoes the characteristic cycle of formation at telophase and disappearance at prophase.

The introduction of new embedding media and techniques allowed a better analysis of the nucleolar organization. Thus four principle components can be recognized:

1. A *fibrillar portion* approximately 50 Å in diameter and upto 300-400 Å long (*Marrinozzi*, 1963). In some cases these fibrils can be seen to have a double stranded structure (Terzakis 1965). These structures were also described as tubular elements of 50 Å diameter.

2. A *granular* portion composed of dense granules with a diameter averaging 150-200 Å, more or less numerous along and between the strands of the fibrillar network (*Marrinozzi*, 1963).

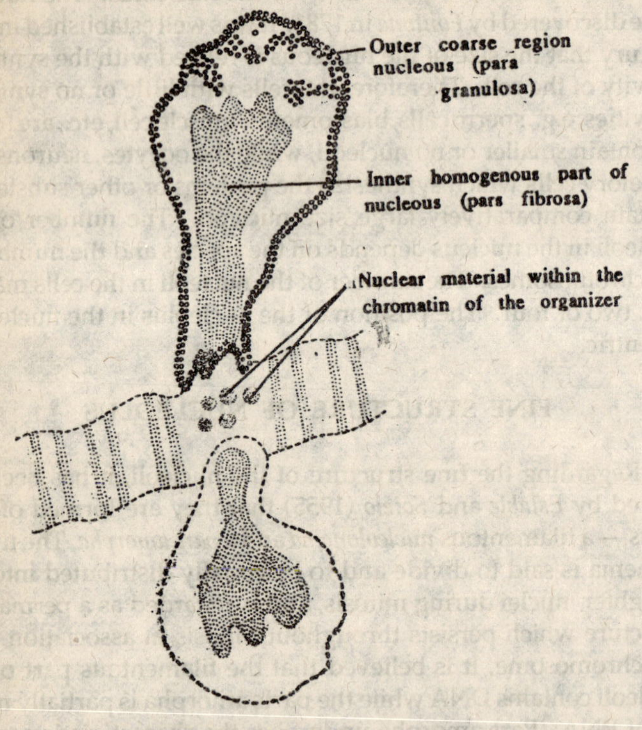

Fig. 9.5. Diagram of a salivary gland nucleolus in Smittia

3. An *amorphous* region of low electrondensity, found in some nuclei (*Terzakis* 1965) made of protein.
4. The *nucleolar associated chromatin* situated around the nucleolus and frequently having intra-nucleolar ramifications.

The existance of the four nucleolar components seem to be constant in vertebrate cells, but their respective amounts or quantities may vary.

Chemistry. Cytochemical studies indicate that 5 to 10 per cent of the nucleolus is RNA; the rest being the protein. The main protein components are phosphoproteins. No histones have been found in isolated nucleoli. There are evidence suggesting the presence of orthophosphate which may serve as a precursor of the RNA phosphorus. Little is known about the enzyme contents of the nucleolus. However, the presence of acid phosphates, nucleoside phosphorylase and NAD+ synthesizing enzymes have been shown. RNA methylase has also been localized in the nucleous of certain cells. The DNA is absent. Nucleolus may be surrounded by a ring of Feulgen-positive chromatin which actually represents the heterochromatic regions of the chromosomes.

Biogenesis of Nucleolus or Nucleolar Cycle. The nucleolus as an organized body is lacking in continuity. It disappears at the beginning of cell division (prophase) and reappears at the end of cell division in telophase stage. A nucleolus is formed at a definite region by one or more chromosomes of a haploid set of chromosomes. Such chromosomes are known as nucleolar chromosomes. Majority of diploid species possess two nucleolar chromosomes in each diploid or somatic cell. But in man chromosomes numbering 13, 14, 15, 21 and 22 participate in the formation of nucleolus. The specific region of these chromosomes active in nucleolar formation is known as nucleolar organizer or nucleolar zone. Very often but not always, it is marked by secondary constriction. The nuclear organizer carries genes for 18S and 28S ribosomal RNA.

The secondary constriction with nucleolar organizer is morphologically different from other secondary constriction. In pachytene stage of *Zea mays*, a darkly stained nucleolar organizing body is associated with the nucleolar zone.

Types of nucleoli. On the basis of distribution of ribonucleoprotein granules and fibrils three types of nucleoli can be distinguished (*Wilson*).

(1) Nucleoli with nucleolonemas, which are found in most cells called *plasmosomes*. (2) Compact nucleoli without nucleolonemas, which have been described in the salivary gland of sciarids and in the protozoan *Tetrahymena pyriformis*. In these nucleoli the ribonucleoprotein granules and fibrils are uniformly distributed. (3) Ring-shaped nueleoli with ribouncleo-protein granules and fibrils present only in the peripheral region (peripheral nucleolonema) have been reported in endothelial cells, smooth muscle

cells and lympho-sarcoma cells. In these nucleoli the central region consists largely of chromatin.

FUNCTION

RNA Production. The nucleolus is one of the most active sites of RNA synthesis. It produces about 70-90 per cent of cellular RNA in many cells. It is the source of ribosomal RNA (rRNA). The chromatin in the nucleolus contains genes or ribosomal DNA (rDNA) for coding ribosomal RNA. The fibrils represent the origin of ribosomal RNA, and the granules the next stage. The granules in turn are the precursors of ribosomes. The nucleolus thus makes ribosomal precursors, rather than whole ribosomes.

CHROMATIN —> FIBRILS —> GRANULES —> RIBOSOMES
(Containing DNA) (containing RNA) (containing RNA)

The nucleous may also produce some types of messenger RNA (mRNA), and at least one type of low molecular wight RNA.

ii.Protein synthesis. *Maggio* (1960) and others have suggested that protein synthesis takes place in the nucolus. If this is true then the ribosomal proteins are produced in the nucleolous. Other studies, however, suggest that ribosomal proteins are syntesized in the cytoplasm.

iii. Ribosome formation. In eukaryotes the gene coding for RNA contains a chain of at least 100 to 1,000 repeating copies of DNA . This DNA is given off in the form of loops from the chromosomal fibre. The DNA loops are associated with proteins to form nucleoli.

The DNA serves as a template for 45S rRNA. Half the 45S rRNA is broken down to forth 28S and 18S rRNA. The other half is broken down further to nucleotide level. Within the nucleolus the 28S rRNA combines with proteins made in cytoplasm to form the 60S ribosomal subunit. The 18S rRNA also associates with proteins to form the 40S subunit of ther ibosome.

iv. Chromatin network. The chromatin appears as thread-line, coiled and elongated structure. These are stained with basic dyes like Feulgen's stain, acetocarmine etc., that is why these are termed as *chromatin fibers* or *chromatin substance (Gr., Chrome* = colour, *soma* = body). These are visible during interphase stage. During cell-division they become thick ribbon - like structures known as *chromosomes*. A detailed account on the chromosomes is given in chapter No.13.

iv. Chromatin network: The chromatin appears as thread like coiled and elongated structure. These are stained with basic dyes like Feulgen's stain, aceto carmine etc., that is why these are named as chromatin fibres or chromatin substance (Gr. Chrome = colour, soma = body). These are visible during interphase stage. During cell division they become thick ribbon like structures known as chromosomes. A detailed account on the chromosomes is given in chapter No. 13.

Molecular Biology

1

NUCLEIC ACIDS

Friedrich Miescher in 1868 isolated a material from pus cells by digesting them for weeks with dilute HCl and called this material as nuclein. *Hoppe Segler* and his co-workers confirmed the work of *Miescher* and also proved the presence of nuclein in yeast and the erythrocytes of the birds and reptiles and various other tissues. The term *nucleic acid* was introduced by *Altmann*.. *Albrechi Kossel, P.A. Levine* and *Walter Jones* described the chemical nature of nucleic acid. According to them the nucleic acid is composed of phosphoric acid, a sugar and nitrogenous bases. *Franklin W. Stahl* presented first evidence that nucleic acid forms the genetic material. *Chargaff* (1951) described the occurrence of nitrogenous bases in equal proportions. *Dotty* (1961) has empahsized much on the physical properties of DNA. In 1962 *Willkins, Watson* and *Crick* proposed a model to explain the double helicular structure of DNA. They also shared the Nobel Prize for the same.

DEOXYRIBONUCLEIC ACID OR DNA

DNA is found in the cells of all living organisms except plant viruses, where RNA forms the genetic material and DNA is absent. In bacteriophages and viruses there is a single molecule of DNA, which remains coiled and is enclosed in the protein coat. In bacteria, mitochondria and plastids of eukaryotic cells DNA is circular and lies naked in the cytoplasm. In the nuclei of eukaryotic cells DNA occurs in the form of long spirally coiled and unbranched threads. The number of DNA molecules is equivalent to the number of chromosomes per cell. In them DNA is found in combination with proteins forming nucleoproteins-the *chromatin* material and is enclosed in the nucleus.

DNA is a polymer, the monomeres of which are the deoxyribonucleo-side monophosphates. Most DNA have high molecular weight, varying from 10^6 to 10^9 or more. Chemical analysis of DNA molecules from different kinds of organisms suggest that in one kind of DNA the number of adenine (A) nucleotides was always the same as the number of thymine (T) nucleotides. Similarly the number of guanine (G) nucleotides was always the same as the number of cytosine (C) nucleotides. This evidence suggests that nucleotides occur in pairs in the DNA molecule. Further, quantity of A present in one organism's DNA (and is varies from species to species) is equal precisely to the amount of T. Similarly the amount of G present is always equal to the amount of C.

PHYSICAL STRUCTURE OF DNA

According to the model proposed by *Watson* and *Crick*, the DNA contains two polynucleotide chains running antiparallel and twisted around each other in the form of a regular double helix. The diameter of the helix is about 20 A° and each chain makes a complete turn every 34 A°. Each chain is polynucleotide in which the sugar of each nucleotide is linked by a phosphate group to the sugar of the adjajcent nucleotide. There are 10 nucleotides on each chain in every turn of the helix. The two helices are coiled in such a way that they cannot be separated without unwinding. The two chains of a helix are of opposite polanty. If one chain runs in 3'-5' direction, then the other will run as 5'-3' direction.

The molecular weight for purified DNA is found in the range 1000,000 to 120 x 10^6. The amount of DNA in a mammalian cell corresponds to about 25,000 molecules of molecular weight 120 x 10^6, a total of about 10,000 million nucleotides.

MOLECULAR STRUCTURE OF DNA

The DNA molecule is a polymer consisting of several thousand pairs of nucleotide monomers. Each nucleotide consists of the pentose sugar, *deoxyribose*, a *phosphate* group and a *nitrogenous base*, which may be either a *purine or a pyrimidine*.

(1) Deoxyribose suguar, *Levine* (1909) identified ribose sugar as a main constituent of mucleic acid structure. *Mori* (1929) isolated sugar from the guanine nucleoside and showed that it is deoxyribose suguar. It is pentose type which in DNA molecule shows the absence of one oxygen molecule from carbon-2 position of ribose sugar. Both deoxyribose and ribose (pentose sugars of nucleic acids) have a pentagonal ring with five carbons among which two (i.e. 3' and 5') are attached to phosphoric acid and three (1') to the base. This suguar is called *deoxyribose* and it simply acts as a support column to which bases are attached.

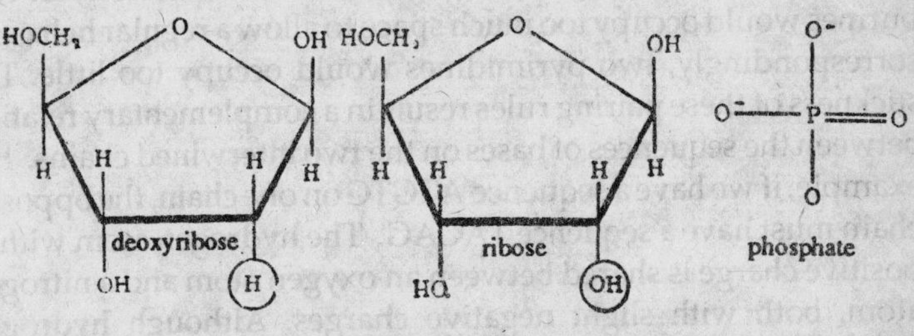

Fig. 1.1 Pentose Sugar.

(2) Phosphate. In the DNA strand the phosphate groups alternate with deoxyribose. Each phosphate group is joined to carbon atom 3' of one deoxyribose and to carbon atom 5' of another. Thus each strand has a 3' end and a 5' end. The two strands are oriented in opposite directions. The 3' end of one strand corresponds to the 5' end of the other. Consequently the oxygen atoms of deoxyribose point in opposite directions in the two strands. *Phosphodiester bonds* are formed between the sugars of two different nucleotides and a phosphate group.

(3) Nitrogenous Bases. The nitrogenous bases of nucleic acid are of two types: *Purine* and *Pyrimidine.* Purine bases comprise mainly adenine (A) and guanine (G) which are common to both DNA and RNA while pyrimidine bases comprise cytosine (C) and thymine (T) in DNA and in the cases of RNA, thymine (T) is replaced by uracil (U).

These bases are arranged linearly as the back bones of chains which (back bones) are composed of alternating sugar and phosphate. The bases have specific way of combining, if C is found in one chain G will be opposite to it and in other if A is on one T must be on the other. Or in other words adenine (A) is always paired with thymine (T) and guanine (G) with cytosine (C).

Among bases A-T and G-C, two hydrogen bonds are formed between A and T and three hydrogen bonds are formed between C and G. This hydrogen bond formation precludes A-C or G-T pairs. Only these arrangements A-T and G-C are possible, for two purines would occupy too much space to allow a regular helix and correspondingly, two pyrimidines would occupy too little. The stickness of these pairing rules result in a complementary relation between the sequences of bases on the two interwined chains. For example, if we have a sequence ATGTC on one chain, the opposite chain must have a sequence TACAG. The hydrogen atom with it positive charge is shared between an oxygen atom and a nitrogen atom, both with slight negative charges. Although hydrogen bonds are weak, the fact that there are so many gives stability to the DNA molecule. The weak hydrogen bonding enables the two strands of the DNA to separate during replication.

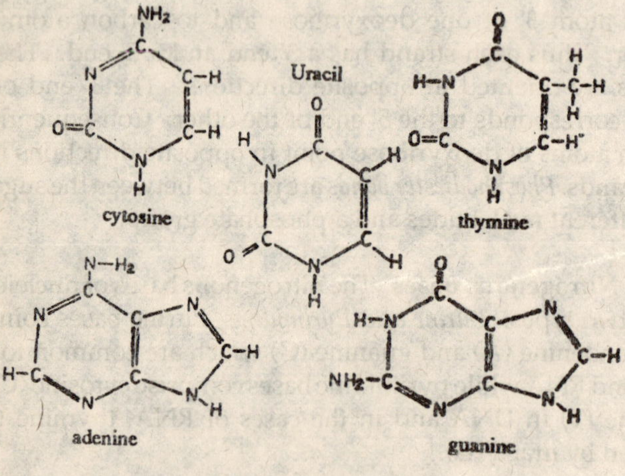

Fig. 1.2. Common nitrogenous bases of nucleic acids.

The bases are joined to the pentoses by N-C *glycosidic bonds.* For the purine, the glycosidic bond is between the C_1 position of the pentosoe sugar and the N_9 position of the bases. For the pyrimidines the linkage joins the C_1 and N_3 positions.

Four nitrogen bases, nucleosides and nucleotides of DNA molecule.

Nitrogen base	*Base+deoxyribose =deoxyribonucleo-side*	*Deoxy ribonucleoside +Phosphoric acid= Deoxy ribonucleotide*	*Abbreviaion for nucleotide*
1. Adenine (A)	Deoxyadenosine	Deoxyadenylic acid (Deoxyadenosine monophosphate)	3'-dAMP
2. Guanine (G)	Deoxyguanosine	Deoxyguanylic acid (Deoxyguanosine monophosphate)	3'-dGMP
3. Cytosine (C)	Deoxycytidine	Deoxycytidylic acid (Deoxycytidine monophosphate)	5'-dCMP
4. Thymine (T)	Deoxyhymidine	Thymidylic acid (Deoxythymidine monophosphate)	5'-dTMP

Nucleosides and nucleotides. A sugar molecule and a nitrogenous base form a *nucleoside,* and a nucleoside plus a phosphate group form a *nucleotide.* In other words a nucleoside is a base-sugar combination and a nucleotide is a nucleoside phosphate. The nucleotides of RNA are called ribonucleotides, and those of DNA deoxyribonucleotides. Ribonucleotides contain the sugar ribose, and deoxyribonucleotides the sugar deoxyribose.

The nucleosides are usually abbreviated as A,T,G or C, with d- as a prefix for deoxy nucleosides (e.g. dG—is the abbreviation for deoxy gnanosine.

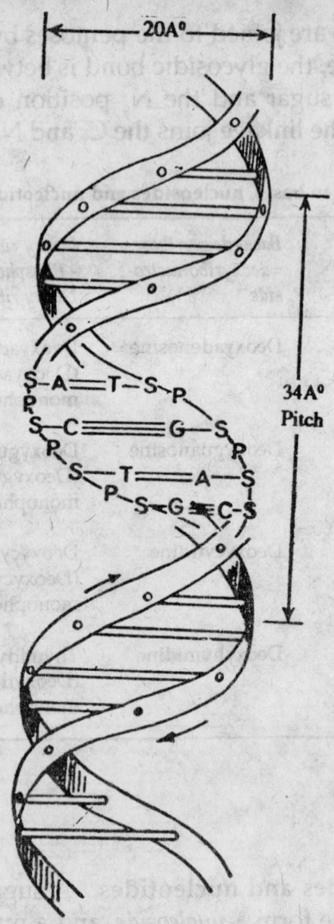

Fig. 1.3. The Watson-Crick base pair in DNA, Adenime-Thymine, and Guanine-Cytosine.

Showing amount of various bases in different tissues.

S.No.	*Source*	*Adenine*	*Guanine*	*Cytosine*	*Thymine*	$\frac{A+T}{G+C}$
1.	Human liver	30.0	19.5	19.9	30.3	1.53
2.	Human sperm	30.7	19.3	18.8	31.2	1.62
3.	Hen red cells	28.8	20.5	21.5	29.2	1.38

cont...

4.	Rat bone marrow	28.6	21.4	21.5	28.4	1.33
5.	Herring sperm	27.8	22.2	22.6	27.5	1.23
6.	*Paracentrotus* lividus (sea urchin) sperm	32.8	17.7	18.4	32.1	1.85
7.	Salmon	29.7	20.8	20.4	29.1	1.43
8.	Wheat germ	26.5	23.5	23.0	27.0	1.19
9.	Yeast	31.3	18.7	17.1	32.9	1.79
10.	*Diplococcus pneumoniae*	29.8	20.5	18.0	31.6	1.59
11.	K-12 *Escherichia coli*	26.0	24.9	25.2	23.9	1.00
12.	*Mycobacterium tuberculosis*	15.1	34.9	35.4	14.6	0.42
13.	Bacteriophate T_2	32.5	18.2	16.7	32.6	1.86

Structural Variation in DNA. The double helicular nature of the DNA has been proved by a number of workers using the isotope and besides this single stranded DNA and circular shaped DNA, having the same chemical composition have been observed. Thus after the discovery of such abnormal variety of DNA, one can place them under the following headings :-

(1) Double stranded DNA
(2) Single stranded DNA
(3) Circular DNA

(1) Double Stranded DNA. This is the common DNA present in all the living organisms. These contain two polynucleotide chains running antiparallel and twisited around each other in the form of a regular double helix. The detailed structure of this type of DNA has already been explained.

(2) Single Stranded DNA. At first it was thought that all DNA molecules are double stranded except during replication, when small portion near the Y regions are temporarily in a non-hydrogen bonded, single stranded form. Many people were surprised, therefore, when conclusive experiments revealed that the DNA of several groups of small bacterial viruses exists normally as single stranded molecules. this single stranded DNA is having the same chemical composition as we find in the double stranded DNA.

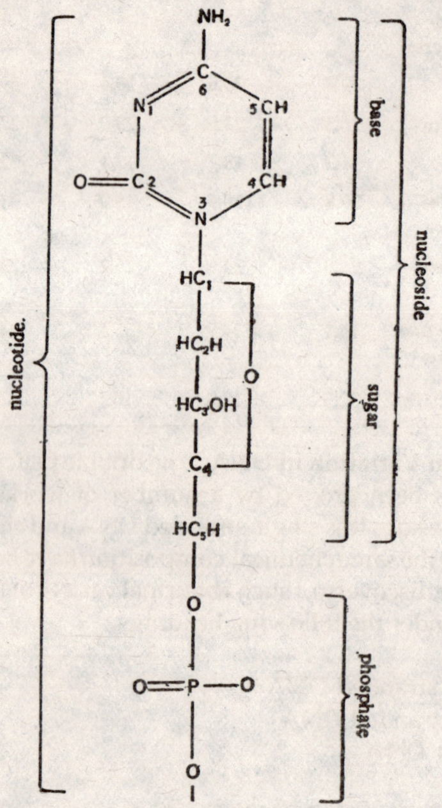

Fig. 1.4 Chemical structure of a nucleotide and a nucleoside.

(3) Circular Shaped DNA. The circular form of the DNA has been observed recently in polyma virus. In *E. coli* chromosome (DNA molecule), the circular shaped DNA has also been seen. The linear molecule of the DNA can be converted into the circular form but we do not know the chemistry of converting a linear molecule of DNA into circular form. When the phage — DNA molecule is isolated from the free phage, it is linear in shape. However, by controlled heating and recooling it can be reversibly converted to a circular form.

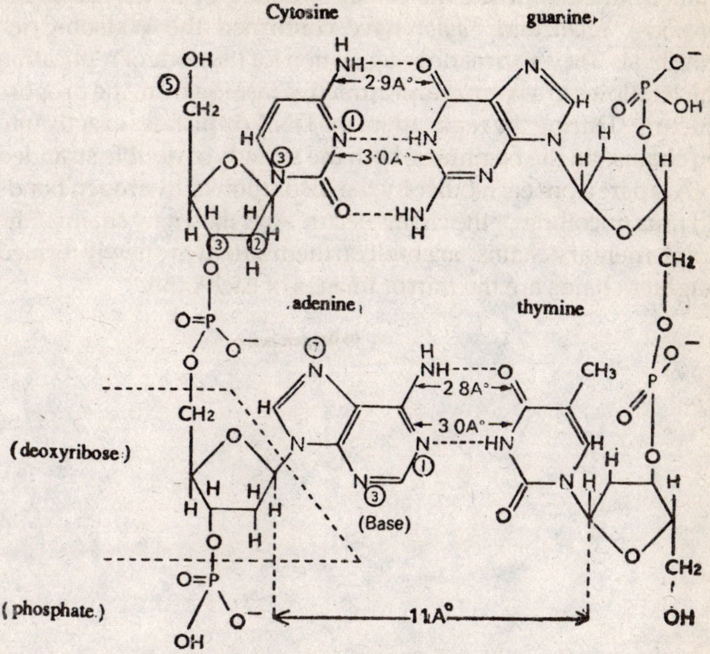

Fig. 1.5. Segment of a DNA molecule.

Z-DNA OR LEFT HANDED DNA

On the basis of the arrangement of pentose sugar forming chains of DNA two forms of DNA have been reported. Usually the sugar chains has the pentose sugar with ascending sequence of carbon atoms. This is the right handed DNA or B-DNA. Recently in 1979, another form of DNA having pentose sugar with descending arrangement of carbon atom has been reported and named Z-DNA or left handed DNA.

BIOLOGICAL REPLICATION OF DNA

Study of replication of DNA is one of the interesting aspect of molecular control of heredity. Various study of the duplication of genetic material was presented from time to time in different organisms. But most of them are discarded because no concrete ideas have been proposed till *Watson* and *Crick* proposed a detailed scheme for the molecular structure of DNA. Later on, *Korenberg, Stahl* and *Taylor* have confirmed the Watson-Crick hypothesis. They also made a suggestion for its mode of replication which follows in a natural and attractive fashion from the propose structure. During the replication, the DNA duplicates exactly into two chains. In the beginning both the strands of double stranded DNA, apart from each other by the disolution of hydrogen bonds and thus uncoiling of the chains occur. And then new chains, "the complementary chains" are built on them so that the newly formed daughter chains are the mirror images of each other.

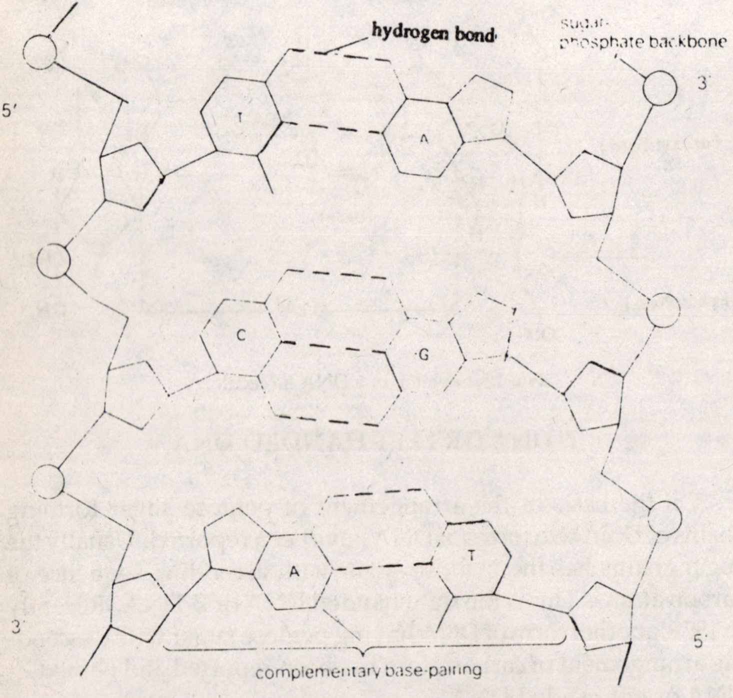

Fig. 1.6. Showing antiparallel nature of back bones of DNA.

Mechanism of DNA Replication. The entire process of DNA replication involves following steps in *E.coli:*

1. Recognition of the initiation point. Replication of DNA begins at a specific point, called initiation point. Specific initiator proteins are required to recognise the initiation point on DNA.

The initiator protein along with DNA directed RNA polymerase initiates the synthesis of RNA primer for the formation of new DNA chain.

2. Unwinding of DNA. The unwinding proteins bind to the nicked strand of the duplex and open up a loop or buble, separating the two strands of DNA duplex.

3. RNA priming. The DNA directed RNA polymerase now synthesizes the primer strands of RNA (*RNA primer*). The priming RNA strands are complementary to the two strands of DNA and are formed of 50 to 100 nucleotides.

4. Formation of DNA on RNA primers. The new strands of DNA are formed in the 5'-3' direction from the 3'-5' template DNA by the addition of **deoxyribonucleotides** to the 3' end of RNA primer. The addition is affected by DNA polymerase III in the presence of ATP. The unwinding proteins separate the duplex strands ahead of the replication fork.

The leading strand of DNA synthesized in 5'-3' direction. The following strand of DNA is formed in its opposite direction. The DNA strands are synthesized in short segments, consisting of 1,000 to 2,000 nucleotides. These segments are called *Okazaki fragments*.

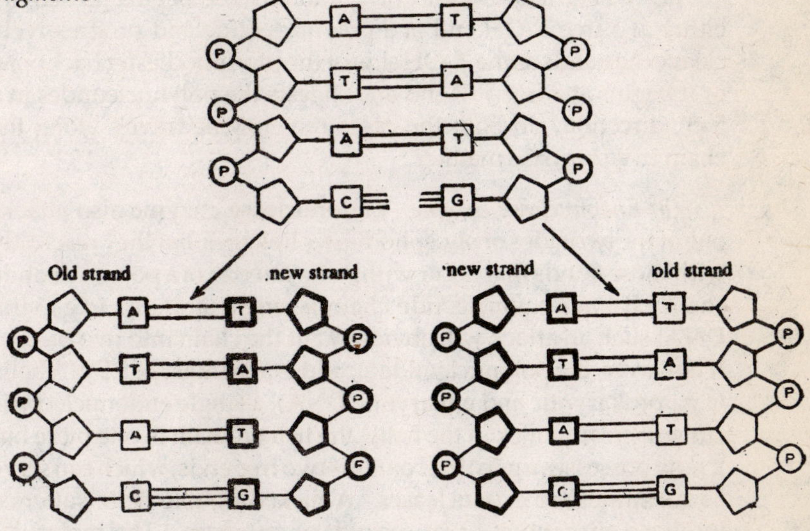

Fig. 1.7. Process of DNA duplication.

5. Excision of RNA primers. Once a small segment of an Okazaki fragment has been formed, the nucleotides of RNA primer are removed from the 5' end one by one by the action of 5'-3' exonuclease activity of DNA polymerase-I.

6. Joining of Okazaki fragments. The gaps left between Okazaki fragments are filled with complementary deoxyribonucleotide residues by DNA polymerase-I. Finally the adjacent 5' and 3' ends are joined by *DNA-ligase.*

In eukaryotic cells, the mechanism of DNA replication is expected to be more complex than in prokaryotes. The replication of eukaryotic DNA begins at multiple points of origin. Their RNA primer is formed of about 10 nucleotides and the Okazaki fragments are much shorter (about 100 to 150 nucleotides).

Enzymes for DNA synthesis. Different prokaryotic and eukaryotic cells have been formed to contain three kinds of enzymes that act on DNA namely nucleases, polymerases and ligases.

1. Nuclease Enzymes. These enzymes attack on the DNA molecules directly. There are two type of nuclease enzyme:

(a) Exonuclease enzyme. The exonuclease begins its activity either at a free 3'-OH end of a polynucleotide and progressively cleave the bands as the 3'-OH side of the phosphodiester back bone or it begins at a free 5'-P end and digests the polynucleotides in a 5'-3', direction. In both the cases the enzyme travels along the chain in a stepwise manner.

(b) Endonuclease enzyme. Endonuclease enzyme also attacks one of the two sides of phosphodiester linkages, but they react only with those bonds that occur within the interior of a polynucleotide chain. If the polynucleotide chain is single stranded (e.g., viral DNA) such an attack will obviousy cut the chain into two pieces. If however, the polynucleotide strand is a member of a DNA helix (e.g., prokaryotic and eukaryotic DNA), a single endonucleolytic cut will create a nick in the helix; the helix remain in one piece but it now possesses a gap that contains two free ends, which can serve as substrates for exonucleases. A nicked double helix suffers a localized disruption of its secondary structure. The molecules becomes free to bend or rotate around its intact strand and the two

broken ends are free to dangle. The increased molecular motion in the region of the nick will very likely interrupt hydrogen bonding between bases in the vicinity of the nick, thus effecting a limited "unraveling" of the helix.

2. DNA Polymerase. For many years, *Korenberg polymerase* was believed to be the enzyme responsible for the replication of the *E.coli* chromosome. But recently *Delucia* and ***Cairns*** isolated a true replicase from *E.coli* and named as *DNA polymerase.* The polymerase catalyses the formation of a polymer. The synthesis of a new complementary chain becomes possible in the presence of polymerase enzyme. There are three categories of DNA polymerase enzymes:

DNA polymerase I. Discovered by *Korenberg* in 1955 and has been studied in *E.coli.* It is believed to take part in the repair of DNA. DNA polymerase I is a single polypeptide chain with a molecular weight of about 109,000. There may be as many as 400 molecule of DNA polymerase I in *E.coli.*

DNA polymerase II. It is also made up of a single polypeptide chain having a molecular weight of about 90,000. The number of DNA polymerase II molecule is about 40 in *E.coli.* This enzyme can elongate Okazaki segments even in the absence of polymerase I.

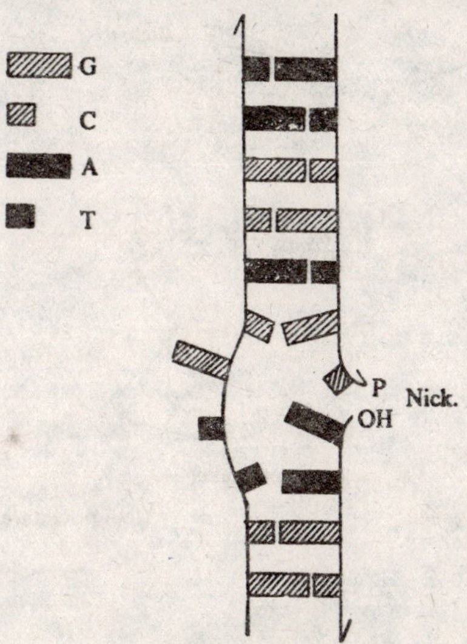

Fig. 1.8. A nicked duplex DNA molecule such as is formed by an endonuclease enzyme.

DNA polymerase III. It is considered to be a true replicase of *E.coli.* It consists of two polypeptide chains with molecular weight of 140,000 and 40,000. It is most effective and can polymersize about 15000 nucleotides per minute in *E.coli.*

3. DNA Ligases. DNA ligase enzymes are capable of catalyzing phosphodiester bond formation between free 3'-OH and free 5'-P groups of a nick of DNA which is created by endonuclease enzyme, thereby restoring an intact DNA duplex. Many DNA ligases have already been discovered. The ligase enzyme from *E. coli* requires the presence of oxidized nicotinamide adenine dinucleotide (NAD+) a cofactor, whereas, the ligase enzyme specified by T_4 bacteriophage requires ATP to bring about the joining reaction.

RNA primers in DNA replication. Short segments of RNA

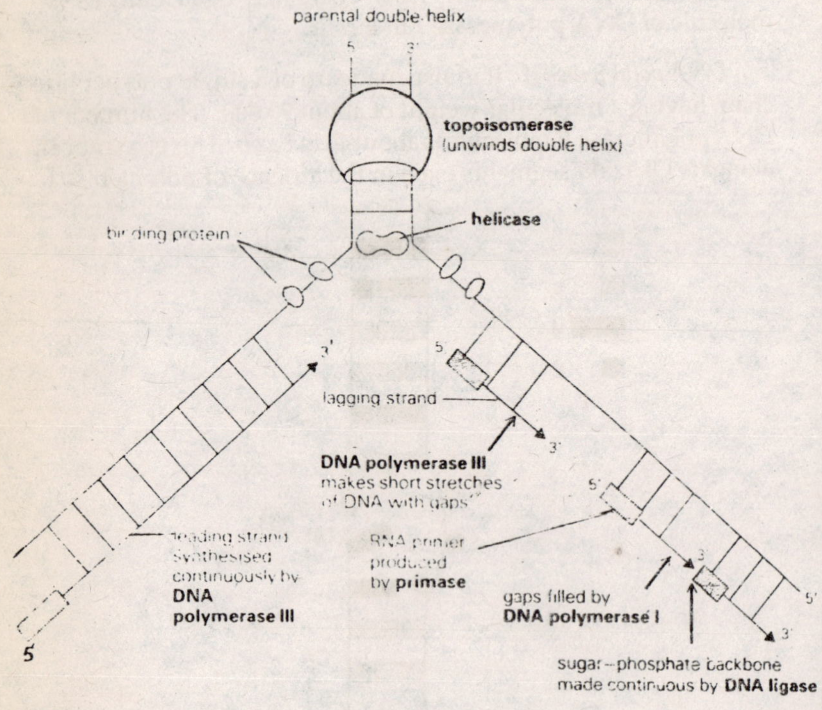

Fig. 1.9. Discontinuous DNA replication

are first synthesized before actual DNA replication starts. These RNA segments are later excised and filled with DNA with the help of enzyme DNA poymerase I. It was found that if RNA synthesis is stopped by a drug rifampicin, DNA replication stops thus proving the role of RNA primers in DNA replication. There are several other evidences which established this point.

Types of replication. Three different types of replication of DNA have been discovered :

(1) Semiconservative
(2) Conservative
(3) Dispersive

(1) Semiconservative. Here the replication of DNA involves the unwinding of the double helix, but no rupture of the separated polyuclotide strands. Thus the primary DNA is conserved during the replication process. According to this mechanism, the unwinding of the original strands would be accompanied or followed by the guided synthesis of the complementary strands of each of the two separatedpolynucleotidestrands. The linearly assembly, catalyzed by enzymes, of the nucleotides of the complementary sequence would be guided by their pairing with the Watson-crick partanres onthe original strands. In this manner, the proper nucleotide sequence would be automatically assumed. The DNA helix would thereby regenerated each of the strand of the original helical duplex uniting with its freshly synthesized complement to form a total of two new double stranded structures. The semiconvervative model thus predicts that entire polynucleotide strands of the parental DNA will be passed on to the progeny in intact form. Each molecule of progeny DNA will receive either one half or none of its nucleotides form the parental DNA.

(2) Conservative. According to this mechanism both the primary and secondary structure of the parental DNA are conserved. Thus the replication process would involve neither the rupture of the individual strands nor the unwinding of the helical duplex. The details of these propose that the sequences of hydrogen bonded base pairs, rather than individual bases, serves the genetic determinant. According to this picture, particular base pairs might preferentially bind specific nucleotides and determine their sequential position in the daughter polynueleotide.

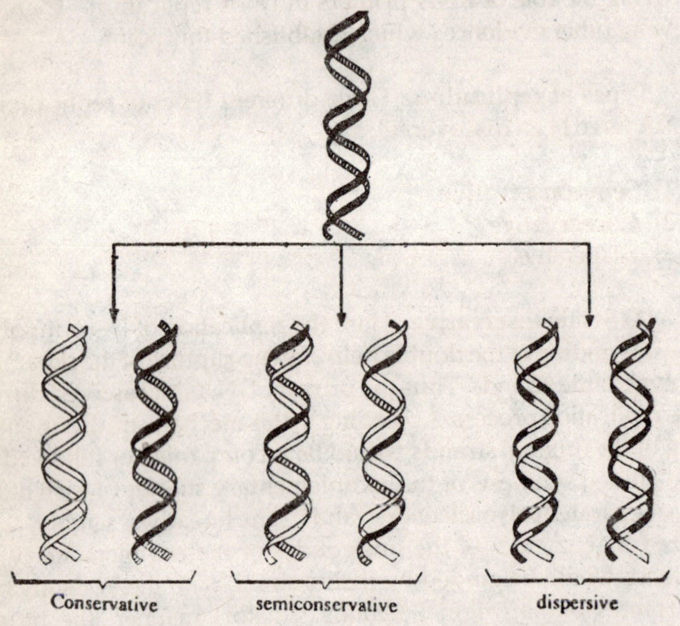

Fig. 1.10 A diagram illustrating three possible modes of DNA replication.

The **convervative** model allows for no redistribution of parental DNA among the progeny. The original DNA is transferred as an intact unit or not at all.

(3) Dispersive. Into this class fall all mechanisms which postulate a general break up of the parental DNA and its more or less uniform distribution among the progeny. It is difficult to propose a model of this type which can possibly allow the preservation of nucleotide sequence. Moreover, the existing experimental evidence is uniformly inconsistent with this kind of scheme.

Hybrid DNA. When double helical DNA molecules are heated above physiological temperature (to near 100°C), their hydrogen bonds break and the complementary strands often separate from each other (*DNA denaturation or melting*). If cooled slowly, the two complementary stands can meet and reform the normal double helix. This process of reunion is called *denaturation* or annealing. This ability to renature DNA molecules permits as to show that artificial hyrid DNA molecules can be formed by slowly cooling mixture of denatured DNA from two species. For example hybrid molecules can be formed containing one strand from man and one from a mouse. Only a fraction (25%) of the DNA strands from a man can form hybrids with mouse DNA. This is, of course not surprising since it merely means that some genes of a man are very similar to those of a mouse, whereas others have quite different nucleotide sequences. It now appears that this molecular technique may be quite useful in establishing the genetic similarity of the various taxonomic groups.

EVIDENCES IN SUPPORT OF SEMICONSERVATIVE REPLICATION OF DNA

1. Meselson and Stahl's Experiment

(i) *Meselson* and *Stahl* (1958) cultured a species of bacteria (*Escherichia coli*) in a culture medium containing N^{15} isotopess of nitrogen. After these had replicated for a few generations in that medium both the strands of their DNA contained N^{15} as constituent of purines and pyrimidines. When these bacteria with N^{15} were transferred in cultural medium containing N^{14}, it was found that DNA separated from fresh generation of bacteria possesses one strand heavier than the other. The heavier strand represents the parental strand and lighter one is the new one synthesized from the culture indicating semiconservative method of DNA replication.

(ii) Density determination experiments were also conducted. The DNA of parental generation (labelled with N^{15}) was found to be heaviest. In first generation it was lighter than the first one. In second generation two bands were observed indicating the presence of DNA with two different densities, as is expected according to semiconservative method of DNA replication. These two bands were of equal intensity in the second generation. In the subsequent generations the intensity of light density bands gradually increased and the intensity of hybrid density band gradually decreased.

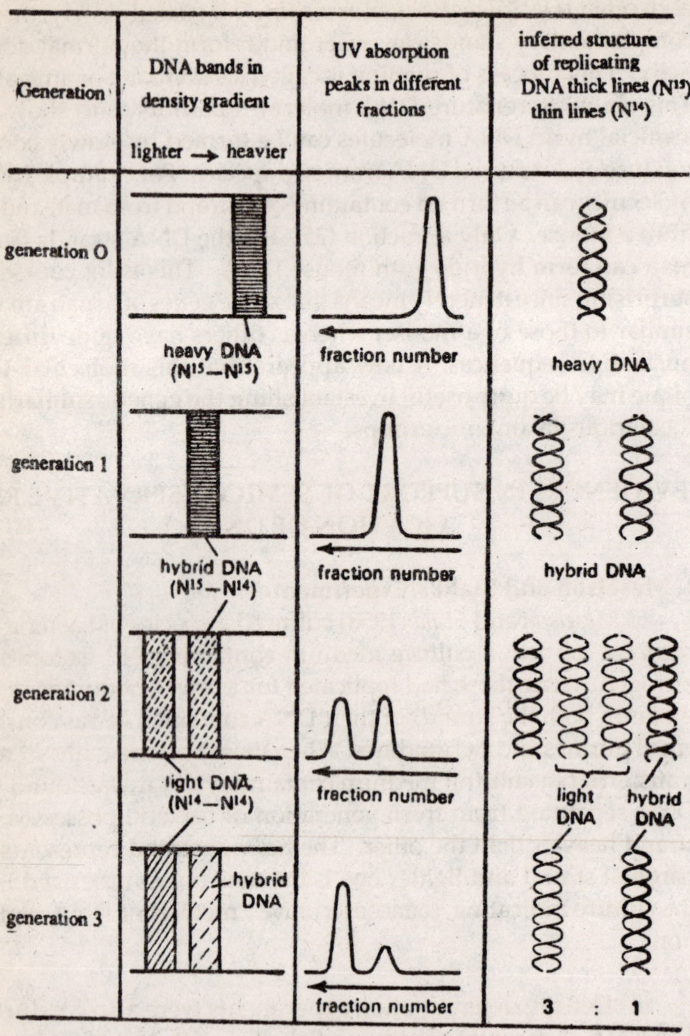

Fig. 1.11 Experiment of Meselson and State in support of Semiconservative Method of DNA Replication

2. Cairns Autoradiography Experiment. *J. Cairns* demonstrated the semiconservative type of replication by using a technique of autoradiography as given in the following lines :

In autoradiography technique, the material is first supplied with a suitable radioactive material like tritiated thymidine (H^3-TdR;H^3 is heavy isotope of hydrogen and it replaces normal hydrogen in thymidine to give rise to tritiated thymidine). Tritiated thymidine is used since this will selectively label only DNA and will not label RNA, since thymine base is absent in RNA. The tritiated thymidine gets incorporated into DNA and replaces ordinary thymidine. The material is then sectioned or else the cells may be broken down to release the intact bacterial chromosome on slides. These slides are then covered by photographic emulsion and stored in the dark. During this storage the particles emitted by tritiated thymidine will expose the film, which can be developed. This photograph will then show the regions of the presence of tritium and thus indirectly the presence of labelled DNA.

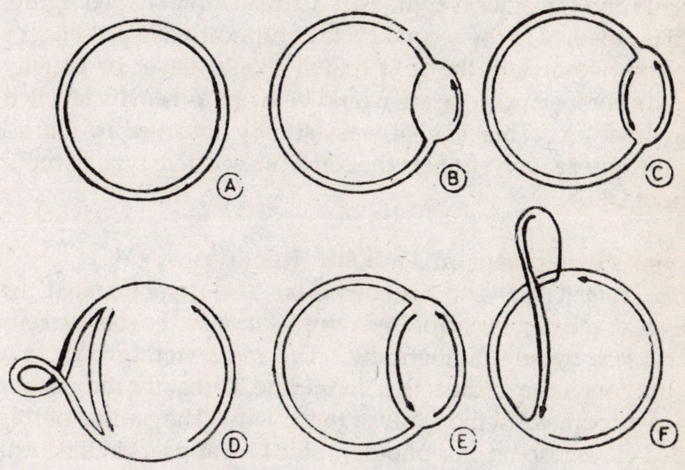

Fig. 1.12. Cairn s model for circular DNA replication.

Using this above technique, the replication of DNA could be easily followed by *J. Cairns* and the results were reported in 1963. During incorporation of tritiated thymidine, autoradiographs could be prepared at regular known intervals. Autoradiographs from this replicating material prepared at regular known intervals demenostated semi-conservative mode of replication. It would be expected that in regions, where one cycle of replication of DNA has been completed, the density of dots will be higher than in the region where the replication has not taken place. The lighter density of dots is considered to indicate that only one of the two strands is labelled, while a heavier density of dots will indicate that both strands are labelled. Such a situation was actually observed. The rate at which the replication proceeds could also be worked out by measuring the length of DNA undergoing replication in a known interval of time. The generation time was worked out by *Cairns* as 30 minutes in *E. coli.* The length of the chromosome was worked out to be about 1 mm. The rate of replication as obvious would be approximately 30μ to 40μ per minute (1 mm=1000μ).

Figure 1.12 indicates that after replication, one of the two strands in the daughter DNA molecules is derived from the parent molecule and the other is synthesized afresh. In 0 shaped figure, which is obtained in the second cycle of replication in presence of label, the two arcs in the split region would never be equally labelled. For instance, one arc would be twice as heavily labelled as the other arc. This is what was actually observed by *Cairns.* Thus the observation support the semiconservative type of replication of DNA.

3. Taylor's Experiment on *Vicia faba* Root tips

J.H.Taylor (1957) and his coworkers also demonstrated the semiconservative method of DNA duplication in the root tip cells of *Vicia faba* by autoradiography. The roots were grown in a medium containing radioactive thymidine, so that the radioactivity is incorporated in the DNA of these cells. The outline of this labelled chromosome on a photographic film appears in the form of scattered black dots of silver grains. When these root tips with labelled chromosomes were transferred to the unlabelled medium containing colchicine and studied for radioactivity, the following observations were made :

1. In the chromosomes of first generation the radioactivity was found to be uniformly distributed in both the chromatids, because in them the original strand of DNA double helix was labelled with radioactivity and the new one was nonlabelled.

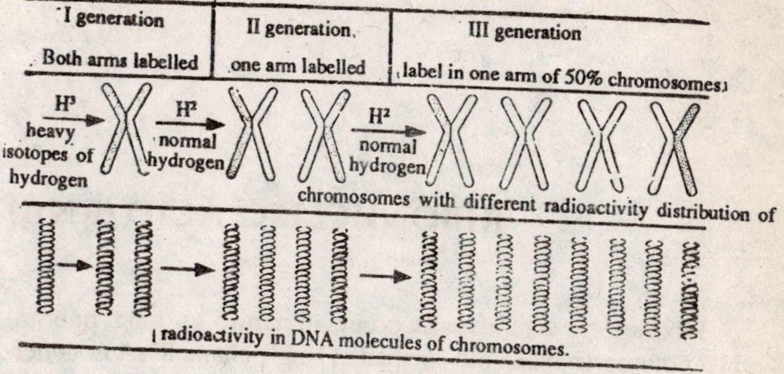

Fig. 1.13. Taylor's experiment on *Vicia faba*.

2. In the chromosomes of second generation only one of the two chromatids in each chromosome was radioactive. This experiment demonstrates the semiconservative method of chromosome replication. But as it is known that each chromatid is composed of only one double helical molecule of DNA, it is the replication of DNA.

BIOLOGICAL SIGNIFICANCE OF DNA

There are four general requirements that genetic material can be expected to fulfil.

(i) That it replicates itself accurately during cell growth and duplication.

(ii) That its structure be sufficiently stable so that heritable changes, mutation occur only very rarely.

(iii) That it has the potentiality to carry all kinds of necessary biological information.

(iv) That it transmits the informations to the cell.

2

RIBONUCLEIC ACID (RNA)

Ribonucleic acid usually occurs in nature as long unbranched polymeric molecule formed of single chain. RNA is generally present in the cytoplasm as well as in nucleolus. *Casperson*(1950) and *Brachet* in 1955 suggested that there is an association between RNA and protein synthesis. A large number of studies have been undertaken to characterise physically the nature and structure of RNA and their biochemical properties and by now we have acquired a lot of knowledge about the various types of RNA and their molecular structures but still there are various gaps to be filled to make a complete picture.

Some plant viruses (e.g., TMV, turnip yellow mosaic viruses, wound tumour viruses, etc.,), animal viruses (e.g., influenza viruses, foot and mouth viruses; rous sarcoma viruses, poliomyelitis viruses reoviruses, etc.) and bacteriophages (e.g., MS_2, etc.) contain ribonucleic acid (RNA) as their genetic material. That is why in these cases it is called the Genetic RNA.

Genetic RNA in Different Viruses

Type of Viruses	*Name of Viruses*	*Type of RNA*
1. Plant viruses	1. TMV	1. Single stranded
	2. Wound tumour	2. Double stranded
2. Aimal viruses	3. Influenza virus	3. Single stranded
	4. Poliomyelities	4. Single Stranded
	5. Reo virus	5. Double stranded
3. Bacteriophages	6. MS_2	6. Single stranded
	7. F_2	7. Single stranded
	8. $r1_2$	8. Single stranded

PRIMARY STRUCTURE OF RNA

RNA usually occur in nature as long unbranched polymeric molecule made up of single chain or helix of polynucleotide strand,Ribnucleic acid is composed of pentose sugars, phosphoric acid and nitrogenous bases. The pentose sugar of RNA is ribose sugar. The sugar forms the back bone along with the phosphoric acid just in a manner studied in DNA.

Phosphroic acid is also one of the constituent of the RNA which along with the pentose sugar forms the back bone, on which the nitrogenous bases are linearly arranged, as shown in the Fig. On the basis of phosphate or phosphoric acid, the chemical constituents of RNA can be written in two ways:

Nitrogenous Base+Rribose Sugar+Phosphate = Nucleotide
Nitrogenous Base + Ribose Sugar = Nucleoside
The nitrogenous bases of ribonucleic acid are of two types :

(i) Purine
(ii) Pyrimidine.

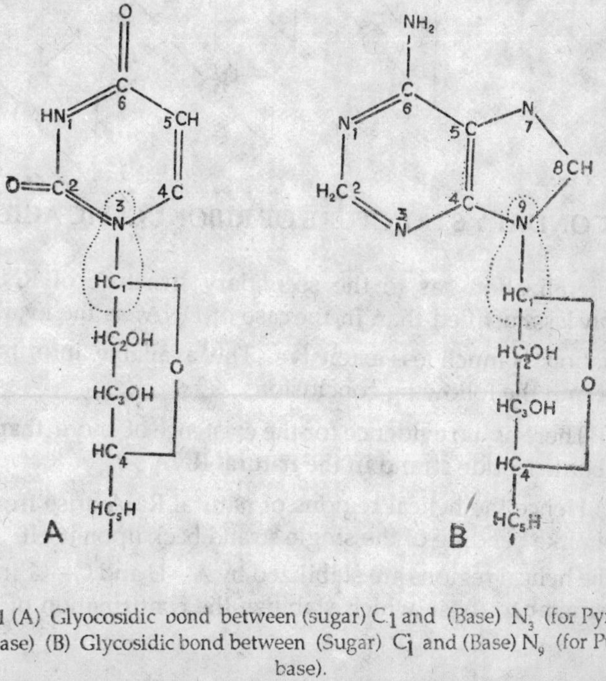

Fig. 2.1 (A) Glyocosidic oond between (sugar) C_1 and (Base) N_3 (for Pyrimidine base) (B) Glycosidic bond between (Sugar) C_1 and (Base) N_9 (for Purine base).

Purine bases comprise mainly adenine (A) and guanine (G) while pyrimidine bases comprise cytosine (C) and uracil (U).

These bases are joined to the pentoses by N-C *glycosidic bonds.* For the purine bases the glycosidic bond is between the \C_1 position of the pentose sugar and the N_9 position of the base. for the pyrimidines, the linkage joins the C_1 and N_3 positions as shown in figure given below :

The bases are arranged on the back bone of the chain which is composed of alternating sugar and phosphate. The bases are attached to the ribose sugar in the same way, the bases in DNA are attached. The arrangement of the bases on the back bone is shown in the following diagram:

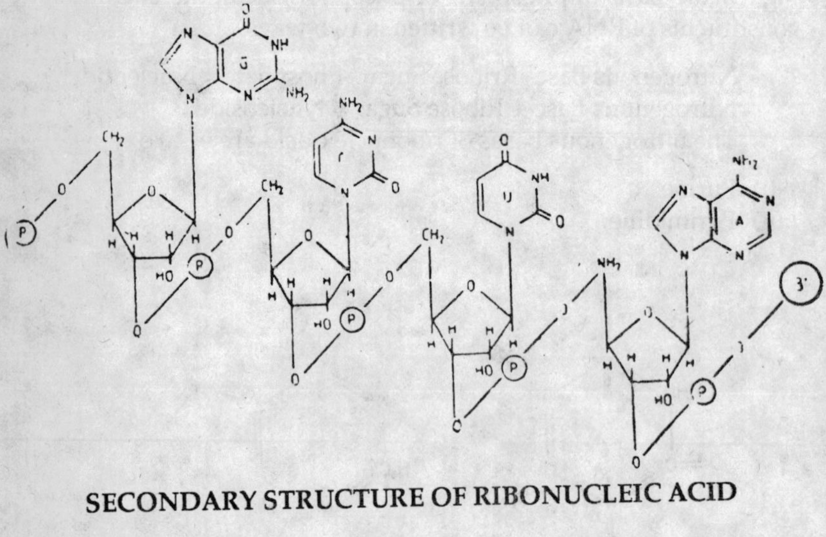

SECONDARY STRUCTURE OF RIBONUCLEIC ACID

Generalization as to the secondary structure of RNA is probably less justified than in the case of DNA, as the available information is much less extensive. The available information does permit the following conclusions :

(1) There is no evidence for the existence of more than one polyribonucleotide strand in the natural RNA's

(2) Hence the helical regions of natural RNA arise from the hair pin like bending of the single strand back upon itself.

(3) The helical regions are stabilized by A—U and C—G interactions similar to those which stabilize the confirmation of DNA.

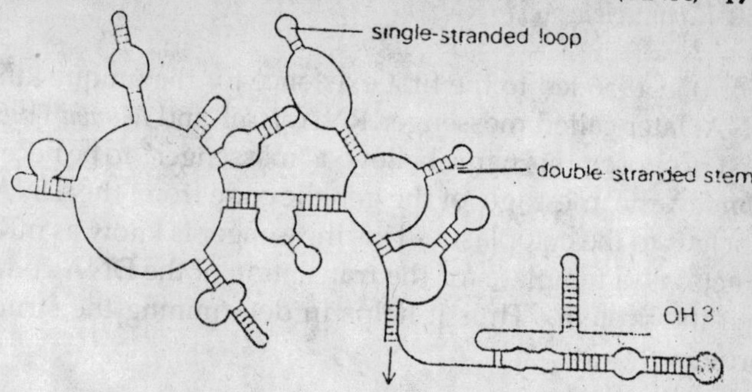

Fig. 2.2. Showing the Secondary structure of RNA.

However, the irregular base composition of RNA does not allow the incorporation of the entire molecule into double perfect helic of this type, and the helical zone co-exist with the random segments.

(4) Two alternative models for the structure of RNA may be postulated : (a) The non-helical fraction of RNA may take the form of extended amorphous zones separating segments of nearly perfect helical organization. This model pre-suppose that extensive complementary sequences exist within the single strand. These tend to seek each other out to form perfect or nearly perfect, helical regions.

(b) Alternatively, nucleotides which do not participate in the helical organization may occur largely as numerous small loops external to the helically paired structure.

TYPES OF RIBONUCLEIC ACIDS

Four types of ribonucleic acids have been studied and they are as follows :

(1) mRNA
(2) tRNA
(3) rRNA
(4) vRNA

1. Messenger (mRNA) : Studies by *Huxley* and later by *Volkin* and *Astrachan* with T_2 bacteriophage infected (bacterial virus,

E.coli) in 1956 led to the first existence for the unique kind of the RNA, later called messenger RNA. *Jacob* and *Monod* (1961) who first proposed this name believed "messenger" to be necessary to convey the message of the genetic code from the DNA of the nucleus to the cytoplasm. This messenger is know as mRNA and it acts as a template for the translation of the DNA code into a specific protein. Thus it helps in determining the structure of protein.

mRNA molecules exist in a large variety of lengths, depending on the length of the polypeptide chain for which they code. Its molecular weight and sedimention value vary considerably. Generally the life span of mRNA is relatively short, although in some eukaryotic cells there is evidence of some degree of stability.

Further mRNA is always complementry to a portion of strand of DNA, with the exception that uracil replaces thymine. It should therefore hybridize with the DNA from which it was transcribed.

It is now an established fact that when the code has been transcribed from DNA on to mRNA, the later leaves the nucleus passes through the nuclear membrane into the cytoplasm. Here it moves to the ribosomes the site of protein synthesis. mRNA molecules attaches reversibly to the surface of ribosome always binding to the smaller sub-units. The magnesium cation, Mg^{++} is involved in the formation of a complex between mRNA and ribosomes.

Types of mRNA. On the basis of size and the coding two types of mRNA has been described:

(a) *Monocistronic mRNA*. Mostly the mRNA carries the codons of single cistron (i.e., codes for one complete protein molecule) of the DNA. Such mRNA molecule is called monocistronic mRNA. For example, for the synthesis of a polypeptide chain of 300 to 500 amino acid residus, a monocistronic mRNA of *E.coli* contains 900 to 1500 nucleotides in its molecule.

(b) *Polygenic or polycistronic mRNA* : Sometimes a mRNA

molecule carries the codes from several adjacent DNA cistrons and become much longer in size. This type of mRNA is called polygenic or polycistronic mRNA. For example, for the metabolism of the histidine protein the cell synthesizes about 10 specific enzymatic proteins and a mRNA in this case may carry codons for all the 10 enzymes.

INFORMOSOMES

In eukaryons mRNA is associated with protein forming ribonucleoprotein complexes. Some of these complexes remain free in the cytoplasm without being attached to the polyribosomes. These are named as infosrmosomes by *Spirin*. These are very stable and can remain in the cell cytoplam for several days. The stability is attributed by the presence of protein sheath around mRNA molecule. In informosomes proteins and mRNA are found in the ratio of 4:1. These occur in the form of particles of 80S or less.

Since informosomes are very stable, these are used by the cell in protein synthesis only when there is delay in translation. In embryonic cells, genetic apparatus starts functioning only late during organogenesis. Therefore, in early stages of cleavage when there is no rRNA, informosomes govern the process of protein synthesis.

Stability. The cell does not contain large quantities of mRNA. This is because mRNA, unlike others RNAs is constantly undergoing breakdown. It is broken down to its constituent robonucleotides by ribonucleases. In bacteria, mRNA may be so short-lived that while one end is translating protein the other end may be undergoing breakdown. In *E.coli* the avarage half-life of some mRNA is about two minutes.

Eukaryotic cells, on the other hand, contain metabolically stable mRNA. Mammalian reticulocytes are immature RBC which have lost their nuclei but have retained ribosomes. These cells can synthesize haemoglobin for many hours and even days by utilizing the mRNA transcribed by the nuclei when they were present.

2. Transfer Ribonucleic Acid. In the literature, t-RNA molecules have been vasriously termed tRNA, sRNA for soluble RNA, or adaptor RNA, it forms about 10-15% of thse total RNA in most of the existence. Each tRNA contains approximate 80 nucleotides. The soluble or t-RNA forms large varieties of different cells, is homogenous in its molecular size having a molecular weight of about 25000.

The nucleotide sequence of tRNA was first worked out by *Holley et al* (1965) for yeast alanine tRNA. Since then the sequence of about 75 different tRNAs has been established. According to the Holley's leaf model the tRNA is a polunucleotide chain which is folded upon itself to form 5 arms. As a result of the folding the 3' and 5' ends of the chain come near each other. An arm consists of a stem and a loop. Bases are arranged in pairs in arms. There is no base pairing in the loops.

The 3' end of the polynucleotide chain ends in CCA base sequence. This represents site for the attachment of activated amino acid. The5'end of the chain terminates with guanine base. The bent in the chain of each tRNA molecule contains a definite sequence of three nitrogenous bases which constitute the anticodon. It recognizes the codon on mRNA.

Four different regions or special sites can be recognized in the molecules of tRNA. These are:

(I) Amino acid attachment site. It occurs at the 3' end of the tRNA chain and has-OH group of ribose molecule free to pair. This-OH group combines with the specific amino acid in the presence of ATP forming amino-acyl tRNA. It is common to all the tRNA molecules.

(II) Recognition site. It contains a specific base sequence which dictates the attachment of correct amino acid to the tRNA molecule. It matches with the amino acid activating enzymes through which attachment of amino acid to tRNA takes place.

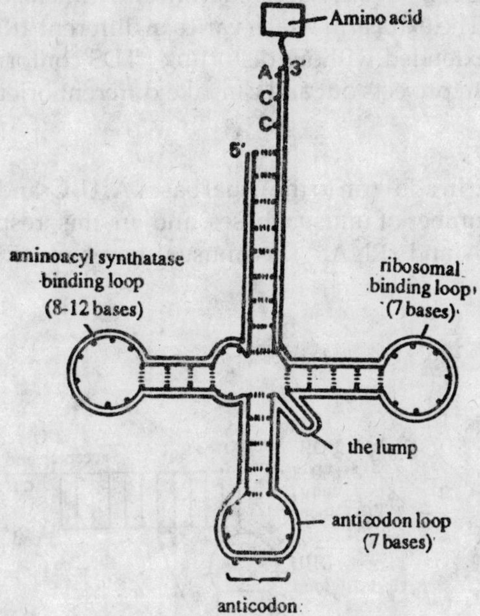

Fig. 2.3. Clover leaf model.

(III) Anticodon or codon recognition site. This site has three unpaired bases (triplet of base) whose sequence is complementary with a codon (triplet) in mRNA. Therefore, it determines the pairing of tRNA with the specific codon (triplet) of mRNA. It is, therefore, the most specific region of tRNA molecule.

(IV) Ribosome recognition site. This helps in the attachment of tRNA to the ribosome. This site is common to all the molecules of tRNA.

Three dimenstional structure of tRNA. In order to understand the stucture-function relationship of tRNA, its three dimensional structure (TDS) should be known. With the availability of tRNA in crystalline form in 1968, TDS of tRNA could be studied through X-ray crystallorgaphy as was done for DNA double helix. About a dozen models for TDS were proposed, but the latest and most acceptable model was proposed in 1973 by *S.H.Kim*. He suggested that TDS of tRNA takes the shape of letter L with a thickness 20 Å. This can be easily derived from two dimensional clover leaf model. The extra arm which varies in different tRNA molecules can be extended without distorting TDS conformation. The CCA stem projects out and can take different orientations.

Unusual bases. In addition to the usual bases A, U, G and C, tRNA contain a number of unusual bases, and in this respect differs from mRNA and rRNA. The unusual bases of tRNA account for 15-20%

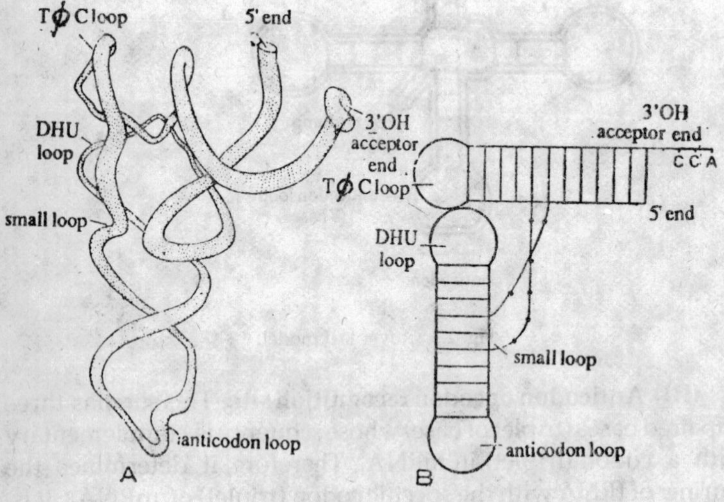

Fig. 2.4. Three dimensional structure of yeast phenylalanine tRNA.

of total RNA of the cell. Most of the unusual bases are formed by methylation (addition of $-CH_3$ or methyl group to the usual bases), e.g. cytosineand and guanine on methylation yield methyl cytosine and methylguanine, respectively. Precursor tRNA molecules transcribed on the DNA template contain the usual bases. These are then modified to unusual bases. The unusual bases are important because theyprotect the tRNA molecule against degradation by RNAse. This protection is necessary because RNA is found floating freely in the cell.

Some of the unusual bases of tRNA are methylguanine (GMe), dimethylguanine (GMe_2), methylcytosine (Me), ribothymine (T) pseudouridine(ψ) dihydrouridine (DHU_2, H_2U, UH_2), inosine (I) and methylinosine (IMe,MeI).

3. Ribsomal Ribonucleic acid or rRNA: Ribosomes are small particles of about 200A° to 250 A° in diameter, and are generally present in the cytoplasm either lying free in the cytoplasm or attached to the **outer** membrane of endoplasmic reticulum or "nuclear membrane". These particles are ribosomes containing about 60% ribonucleic acid or RNA which is ribosomal RNA or rRNA and 40% protein. It is generally agreed that cytoplasmic ribosomes or their subunits are made in the nucleus and are subsequently transferred to the cytoplasm.

However, the mode of their passages across the nuclear membrane is still a matter of controversy.

Even from the morphological evidence, it would appear that the reticular or microvesicular spheres of the nucleus could be engaged in either the synthesis of rRNA, or its assembly, or both.

The finding that hybridization of rRNA takes places with the chromatin associated with the nucleolar region suggests that rRNA is synthesized on the part of the chromosome traversing the nucleous (the nucleolar organizer) or, in the some cases, on DNA detached from the chromosome and associated with the nucleolus.

Ribosomal RNA differs in size and base contents from t-RNA and from other RNA classes of most cells. r-RNA from most organism is relatively rich in guanine and cytosine, and it lacks many of the rare bases found in tRNA, although some methylated bases are present.

The function of rRNA in protein synthesis is not yet completely clear. The unpaired bases in the molecule may bind mRNA and tRNA to ribosomes possibly by Mg^{2+} linkages between phosphate groups on the two molecules.

Ribosomal RNA also gives some evidence for developing the double helical structure.

4. Virual RNA (vRNA) : Viruses may contain either DNA or RNA. However, each particular virus generally contains nucleic acid of only one type. Some examples of RNA viruses are influenza, turnip yellow mosaic, tomato bushy stunt, tobacco necrosis, and the particularly well studied tobacco mosaic virus (TMV).

REPLICATION OF RIBONUCLEIC ACID

At first it was difficult to apply the rules of DNA replication to RNA replication, because less is known about the macromolecular structure of DNA, but with the basic principles of the template theory laid down, the synthesis of RNA became accessible to further investigation.

As discussed above the four various kinds of RNAs, which are structurally alike, but differ considerably in molecular weight and are distributed in different parts of the cell, are replicated or biosynthesized as follows :

Biosynthesis of rRNA. rRNA although present in ribosomes is formed inside the nucleus. DNA associated with the nucleolus is responsible for coding rRNA. This part of DNA is known as nucleolar organizer. In bacteria about 10-200 cistrons are concerned with the rRNA syntehsis, whereas in higher organisms 200-2000 tightly clustered rDNA cistrons are involved in rRNA synthesis.

The two types of rRNA (28S and 18S) are transcribed from the nucleolar DNA as a single elongated unit of 45S. Inside the nucleus, the 45S RNA is methylated and complexed with protein. Finally, via a number of steps it is cleaved into 32S and 18S segments. The 18S RNA gets associated with basic proteins to form the small subunit of ribosomes. The 32S segment is further severed and finally change to 28S RNA. This 28S RNA also gets associated with proteins and forms the large subunits of ribosome. These units then come out into the cytoplasm.

The 5S RNA has a extrancleolar origin, transcribed from genes located outside the nucleolar organizer. It gets associated with each large ribosomal subunit. The function of 5S RNA is unknown.

Biosynthesis of mRNA. The existence of a short lived type of RNA was predicted on theoratical grounds by *F. Jacob, J. Monod,* and associates. The name messenger RNA was used to describes a form of RNA that would be made in the cell nucleus, but would be transferred to the cytoplasm during protein synthesis. During protein synthesis, the amino acid sequence was determined by DNA which is mainly in the nucleus. The information from DNA in the form of a specific sequence of bases had to be transferred some how to the cytoplasm.

The notion of a mRNA demanded that DNA acts as template for RNA synthesis. The principle of base pairs still applies here, because uracil in RNA has the same dimension as theymine in DNA, and one can substitute for the other. In this manner a DNA strand could function as template for RNA synthesis.

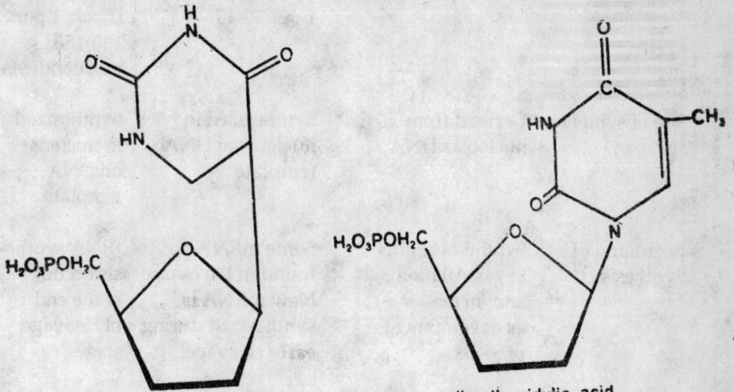

pseudo uridylic acid

ribo thymidylic acid

Fig. 2.5 Showing the structural formula of Pseudo-Uridylic acid and Ribo-thymidylic acid.

A –	T –	T –	G –	A –	C	DNA
|	|	|	|	|	|	
U –	A –	A –	C –	U –	G	m RNA

Biosynthesis of Transfer RNA. It is of low molecular weight. The structure of tRNA has been explained already. Although the details of its synthesis are not known. It is known that tRNA is synthesized on DNA templates by steps similar to those of the other types of RNA.

Table 2.2. Comparison of the different types of RNA

	Ribosomala RNA (tRNA)	Messenger RNA (mRNA)	Transfer RNA (tRNA)
Percentage of total RNA of cell	80%	3 to 5%	10 to 20%
Sedimentation Coefficient	28S,18S,5.8S,5S 23S,	8S 16S,	3.8S 5S
Number of nucleotides	5S RNA: 120 nucleotides 16-18S RNA : 1,600 to 2,500 nucleotides. 23-28S RNA : 3,200 to 5,500 nucleotides	*E.coli*: 900 to 1,500 nuciotides	73 to 93 nucloetides.
Molecular weight	23S RNA : 1.1 x 10^6 30S RNA : 0.55 x 10^6	500,000	25,000-30,000
Unusual bases	Small amount of methylated bases.	Small amount of unusual bases. 1 per 30-40	High content unusual bases. (*E.coli*: 1 per 100-150 nucleotides).
Site of syntehsis	Derived from nucleolar DNA	Synthesized in nucleus on DNA template.	Synthesized in nucleus on DNA template.
Beginning of Synthesis	Synthesis begins at gastrulation, and increases as development proceds.	Some mRNA is found in the ovum. New mRNA is synthesized during early cleavage.	tRNA synthesis occurs at the end of cleavage stages.
Function	Unpaired bases may bind mRNA and tRNA to ribosomes.	Conveys genetic information from DNA of chromosomeswhere it takes part in protein synthesis	Adaptor for attaching amino acids to mRNA template.

Table 2.3 Comparison between DNA and RNA

Deoxyribonucleic acid	*Ribonucleic acid*
1. DNA is the usual genetic material	1. RNA is the genetic material of some viruses.
2. DNA is usually double-stranded, (In certain viruses DNA is signle stranded,) % 174).	2. Most cellar RNA is single stranded. (Some viruses e.g., reovirus, have double stranded RNA).
3. The pentose sugar is deoxyribose	3. The pentose sugar is ribose.
4. The common organic bases are adenine, guanine, cytosine and thymine.	4. The common organic bases are adenine, guanine, cytosone and uracil.
5. Base pairing : adenine pairs with thymine and guanine with cytosine	5. Adenine pairs with uracil and guanine with cytosine.
6. Pairing of bases is throughout the length of the molecule.	6. Pairing of bases is only in the helical region.
7. There are fewer uncommon bases.	7. There are more uncommon bases.
8. DNA is only of one type.	8. There are three types of RNA, messenger RNA, ribosomal and RNA transfer RNA.
9. Most of the DNA is found in the chromosomes. Some DNA is also found in the cytoplasm e.g. in mitochondira and chloroplasts.	9. Messenger RNA is formed on the chromosomes, and is found in the nucleolus and cytoplasm. rRNA and tRNA are also formed on the chromosomes, and are found in cytoplasm.
10. Denaturation (melting) is partialy reversible only under certain conditions of slow cooling (renaturation).	10. Complete and practically instantaneous reversibility of the process of melting.
11. DNA on replicaticnforms DNA, and on transcription forms RNA.	11. Usually RNA does not replicate or transcribe. (In certain viruses RNA can synthesize an RNA chain).
12. Genetic messages are usually encoded in DNA	12. The usual function of RNA is translating message encoded in DNA into proteins.

13. DNA consists of a large number of nucleotides, up to 4.3 million.	13. RNA consists of fewer nucleotides, upto 12,000.

Several aspects of tRNA merit some comment. One is that all tRNA types so far isolated contain the same sequence of bases at one end of the molecule, cytosine-cytosine-adenine (C-C-A). An other irteresting observation is that in tRNA one invariably finds nucleotides not yet described: **pseudo**-uridylic acid and **ribothymi**dylic acid.

The presence of the two bases present a problem. If synthesis of tRNA proceeds by the same mechanism as other types of RNA, the enzymes involved in tRNA synthesis must be assumed to have unique specificity for the two new nucleotides. A more attractive idea is that tRNA is formed from the familiar four nucleotides, and by enzymatic modification of selected uridylic acid units in the tRNA, the new nucleotides, are formed. Pseudo-uridylic acid could be the product of an isomerization reaction of tRNA. Ribothymidylic acid is known to be formed by methylation of uridylic acid present in tRNA. The characteristic terminal —C-C-A sequence is belived to be added enzymatically after tRNA is already made.

3

PROTEIN SYNTHESIS

The proteins are highly organized and complex structures. The proteins have significant role in the structural and functional organisation of the cell. The structural proteins constitute various cellular components and some extracellular parts such as cuticle and fibres, etc. The functional (e.g., enzymatic and hormonal) proteins control almost all metabolic, biosynthetic, bioenergetic, growth regulating, sensory and reproductive activities of the cell. All the proteins which are required by the cell for its different purposes are synthesized by the cell itself intracellularly.

Chemically, proteins are polymers of amino acids. The amino acids molecules are linked together in linear fashion forming long polypeptide chain. The adjacent amino acid are joined together by covalent peptide bond between the carboxy group of one amino acid and the amino group of the other. DNA initiates the mechanism since it carrys the genetic message for protein synthesis. This genetic message from one DNA strand is transferred to a complementary strand of messenger RNA; mRNA then passes out of the nucleus and carry the message to the ribosomes where it is used to synthesize the particular type of protein molecule. The first step is called *transcription* because it involves copying of the genetic information from DNA into mRNA which transmits the coded information from DNA to ribosomes, the site of protein synthesis. The second step is termed as *translation* as it involves the *translation* of the information encoded on mRNA with newly synthesized protein molecule.

CENTRAL DOGMA & REVERSE CENTRAL DOGMA

It is a sort of relationship between DNA, RNA and protein. It details with the flow of genetic information and can be studied under the following heads:

1. One way flow of informations. *Crick* (1958) suggested that DNA transmits the genetic informations for protein synthesis by transcribing mRNA (transcription) and other types of RNAs. These RNAs then translate the nucleotide sequence into the sequence of amino acids (translation). This is known as one way flow of information or central dogma.

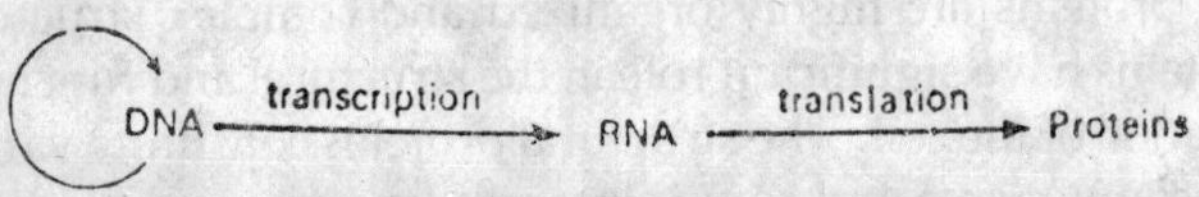

2. Circular flow of information. *Barry Commoner* (1968) suggested circular flow of information. The DNA transcribes RNA (mRNA, tRNA etc.), RNA translates the information into protein, protein then directs the synthesis of RNA and RNA dictates the synthesis of DNA.

3. Inverse flow of information. *Temin* (1970) has described the presence of an enzyme-*RNA dependent DNA polymerase*, which controls the synthesis of DNA from a single strand of RNA. *D. Baltimore* (1970) has described the presence of this enzyme in certain RNA tumour viruses. In tumour viruses the RNA is genetic RNA but in certain cases the nongenetic RNA synthesized under the control of DNA may also control the synthesis of DNA by inverse flow of information. This is known as central dogma reverse.

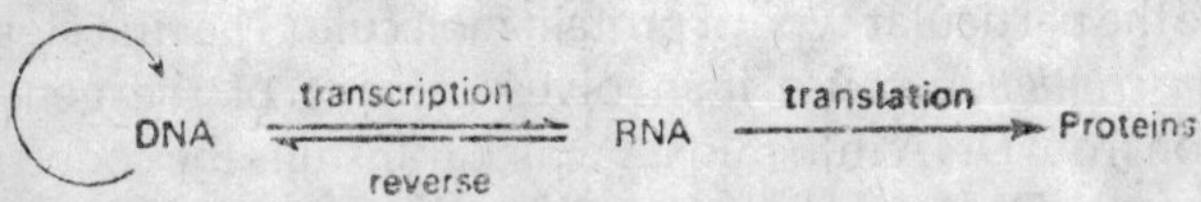

(*Dr. H. Temin, Dr. Baltimore* along with *R. Dulbecoo* received Nobel Prize in Medicine for 1976).

Role of amino acids. Amino acids are the units from which the protein molecules are made. In the cytoplasm of every cell a number of amino acids are present. Out of these 20 amino acids stake the important part in protein synthesis. Amino acids are as given below :-

Table 3.1 Structure of the Common amino acids

Name	Symbol	Structure
Glycine	Gly	$H-\underset{^{+}NH_3}{\overset{H}{\underset{\mid}{\overset{\mid}{C}}}}-C{\large\substack{\nearrow O \\ \searrow O^-}}$
Alanine	Ala	$CH_3-\underset{^{+}NH_3}{\overset{H}{\underset{\mid}{\overset{\mid}{C}}}}-C{\large\substack{\nearrow O \\ \searrow O^-}}$
Valine	Val	$(H_3C)_2HC-\underset{^{+}NH_3}{\overset{H}{\underset{\mid}{\overset{\mid}{C}}}}-C{\large\substack{\nearrow O \\ \searrow O^-}}$
Leucine	Leu	$(H_3C)_2CH-CH_2-\underset{^{+}NH_3}{\overset{H}{\underset{\mid}{\overset{\mid}{C}}}}-C{\large\substack{\nearrow O \\ \searrow O^-}}$
Isoleucine	Ileu	$(H_3C-H_2C)(H_3C)HC-\underset{^{+}NH_3}{\overset{H}{\underset{\mid}{\overset{\mid}{C}}}}-C{\large\substack{\nearrow O \\ \searrow O^-}}$
Serine	Ser	$HO-CH_2-\underset{^{+}NH_3}{\overset{H}{\underset{\mid}{\overset{\mid}{C}}}}-C{\large\substack{\nearrow O \\ \searrow O}}$
Threonine	Thr	$(HO)(H_3C)CH-\underset{^{+}NH_3}{\overset{H}{\underset{\mid}{\overset{\mid}{C}}}}-C{\large\substack{\nearrow O \\ \searrow O^-}}$
Phenylalanine	Phe	$C_6H_5-CH_2-\underset{^{+}NH_3}{\overset{H}{\underset{\mid}{\overset{\mid}{C}}}}-C{\large\substack{\nearrow O \\ \searrow O^-}}$ (benzene ring drawn as HC, C–C, C=C with H atoms)

Name	Symbol	Structure
Tyrosine	Tyr	$HO-C_6H_4-CH_2-CH(^{+}NH_3)-COO^-$
Tryptophane	Try	$C_8H_6N-CH_2-CH(^{+}NH_3)-COO^-$
Cystine	$(CyS)_2$	$^{-}OOC-CH(^{+}NH_3)-CH_2-S-S-CH_2-CH(^{+}NH_3)-COO^-$
Cysteine	CySH	$HS-CH_2-CH(^{+}NH_3)-COO^-$
Methionine	Met	$CH_3-S-CH_2-CH_2-CH(^{+}NH_3)-COO^-$
Proline	Pro	$H_2C-CH_2-CH_2-\overset{+}{N}H_2-CH-COO^-$ (ring)
Hydroxyproline	Hypro	$HO-HC-CH_2-CH-\overset{+}{N}H_2-CH_2$ (ring), $-COO^-$
Aspartic acid	Asp	$^{-}OOC-CH_2-CH(^{+}NH_3)-COO^-$

Glutamic acid	Glu	$^{-}O(O{=})C-CH_2-CH_2-C(H)(^{+}NH_3)-C(=O)O^-$
Asparagine	Asp-NH_2	$H_2N-C(=O)-CH_2-C(H)(^{+}NH_3)-C(=O)O^-$
Glutamine	Glu-NH_2	$H_2N-C(=O)-CH_2-CH_2-C(H)(^{+}NH_3)-C(=O)O^-$
Histidine	His	$HC{=}C-CH_2-C(H)(^{+}NH_3)-C(=O)O^-$ (ring: N, NH, C–H)
Arginine	Arg	$(H_2N)(H_2N)C-NH-CH_2-CH_2-C(H)(^{+}NH_3)-C(=O)O^-$
Lysine	Lys	$\overset{+}{H_3}N-CH_2-CH_2-CH_2-CH_2-C(H)(^{+}NH_3)-C(=O)O^-$

The amino acids are distributed through out the cytoplasm, which are collected by specific tRNAs bring the amino acids to the actual site of protein synthesis i.e. to ribosomes where the synthesis of protein takes place.

ROLE OF mRNA DURING SYNTHESIS OF PROTEIN

According to *Jacob* and *Monod* (1961) mRNA conveys necessary message of genetic code from the DNA of the nucleus to the cytoplasm. It acts as template for the translation of the DNA code into specific protein. It is formed from DNA during repliclation with similar base composition. The evidence that DNA is the main source from which RNA is synthesized can be received by using deoxyribonuclease, which ceases protein synthesis. The inhibition of protein synthesis is due to a fact, that mRNA is not formed in the absence of DNA as it is digested by the enzyme. *Hall* (1961) further gave similar evidence regarding the formation of mRNA from DNA.

Messenger RNA molecules necessarily exist in a large variety of lengths, depending upon the length of the polypeptide chain for which they code. There are very few polypeptide chains which contain less than 100 amino acids, and so very few molecules which contain less than 300 nucleotide units, the length of mRNA which carries information necessary to determine the complete polypeptide chain of a protein molecule is called a ***cistron***, as postulated by *Benzer*. Some mRNA molecules are able to carry information for the synthesis of more than one protein molecule. Such types are known as polycistronic. The average life time of mRNA molecules is variable. In bacterial cell mRNA molecules exist for few minutes at 37° C, after which they are broken down into its components by enzymes. In the case of mammalian reticulocytes the mRNA are long lived. There is then considerable variation in average lifetimes of mRNA molecules.

While studying the impact of radioactive substances on the incubated cells, it has been observed that he labelled material is first incorporated into the nuclear RNA and then appears in the cytoplasmic RNA. This indicates that when the code has been transcribed from DNA into mRNA, the latter leaves the nucleus. In the cytoplasm it reaches to the site of protein synthesis, the ribosome. The mRNA molecule attaches reversibly to the surface of the ribosome. The attachment is manifested by Mg++ (magnesium cation) and finally a complex is formed, between mRNA and the ribosome.

Role of tRNA. It is also called as soluble RNA. This particular nucleic acid is present in the cytoplasm in sufficient amount and the main role of tRNA is to pick up the amino acid from cytoplasm and bring to the site of protein synthesis on the ribosome. As already stated that a number of amino acids (20) are present in the cytoplasm and for every specific amino acid there is one specific tRNA, so there are different specific tRNA molecules. A specific adopter enzyme (an-amino-acyl tRNA synthetase) is required to couple each amino acid to its specific tRNA.

The part of tRNA which becomes attached to its particular amino acid appears to be same for all sorts of tRNAs. This limb is the 3' end of the molecule, terminating in the sequence of three bases-Cytosine-Cytosine-Adenine. Another 5' end of the molecule terminates in the base guanine. This sequence only enables amino acid to be attached at particular site.

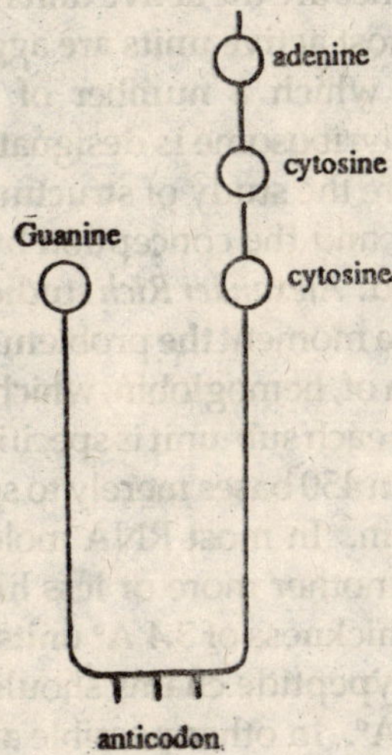

Fig. 3.1 Structure of tRNA molecule.

The process by which the amino acids become attached to the tRNA is quite complicated. ATP provides energy which is required during the process. The link formed between the amino acid and transfer RNA is a covalent bond between the carboxyl group of the amino acid, and the ribosome of the terminal adenine nucleotide of the tRNA. Thus there are three components necessary for the reaction :

(i) a specific amino acid
(ii) a specific enzyme, and
(iii) a specific tRNA.

The reaction can be shown by the following equations:

(i) Amino acid + ATP + Amino acyladenylate —> Enzyme bond Amino acid adenylate + 2P

(ii) Enzyme bound Amino acid adenylate + uncharged tRNA —> charged tRNA + Enzyme + amino acid complex.

POLYRIBOSOMES AND THEIR ROLE IN PROTEIN SYNTHESIS

The 70S free ribosomes are the active units in protein synthesis in a normal cell. The most active units are aggregates containing a mRNA molecule to which a number of 70S ribosomes are attached. The name polyribosome is designated to this assembly line of ribosomes. Before the study of structure of polyribosomes let us know the history and the conception by which the idea of polyribosomes appeared. *Alexander Rich* studied and expressed in his words "consider for a moment the problem of synthesizing one of the polypeptide chain of, hemoglobin, which contains about 150 amino acid sub-units. If each sub-unit is specified by a triplet code, the m-RNA must contain 450 bases merely to specify the sequence of sub units in one chain. In most RNA molecules the bases are stacked on top of one another more or less like a pilo of pennie. Since the bases have a thickness of 3.4 A° units, the mRNA strand for the hemoglobin polypeptide chains should have a molecular length of at least 1,500 A°. In other possible arrangements of the RNA molecule the length might be almost twice. By comparison, the individual ribosome has a diameter of only about 230 A°, and so we wondered how the long messenger molecule interacted with such a small particle to manufacture a polypeptide chain." Some investigators thought that the RNA chain might be wrapped around the out side of the ribosome,but it was hard to visualize how intimate contact between the two should be maintained. The wrapping proble would be still more difficult for RNA chain 20,000 A° long, which are found in many viruses. Alternative suggestions that the mRNA might come how be coiled inside the ribosomes seemed to present even more formidable topographical problems. It occured to us that proteins might actually be made on groups of ribosomes lined together some how by mRNA. There was already a little evidence pointing in this direction. *Walter Gilbert* of Havard University, as well as other investigators, had found that when a synthetic RNA was added to a cell free system of bacterial ribosomes, the ribosomes would tend to clump together.

Probably the first polyribosomes were studied in mammalian (rabbit) reticulocytes that predominantly synthesize the blood protein hemoglobin contains ribosomes. The negative staining procedure of *Slayter* shows that ribosomes in a polyribosome are separated by gaps of 50 to 150 A° while positive staining with uranyl acetate reveals that the ribosomes are connected by a thin thread 10 to 15 A° in diameter which is about the thickness of a single strand of RNA. From these studies, it is concluded that the over all length covered by a five unit polyribosomes is about 1,500 A°. The space covered by the polyribosome is nearly the same which is needed for mRNA strand in the synthesis of haemoglobin in reticuloytes.

POLYRIBOSOME CYCLE AND ASSOCIATION AND DISSOCIATION OF SUBUNITS

Few years ago it was thought that the various molecules involved in the protein synthesis were bound on the complete ribosome. However, *Mangiarotti and Sclessinger* (1966) have shown that the two sub-units of the ribosome may exist freely and that they associate during the protein synthesis and may dissociate again at the end of the process. *Kalmpfer* (1965) and his associates have shown the essential features of ribosomal cycle as indicated in the figure 3.2.

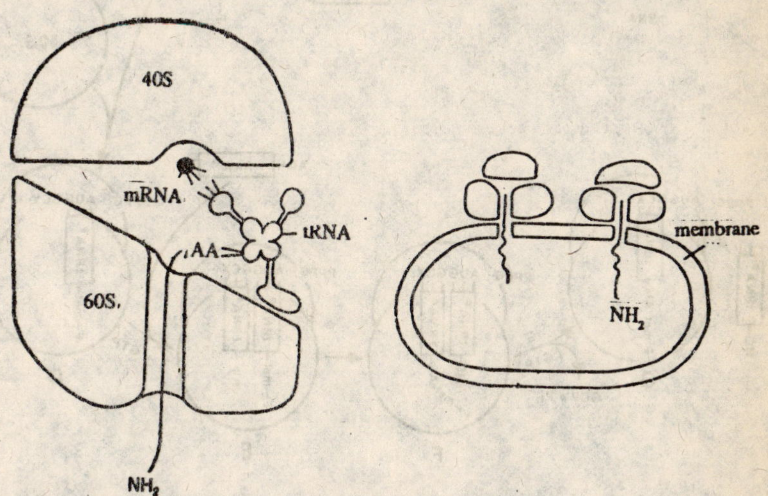

Fig. 3.2. Diagram of ribosome showing the two sub-units and the probable position of mRNA and tRNA.

In this figure, the two different subunits (30 S and 50S in *E. coli* or 40S and 60S in reticulocytes enter in the process at the initiator end and separate at the terminator end after the completion of the cycle. Thus, according to this concept the subunits of different ribosomes could be exchanged during the ribosomal cycle.

The factors which are responsible for the initiation of the 30S particles in the ribosomal cycle, are identified as F1, F2, F3 + ATP. The separation factor is, however, tentatively identified as F2 (*Liptmann*, 1969).

ROLE OF SUBUNITS IN PROTEIN SYNTHESIS

These subunits (30S and 50S or 40S and 60S) perform different types of functions in the process of protein synthesis In *E. coli*,

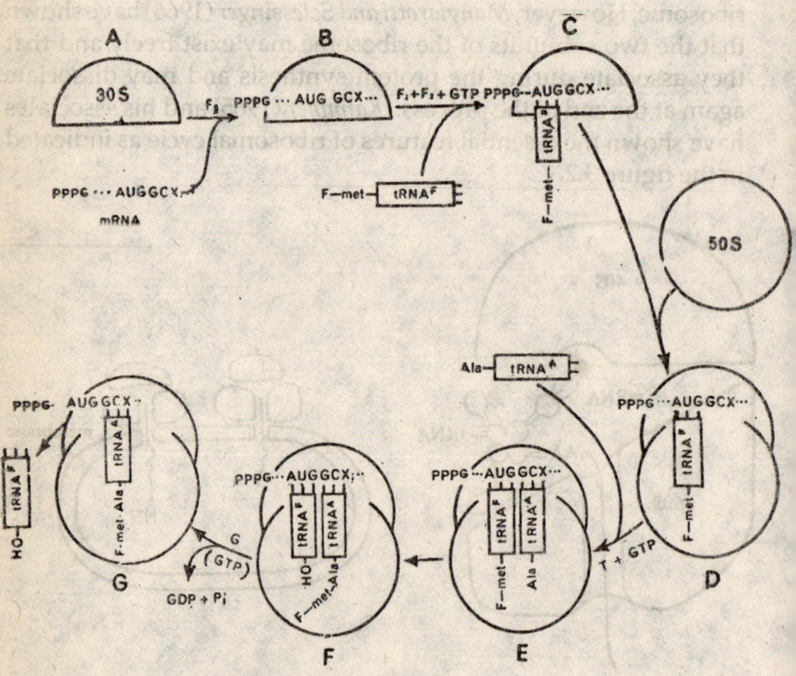

Fig. 3.3. General diagram of the initiation steps in protein synthesis.

mRNA binds to the 30S subunit for the reading of genetic message. In first step small 30S sub-unit binds with the first codon of the mRNA to form the so called initiator complex (*Nomura* and *Lowry*, 1967). The successive steps would be the binding of the first amino acyl-tRNA and then the coupling of the other subunit (50S) as shown in the figure 3.3.

In *E.coli* it has been demonstrated that the first aminoacyl tRNA which initiates the synthesis of protein is quite specific because it contains a formyl (-CHO) derivative of methionine which is coded by AUG codon. This codon is always present at the beginning of all the mRNA molecules. In the protein synthesis the peptide chain always grows from the free terminal end of -NH_2 group towards the-COOH end. Therefore, the function of formyl methionine-tRNA (F-met-tRNA of the figure) is to ensure that proteins are synthesized in that direction. In F-met-tRNA, the NH_2 group is blocked by the formyl group leaving only the -COOH available to react with the -NH_2 of the second amino acid. Thus, in this way the synthesis follows in only correct direction and sequence.

The 50S subunit contains the enzyme peptidyl transferase or peptide synthetase, which is essential in the formation of peptide bond (*Haenni*, 1969). The other function of the 50S subunit is to provide two binding sites for the two tRNA molecules. These two sites should be next to each other in order to permit the formation of the peptide bond. However, it is possible to envision process of protein synthesis as a continual entrance of aminoacyl tRNA on 30S unit of the ribosome and exist of the tRNA molecules from the 50S sub unit after giving after aminoacids to the developing polypeptide chain.

MECHANISM OF PROTEIN SYNTHESIS

The mechanism of protein synthesis has been investigated most thoroughly in bacteria (usually *E. coli*), therefore, the process of protein synthesis of *E. coli* which contains 70S ribosomes will be described in more detail and then this will be discussed in relation to our present knowledge of protein synthesis on 80S ribosomes of plants and animals.

Protein synthesis consist of two main events :

(I) Transcription
(II) Translation

(I) Transcription. The formation of m-RNA is called transcription. During the process an enzyme-RNA polymerase is needed. The enzyme is then attached to the DNA at the initiation site, where a short segment of the DNA molecule is opened up. The complementary nucleotides developed from one of the DNA strands, form m-RNA. The RNA polymerase moves along the DNA strands, and the growing m-RNA strand is peeled off till a termination site is reached.

The enzyme RNA polymerase consists of five different polypeptide chains, of which four collectively form the core enzyme while the fifth is called the sigma σ chain. They are given below.

(1) Core enzyme.
 (a) β^1 having mol. weight 1,60,000.
 (b) β having mol. weight 1,50,000.
 (c) α having mol. weight 40,000.
 (d) α having mol. weight 10,000.

(2) Sigma factor (σ) having mol. wt. 90,000.

The sigma chain recognizes start signals along the DNA molecules. A specific protein called the rho (ρ) factor (mol. wt. 60,000) stops the formation of the RNA chain. Once RNA synthesis is initiated, the sigma factor dissociated and core enzymes bring about elongation of mRNA.

The mRNA makes its way through the pores in the nuclear membrane to the cytoplasm to start the next stage which is translation.

(II) Translation. It involves the translation of the language of DNA into the language of protein i.e. the formation of protein takes place under the control of mRNA. This process can be studied under the following heads:

(1) Activation of Amino acids. The first step in protein synthesis is the activation of amino acids with ATP (Adenosine triphosphate). The reaction is catalysed by a specific enzyme *amino acyl synthetase* and by this the first product is formed which is the amino acid adenylate in which the energy is consumed for the requirement of the next step. The reaction can be shown by equation as follow:

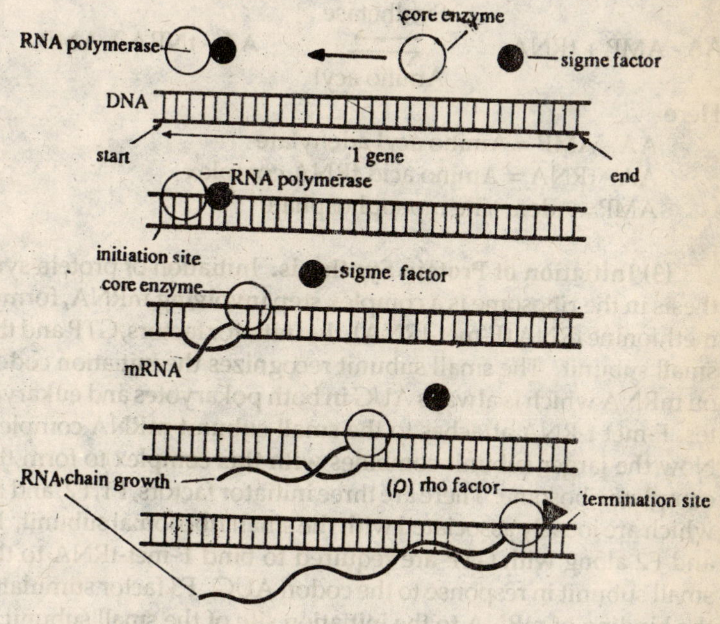

Fig. 3.4. Showing transcription

Amino acid + ATP + Amino acyl synthetase ——>
Enzyme bound amino acid adenylate + 2P.

or

$$AA + ATP \underset{\text{Synthetase}}{\overset{\text{Amino acyl}}{\rightleftharpoons}} AA - AMP + 2P$$

(2) Attachment of Activated Amino Acid with tRNA. Here in this step the activated amino acids are attached with the tRNA. The adenylate remains bounded to the enzyme until it is transformed to the tRNA and this transfer is again catalysed by the same enzyme. The link formed between the amino acid and tRNA is a covalent bond between the carboxyl group of the amino acid and the ribose of the terminal adenine nucleotide of tRNA. The reaction is as shown below:

$$\text{AA - AMP + tRNA} \underset{\text{Amino acyl}}{\overset{\text{Synthetase}}{\rightleftharpoons}} \text{AA - tNRA + AMP}$$

Here

AA - AMP = Amino acyl adenylate
AA - tRNA = Amino acid tRNA complex
AMP= Adenosine monophosphate

(3) Initiation of Protein Synthesis. Initiation of protein synthesis in the ribosome is a complex step involving mRNA, formyl methionine tRNA (F-met-tRNA), the initiator factors, GTP and the small subunit. The small subunit recognizes the initiation codon on mRNA which is always AUG in both pokaryotes and eukaryotes. F-met t-RNA attaches to the small subunit-mRNA complex. Now the larger subunit combines with this complex to form the complete ribosome. There are three initiator factors, F1, F2, and F3 which are loosely associated with the small ribosomal subunit. F1 and F2 along with GTP are required to bind F-met-tRNA to the small subunit in response to the codon AUG. F3 factor stimulates the binding of mRNA to the initiation site of the small subunit.

In eukaryotes, met-t-RNA is involved instead F-met-tRNA. Secondly in them the initiation factors are M1, M2 and M3 which are homologous to F1, F2, and F3 of prokaryotes.

(4) Chain Elongation. It involves the following four sub phases :

(i) Elongation factors. Elongation of the polypeptide chain requires elongation factors (EF). These are EF-Tu, EF-Ts and Ef-G in prokaryotes and EF-1 and dEF-2 in eukaryotes.

(ii) Binding of aminoacyl-tRNA to the A site. The second amino acid-tRNA complex (ala-tRNA) now occupies the acceptor site (A site) of the 50S subunit of the ribosome.

(iii) Peptide Bond Formation. The next step include the formation of a peptide bond between the amino acid and the growing polypeptide of F-met-tRNA, if the initiation has just been completed. The polypeptide chain is transferred from its position at he P site to the aminoacyl tRNA, located at the A site.

In the reaction, the polypeptide is first cleaved from the tRNA at the P site and becomes attached to the aminoacyl-tRNA at the A site. In the process, the bond formation is mediated by an enzyme *peptidyl transferase* which is located in the 50S subunit between P and A sites. GTP is hydrolyzed to GDP + inorganic phosphate. The energy released during hydrolysis may have a warping effect on the ribosome so that peptidyl-tRNA can be aligned for bond formation between the polypeptide and the amino acid (*Kurland*, 1972).

(iv) *Translocation of Polypeptide.* The next step comprise the discharge of unloaded tRNA from the P site. This translocation of the polypeptide from the A site to the P site requires the supernatant G factor, which is a ribosome-dependent GTPase. GTP is also required. As translocation occurs, the peptidyl-tRNA is moved from the A site to the P site, and the mRNA moves one codon. The uncharged tRNA from the P site is discharged. The role played by the G factor is that by reacting with GTP to produce energy which might be converted to mechanical energy, resulting in translocation and movement of mRNA.

(5) Chain termination. The polypeptide chain elongates, until a termination codon on mRNA is reached. This may be UAA, UAG or UGA. The termination codon provides signals to the ribosomes for the attachment of release factors. In prokaryotes there are three release factors, RF-1, RF-2, and RF-3. RF-1 recognizes the termination codons UAA and UAG. RF-2 recognizes UAA and UGA. RF-3 (stimulatory factor) stimulates the binding and release of RF-1 and RF-2 from the ribosome. In eukaryotes a single release factor (RF) recognizes all three termination codons.

The release factors interact with peptidyl transferase, and cause hydrolysis of the polypeptide chain at the site thus the chain is released from the tRNA molecule. The residual tRNA is discharged from the P site. The ribosome dissociates into 30S and 50S subunits. The polypeptide chain may undergo further processing, like cleavage of the formyl residue and internal cleavage. Secretory polypeptide pass through a tunnel between the two ribosomal subunits into the endoplasmic cisterna. Structural proteins are incorporated into the cell membrane.

Inhibitor of Protein Synthesis. Antibiotic, *chloramphenicol,* have long been known to be the inhibitor of protein synthesis. They appear to function in the transfer reaction at the step of peptide-bond synthesis. Attachment of mRNA to ribosomes seems to occur normally, synthesis seldom proceeds past the di- or tripeptide stage. The inhibitor is probably bound to a specific site on the ribosomes. The another important inhibitor of protein synthesis, is *cycloheximide* not effective in bacteria but seems to function in mammals and further in a similar way as does chloramphenicol.

4

REGULATION OF GENE ACTION OR PROTEIN SYNTHESIS

Genes are arranged in a linear fashion on the chromosomes. The number of genes present on a single chromosome varies from 1000-10,000 depending upon the size of the chromosome. In human being there are 90,000 functional genes. But all genes do not become functional in every cell of the body. Some genes function in one type of cells while some others in other type of cells. This regulation of genes was best described in certain microorganisms such as *Escherichia coli* and in certain higher organisms. *Jacob* and *Monod* proposed *Operon* to explain this sort of gene regulation. Genes show their activities by synthesizing their related proteins. Thus the regulation of gene action or protein synthesis is one and the same thing. The entire mechanism can be studied at three stages.

(i) transcription stage
(ii) translation stage
(iii) at the release of polypeptide chain.

Certain enzymes are produced continuously by an organism regardless of the presence or absence of its substrate in the environment. Such enzymes are called constitutive enzymes and they require no regulation. The constitutive enzymes are generally those that are needed at all times. Thus the enzymes involved with glucose metabolism-enzymes of glycolysis and the hexose monophosphate pathway-are constitutive, and one can imagine that the metabolism of glucose is sufficiently central to the physiology of *E. coli* that these pathways should be continuously functional.

There are certain enzymes which are synthesized in certain specific conditions and require one or other type of gene regulation. For example, the metabolism of less common sugars such as lactose, arabinose, and galactose, is effected by *regulated enzymes*, and it is clearly economical to elaborate such enzymes only on those occasions when their substrates are present. Regulated genes also specify enzymes of most biosynthetic pathways-pathways for the synthesis of amino acids, purines, pyrimidines, and so on-and these enzymes are synthesized according to the demand for their biosynthetic products.

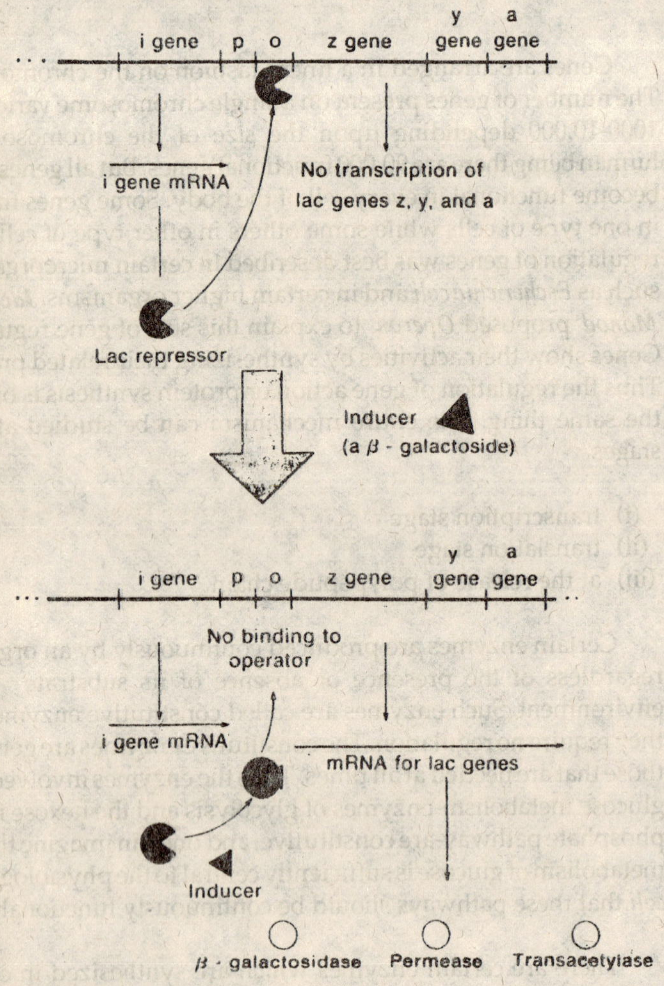

Fig. 4.1. The Jacob-Monod model for the product repression.

Induction & Repression : The substrate whose addition induces the synthesis of an enzyme is called inducer. THe phenomenon involved in the production of new enzyme in the presence of inducer is called induction. For example in ***E. coli*** b galactosidase enzyme hydrolysis the lactose into glucose and galactose. A bacterial culture of ***E-coli*** growing in a medium with glucose produces only minute quantities of the enzyme b galactosidase. On adding inducer (lactose), the production b galactosidase is, however, increased as much as 10,000 times and can easily be detected. The formation of b galactosidase can be slowed down quickly if the lactose is removed. Such an enzyme is called an inducible as adaptive enzyme because its synthesis is induced by the inducer which is lactose in this case. Reverse activities have also been observed in *E. coli.* The amino acid histidine is synthesized from carbohydrate precursors in a culture of bacteria. All enzymes necessary for the synthesis of histidine are produced. If, however, histidine is added to the medium, synthesis of histidine stops. Such enzymes whose synthesis can be checked up by adding repressor are known as repressible enzymes. This phenomenon is called the feedback mechanism

OPERON HYPOTHESIS

Jacob and *Monod* in 1961 forwarded a hypothesis called *Operon hypothesis* to explain the regulating mechanism of expressions of regulated genes at transcriptional level. They analysed the genetic basis for induction and repressions. The hypothesis has the following components.

STRUCTURAL GENES

The structural genes direct the synthesis of cellular proteins though messenger RNA (mRNA) and determine the sequence of amino acids in the proteins synthesized. There are as many structural genes in an operon as there are proteins or polypeptides under common control. Each structural gene may be controlled independently and transcribes a separate mRNA molecule, or all the strucutural genes of an operon may form one long polycistronic or polygenic mRNA molecule. Polygenic RNAs are common in bacteria and bacteriophages. All known eukaryotes, however, contain only a single functional site for initiating protein synthesis.

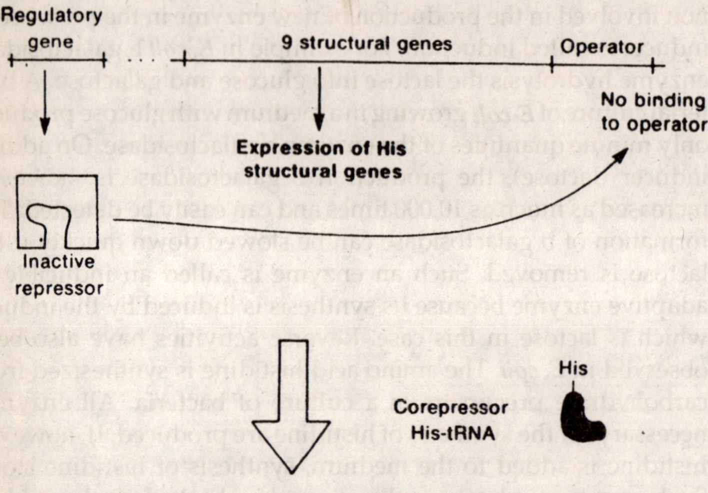

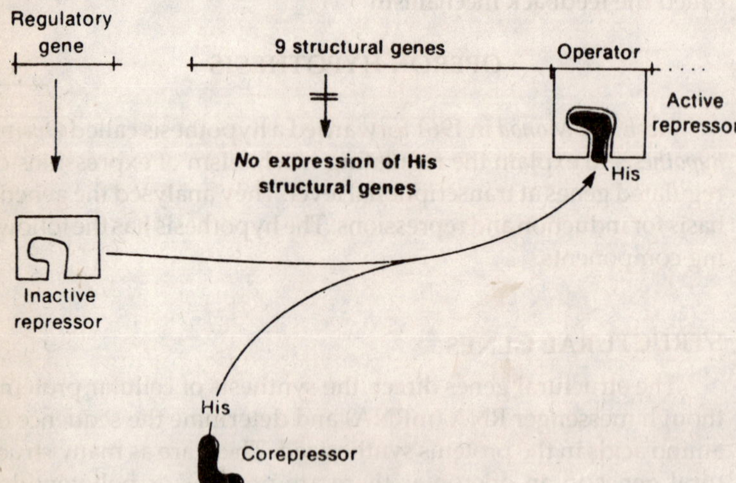

Fig. 4.2. Repression of gene expression in the histidine operon of salmonella typhimurium.

The lactose (lac) operon of the bacterium *Escherichia coli* has been particularly well studied. It is a small segment of a circular

DNA molecule which constitutes most of the genetic material of the bacterium. It has three structural genes, z., y and a which transcribe one long polycistronic RNA molecule. This controls the synthesis of three different proteins (enzymes), B galactosidase, galactoside permease and galactoside transacetylase. These consist of 4, 1 and 2 units, respectively. B galactosidase is the enzyme that splits lactose into glucose and galactose. Galactoside permease facilitates the entry of lactose into the cell. Galactoside transacetylase appears in small quantities upon lactose induction. The initiation codon of structural gene z is TAC (corresponding to AUG of mRNA). It is located 10 base pairs away from the end of the operator gene.

OPERATOR GENE

An operator gene present adjacent to the structural gene and represents a sequence of bases that interacts with a protein. The protein is also called a regulator molecule, and operator-regulator interaction will either prevent or promote transcription of the regulated gene, depending on which operator is being considered. The major distinction between an operator and promotor is that the operator is not normally the site of attachment of RNA polymerase. Instead, it ordinarily lies between the promotor and the beginning of a regulated gene of an operon and thus it comes to influence whether a polymerase is able to progress from its attachment site to the gene itself.

PROMOTOR GENE

While operator is the site of action of repressor, the actual site of transcription initiation is different and is known as promotor gene, which lies to the left of operator gene. It is also believed, therefore, that perhaps RNA polymerase, binds to and moves from the promotor site. The repressor, when attached to operator prevents the movement of RNA polymerase. The presence of the promotor gene was inferred from the mutations at this locus, which were found affect the maximum rate of transcription.

In the recent years, promotor region has been studied in some detail and three sites are proposed (a) catabolite gene activator site

(Cga), (b) initial binding site (ibs) and (c) operator gene (op). It is obvious that operator gene makes a part of promotor region.

Two proteins are known to be involved in the regulation of lactose operon, (i) lac repressor,(ii) catabolite gene activator protein (Cga protein).

While repressor binds to operator site, Cga protein binds to Ca site. Moreover, repressor excercise positive control by checking RNA polymerase to travel through operator. Ca protein exercises positive control. Only when cyclic AMP molecule activates Cga protein, the latter will allow RNA polymerase to bind.

REGULATOR GENE

The activity and working of operator gene depends on the activity of another gene called regulator gene. The regulator gene produces a substance called *repressor substance*. The repressor is an allosteric protein which has affinity of binding with DNA. This substance control the switching on and switching off the operator gene. The activity of this substance in turn depends on the presence orabsence of lactose substrate on which B galactosidase enzyme acts. In the absence of lactose the repressor substance binds with DNA of operator gene thus blocking its transcription to m-RNA. Since no m-RNA is produced, no enzyme is synthesized. In the presence of lactose the repressor binds to the lactose, thus it does not remain free to block the operator gene, which in turn helps in transcribing of m-RNA by structural genes and thus enzymes are synthesized. One regulator gene may control several operons and several regulator genes may control only one operon. This system of regulation and operation is called a ***Regular***.

FEEDBACK INHIBITION

In some cases, the end product of a particular biosynthetic pathway gets accumulated if not utilized. Sometimes such an accumulation may stop further synthesis of this substance. For instance, if *E. coli* cells growing normally are supplied with the amino acid isoleucine, it blocks the activity of the enzyme involved in the first step. This inhibition is due to binding of isoleucine to the enzyme threonine deaminase.

This mechanism of the regulation of enzyme activity is known as feedback inhibition. If the first enzyme is blocked in this case., it may not be necessary to check the other intermediate enzymes, since there will be no accumulation of intermediate products.

The end product in this case perhaps act through allosteric transformation of the enzyme as a result of which the site of activity of the enzyme gets transformed in such a way that it can not perform its catalytic function. This would mean that in feedback inhibition the enzyme does not function, while in repression no mRNA synthesis and hence no enzyme synthesis take place.

Regulation by Cyclic AMP

Lac operon in the case of E.coli has also been found to be regulated by cyclic AMP. Cyclic AMP (cAMP) has been found activating and deactivating the inducible operons at the level of the promotor. Cyclic AMP interact with cyclic receptor protein (CRP) forming the CRP + cAMP complex which binds to the promotor, allowing the RNA polymerase to recognize the promotor, thus enhancing the transcription of the inducible operon. When cAMP levels is low, as in glucose-grown cultures of *E. coli*, the cAMP + CRP will not bind to the promotor of the lac operon consequently protein syntheis will not be "switched on." This can be reversed upon addition of exogenous cAMP in the case of bacterium.

5

GENETIC CODE

Genetic code is a sort of relationship between the nucleotide sequence in mRNA and amino acid sequence in protein molecule. The word "code" has several meanings. Out of them one is "a system of signals communicating". A pertinent example is the Morse code. In this chapter too we are dealing with the code, for messenger RNA having a means for communicating message that directs the combination of amino acids in a specific sequence. *George Gamow* first proposed the coding scheme in 1954.

Several theories were proposed to explain the mechanism by which a particular sequence of nitrogenous bases in DNA by transcribing complementary bases in mRNA determines the position of specific amino acid in the protein molecule. The theory which is widely accepted till now was proposed by *F.H.C. Crick.* The theory holds the existence of a genetic code and its smallest unit which codes for one amino acid is known as *codon.* Thus we see that the code in DNA is copied in the form of mRNA. But since little was known about the base sequences in DNA, the genetic code seemed a remote goal never to be attained. But in few years the genetic code become known as a result of ingenious experimentation mainly in the laboratories of *M.W. Nirenberg, S. Ochoa* and *H.G. Khorana.*

THE GENETIC CODE IS A TRIPLET CODE

DNA contains four kinds of nucleotides (of A, T, G and C), and proteins are synthesized from 20 different types of amino acids. A basic problem regarding the genetic code was: how many bases of DNA specify one amino acid? In a *singlet code* each base or letter would specify one amino acid. Only 4 of the 20 types of amino acids would be coded unambiguously by a *singlet code.* In a two-letter or *doublet code* two bases would specify one amino acid. Here 16 (4 x 4) of the 20 amino

A
G
C
T

singlet code

AA	AG	AC	AT
GA	GG	GC	GT
CA	CG	CC	CT
TA	TG	TC	TT

doublet code

AAA	GAA	CAA	TAA
AAG	GAG	CAG	TAG
AAC	GAC	CAC	TAC
AAT	GAT	CAT	TAT
AGA	GGA	CGA	TGA
AGG	GGG	CGG	TGG
AGC	GGC	CGC	TGC
AGT	GGT	GGT	TGT
ACA	GCA	CCA	TCA
ACG	GCG	CCG	TCG
ACC	GCC	CCC	TCC
ACT	GCT	CCT	TCT
ATA	GTA	CTA	TTA
ATG	GTG	CTG	TTG
ATC	GTC	CTC	TTC
ATT	GTT	CTT	TTT

triplet code

Fig. 5.1. Singlet code, a doublet and a triplet code.

acids can be specified, but there would be ambiguous determination of a number of amino acids. A *triplet* or three-letters code was first suggested by the physicist *Gamow* in 1954. According to the triplet code three letters or bases specify one amino acid. Thus 64 (4 x 4 x 4) distinct triplets of purine and/or pyrimidine bases determine the 20 amino acids. These triplets have been called *codons.* Since there are 64 codons and only 20 amino acids it is obvious that there are many more codons than there are amino acids, i.e. the code is degenerate. Experimental evidence shows that the code is a triplet one and that 61 of the 64 codons code for individual amino acids during protein synthesis.

PROPERTIES OF GENETIC CODE

Following properties of the genetic code have been studied and proved experimentally.

(i) Genetic code is non overlapping : When *Gamow* first proposed the genetic code, he had suggested it to be an overlapping code. No doubt *Crick* had suggested a non overlapping code but the direct experimental evidence for a non-overlapping triplet code was given by *Khorana* and his coworkers in 1965.

On the surface, it appears wasteful for 64 triplets to stand for 20 amino acid, so attempts were made to hypothesize a triplet code in which the code was overlapping and so to reduce the number of codons to about 20. But a lot of shortcomings are there in this proposal. Let us examine the case of lysine, whose codons appear to be AGG and AAA, and that of phenylalanine, whose codons appear to be UUU and UUC since the code letter of these two amino acids ar mutually exclusive, lysine could not follow phenylalanine, or *vice versa,* in any protein; this would constitute a forbidden combinations of amino acids in proteins. Any two or three or so on amino acids combinations are possible. Therefore it can be concluded that the genetic code is non overlapping.

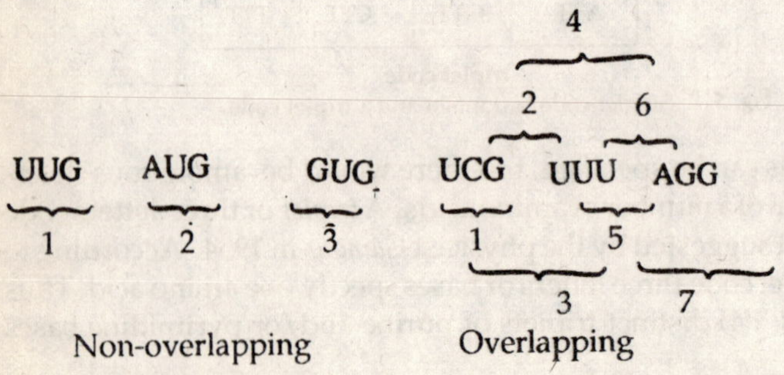

(ii) Genetic code is degenerate : The code contains many synonyms, in that almost all amino acids are represented by more than one codon. For example, the three amino acids-arginine, serine and leucine- each has six synonymous codons. However, for many of the synonym codons specifying the same amino acid the first two bases of the triplet are constant, whereas the third can vary; for example, all codons starting with CC specify proline (CCU, CCC, CCA and CCG) and all codons starting with AC specify threonine. This flexibility in the third nucleotide of a codon may well help to minimize the consequences of errors.

(iii) The Genetic code is commaless : A commaless code means that no punctuations are needed between any two words. in other words, we can say that after one amino acid is coded, the second amino acid will be automatically coded by the next three letters and that no letters are wasted for telling that one amino acid has been coded and that now second should be coded.

(iv) Universality of the Code : The code is based on work on the bacterium *E. coli* but it is valid for other organisms. This important characteristic of the genetic code is called its *universality.* Consider any codon that codes for the same amino acid from the smallest organism to the largest, plant or animal. Thus, UUU codes for phenylalanine and GUC for valine in all living organisms, from *Amoeba* to ape, bacteria to the banyan tree and from cabbage to kings. The genetic code which was first developed in the bacteria about 3 billion (300 crore) years ago has not undergone any change and has been preserved in its almost original form in the course of evolution. In other words, the code is a conservative one.

The best evidence for the universality of the code comes from studies in which amino acid-charged tRNA from *E.coli* was placed with mRNA and ribosomes derived from rabbit reticulocytes. The result was the production of rabbit haemoglobin. Obviously, the bacterial tRNA was able to recognize perfectly the mammalian mRNA for haemoglobin and could work perfectly with mammalian ribosomes. Studies on amino acid sequence of homologous proteins from widely divergent and unrelated species (cytochrome C from man, chicken, several bacteria and yeast etc.) show great uniformity although genetic divergence took place hundreds of millions of years ago. Similarly, studies with synthetic messenger RNAs and binding studies with tRNAs also point towards a universal code, though slight variations occasionally occur. Organisms with high G/C content in the DNA appear geared for more common reading of codons ending in C or G. Their proteins also are relatively rich in amino acids coded by G- and C- rich codons, for example Ala, Arg and Gly and relatively poor in Ile, Lys, Phe and Tyr (see codon table). Certain mutant microorganisms show exceptions to the absolute universality of the code. There are mutants that have acquired ability to read nonsense triplets. However, this accessory ability is only partial and nonsense triplets are nonsense much of the time. Some natural differences may exist among organisms. Initiation of polypeptide chains is encoded differently in bacteria and their bacteriophages (viruses) as compared to higher organisms. Thus, tRNA for cysteine binds well with mRNA triplet UGA (nonsense in bacteria). Biological significance of these observations remains to be seen as there is more to biology than the 64 triplets.

(v) The code has polarity : If a gene is to specify the same protein repeatedly it is essential that the code must be read between fixed start and end points. These points are the initiation and the termination codons, respectively. It is also essential that the code must be read in a fixed direction. In other words the code must have polarity. It is obvious that if the code is read in opposite directions it would specify two different proteins, since the codons would have reversed base sequences.

For example :

	Leu	Ile	Val	Ser ——>
Codon	UUG	AUC	GUC	UCG
<——	Val	Leu	Leu	Ala.

(VI) Initiation codons : The starting amino acid in the synthesis of most protein chains is methionine (eukaryotes) or *N-formyl methionine* (prokaryotes). *Methionyl* or *N-formyl methionine*-RNA specifically binds to initiation sites containing the AUG codon. This codon is therefore called the *initiation codon.* Less often, GUG also serves as the initiation codon in bacterial protein synthesis.

(VII) Non-sense codons. The UAA (also called *ochre*), UAG (also called *amber* because an investigator who studied the properties of this codon belonged to the Bernstein family, and Bernstein means "amber" in German) and UDA codons do not specify any amino acid so, are called *non-sense codons.* They are also called *termination codons*, because, these codons are used by the cell to signal the natural end to translation of a particular polypetide. However, their inclusion in any mRNA results in the abrupt termination of the message of the point of their location even though the polypeptide chain has not been completed.

DECIPHERING OR CRACKING OF GENETIC CODE

Deciphering the Genetic Code : We may here briefly describe the techniques which ultimately resulted in determining the code words for each of the 20 proteinogenic amino acids. Most of our current knowledge of the general nature of the genetic code and of the nucleotide composition and sequences of the various codons has been obtained from the following five main types of experimental approaches.

(1) *The first method* is analysis of the primary structures of the wild type and mutant proteins. In each of the mutant proteins so far analysed a mutant amino acid replaces a particular wild type amino acid. But the data so far accumulated on such amino acid replacements is very meagre and sets restrictions on the genetic code.

(2) *The second method* for establishing the genetic code consists of determining the sequence of nucleotides in the mRNA and also of amino acids in the protein molecules synthesized under its influence. The sequence analysis for proteins is now a standard biochemical technique but unfortunately the determination of the base sequence of large nucleic acid molecules (like mRNA) is yet to be achieved. Biochemists, therefore, adopted indirect methods to crack the genetic code. A cell-free amino acid incorporating system and the polymerising enzyme were known which could polymerise single mononucleoside triphosphates or their mix-

tures to produce long nucleotide chains of randon base sequence. Initial break-through in this direction was achieved by *Nirenberg* and *Mathei* (1961) who adopted the following technique. Using the enzyme *polynucleotide phosphorylase* they prepared a synthetic polyribouncleotide containing only one kind of base and added it to a cell-free amino acid-incorporating system from *E.coli.* In this way they prepared, for example, a poly uracil (UUU...UUU) to which they added different amino acids labelled with C^{14}. They found that this poly-U system specifically stimulated the formation of a polypeptide which contained only the amino acid phenylalanine. The conclusion was drawn that the code word for the amino acid phenylalanine was a sequence of three uracil nucleotides (UUU) in mRNA. This was the first demonstration that synthetic polyribonucleotides could act as a messenger for polypeptide synthesis. Later on, *Nirenberg* and *Ochoa* became deeply involved in this problem. They prepared poly-G, poly-C and poly-A polynucleotides from the riboside diphosphates GDP, CDP, and ADP, and employing the same technique. They observed that these homoribonucleosides stimulated the incorporation of amino acids glycine, prolin and lysine to the corresponding homopeptides respectively. *Crick* had already shown that the code was triplet in nature. It was, therefore, concluded that the base triplets GGG, CCC and AAA coded respectively for the amino acids glycine, proline and lysine.

Later on, mixtures of two or more ribonucleoside diphosphates were used by *Nirenberg* and with the help of the enzyme mentioned above polyribonucleotides were prepared. Thus, using UDP and CDP in the ratio of 3:1, he obtained a polynucleotide which contained the following triplets in the descending order of frequency: UUU, UUC, UCU and CUU. The triplets containing 2Cs and 1U were the least frequent. With such a poly-UC system *Nirenberg* obtained a poly-peptide containing the amino acids phenyalanine and serine in the ratio 3:1. He concluded that the code word for serine contains 2Us and 1C. This method, however, did not give the exact sequence of the three bases. *Ochoa* also used this technique and determined the code words for most of the amino acids. The exact sequence of the three bases for any amino acid was not known because all these polynucleotides had random base sequence. The assigning of the exact triplet for every amino acid was not possible at this stage.

(3) *The Third method.* The determination of the exact base sequence of mRNA triplets which coded for each amino acid was made possible by a later discovery of *Nirenberg* that each trinucleotide (triplet) caused a specific aminoacyl- tRNA to bind to the ribosome and to the specific base sequence of synthetic mRNA. With the help of this elegant technique and using trinucleotides of known sequences, *Nirenberg* and *Lader* (1965) observed that aminoacyl-tRNA could be bound to ribosomes in the presence of specific trinucleotide phosphates (triplet). In the absence of a specific triplet the animo acyl-tRNA could not bind to the ribosome and therefore, passed through the nitrocellulose filter while the tertiary complex containing amino acyl-tRNA-ribosome-mRNA was retained on the filter. Using this technique, *Nirenberg* and his associates tested 64 triplets for binding of the 20 amino acyl-tRNA's. They succeded in assigning 50 out of the 64 codons with their exact base sequences with which each of the amino acyl-tRNAs formed a union. This method was based on the assumption that binding required the same code word as did protein synthesis. This method, however, did not prove to be very satisfactory as binding stimulations observed in a number of cases were very poor and artifactual. Moreover, several authentic codons did not bind the amino acyl-tRNA.

(4) *The fourth method — Khorana's direct method* of confirming the genetic code is the most direct method and was devised by the Nobel Prize winner *Dr. H.G. Khorana.* This method consists in *vitro* chemical synthesis of short segments of DNA of known base sequence with the help of *DNA polymerase.* From this synthetic DNA a polyribonucleotide (RNA) of strictly defined base sequence is transcribed under the catalytic influence of *RNA polymerase.* A polypeptide is then synthesized under the direction of RNA as represented in the following schematic diagram :

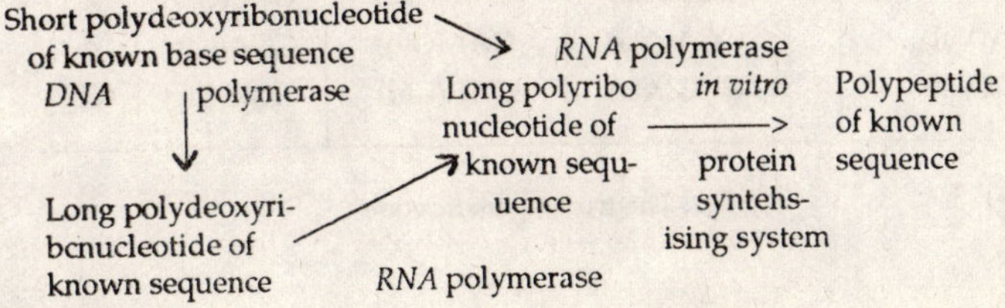

The amino acid sequence of the polypeptide so formed is then determined and correlated with the base sequence of DNA and RNA. These studies of *Khorana* and his co-workers with chemically defined messengers proved very conclusively that (1) the base sequence in DNA specifies the sequence of amino acids in proteins ; (2) the information contained in DNA is conveyed through RNA and (3) the genetic code is triplet and non-overlapping in nature. The results obtained from these polypeptide synthesis in combination with the results obtained from the binding technique of *Nirenberg* and coworkers led to the deciphering and establishment of the genetic code.

SECOND LETTER

FIRST LETTER	U	C	A	G	THIRD LETTER
	UUU(Phe)	UCU(Ser)	UAU(Tyr)	UGU(Cys)	U
	UUC(Phe)	UCC(Ser)	UAC(Tyr)	UGC(Cys)	C
U	UUA(Leu)	UCA(Ser)	UAA(Ochre)	UGA?	A
	UUG(Leu)	UCG(Ser)	UAG(Amber)	UGG(Tryp)	G
	CUU(Leu)	CCU(Pro)	CAU(His)	CGU(Arg)	
C	CUC(Leu)	CCC(Pro)	CAC(His)	CGC(Arg)	C
	CUA(Leu)	CCA(Pro)	CAA(GluN J	CGA(Arg)	A
	CUG(Leu)	CCG(Pro)	CAG(GluN)	CGG(Arg)	G
	AUU(Ileu)	ACU(Thr)	AAU(AspN)	AGU(Ser)	U
A	AUC(Ileu)	ACC(Thr)	AAC(AspN)	AGC(Ser)	C
	AUA(Heu)	ACA(Thr)	AAA(Lys)	AGA(Arg)	A
	AUG(Met)	ACG(Thr)	AAG(Lys)	AGG(Arg)	G
	GUU(Val)	GCU(Ala)	GAU(Asp)	GGU(Gly)	U
	GUC(Val)	GCC(Ala)	GAC(Asp)	GGC(Gly)	C
	GUA(Val)	GCA(Ala)	GAA(Glu)	GGA(Gly)	A
	GUG(Val)	GCG(Ala)	GAG(Glu)	GGG(Gly)	G

Fig. 5.2. The triplet genetic code

By this technique, *Khorana* not only worked out and confirmed the exact sequence of code words for all the amino acids but also clarified the roles of the 5' and 3' terminals of mRNA molecule. He showed that the translation of mRNA proceeded from its 5' hydroxyl end towards its 3' — hydroxyl end. His investigations also led to the artificial production of small segments of DNA molecule, thereby paving the way for the synthesis of artificial genes which could function in a living cell. In 1970, a Japanese student of *Khorana, Dr. Miss Otsuka,* succeeded in chemically linking six nucleotides by attaching an extra phosphoric acid artifically to a nucleotide in addition to the one it already had. By this process *Otsuka* and her coworkers at the Osaka University synthesized alanine tRNA. This synthetic RNA had exactly the same sequence of nucleotides as the one that occurs in natural cells. The same year *Dr. K.L. Agarwal*, another student of *Khorana*, succeeded in making an artificial gene. This gene, however, failed to function in a living cell because it did not possess the necessary "start" and "stop" signals for its functioning. He reported that enough advance had been made towards incorporating these control signals in a synthetic gene. It appears that scientists are very close to synthesizing artificial genes which, when introduced into a cell, could function like a natural gene and alter the heredity of the organism. This had opened the wide but virgin field of genetic engineering with the possibility of finding a cure for genetic disorders of metabolism and of producing organisms to precise specification by introducing artificial genes into the body. But this also carries the risk of artificial genes producing undersirable traits and monstrosities in the organisms in which they are introduced.

(5) Fifth Method. The fifth and final approach in this context involves inference from the results of purely genetical experiments. These included studies on mutant proteins due to the action of certain mutagens in reversing particular kinds of mutation ; others involve incorporating two or more mutations in the same DNA strand and observing the effect on the phenotype. Such observations give us confidence in the genetic code as deduced from in *vitro* experiments. Moreover, extraction of tRNAs from cells and studies of the nucleotide sequence found in certain regions of these isolated tRNAs all converge to give single, consistent picture of the code.

WOBBLE HYPOTHESIS

It is sometimes argued that the third base of a codon is not very important and that specificity of a codon is particularly determined by the first two bases. It has been shown, for instance that the same tRNA can recognize more than one codon differing only at the third position. This pairing is not very stable and is allowed due to wobbling in base pairing at the third position. *Crick*, in 1965 proposed a hypothesis called *Wobble hypothesis* to explain this phenomenon. He discovered that if U is present at first position of anticodon, it can pair with either A or G at the third position of codon. Similar is the case with U and I (Inosine, modified base in tRNA) found in anticodon. The pairing relationships between first base of anticodon and third base of codon are given in Table.

Table 5.1. Wobble pairing.

Anticodon (first base)	*Codon (third base)*
U	A,G
C	G
A	U
G	U,C
1 (Inosine, resembles G)	U,C,A

This kind of wobbling allows economy of the number of tRNA molecules, since several codons meant for same amino acid are recognized by same tRNA. For instance, anticodon IGC can recognize codons GCU, GCC and GCA (coding for alanine); IGA can recognize UCU, UUC and UCA (coding for serine) and IAC can recognize GUU, GUC and GUA (coding for valine).

CONTRIBUTION OF KHORANA

India born biochemist *Dr. Khorana* has devised an ingenious technique for artifically synthesizing mRNA with repeated sequences of known nucleotides. For this valuable contribution he was awarded Nobel Prize in 1970.

By using synthetic DNA, *Khorana* and his coworkers prepared chains of polyribonucleotides with known repeating sequences of two or three nucleotides as follows :

(i) Poly CUC UCU CUC UCU....
(ii) Poly CUA CUA CUA CUA...

In first case CUA and UCU are two codons arranged alternately in the polynucleotide chain. This dictates the formation of a polypeptide chain having two amino acids (leucine and serine) arranged alternatively. The second case is an example of *copolymers chains*. The polynucleotide chain is formed of repeated linkage of codon CUA. This dictates the formation of a polypeptide chain consisting of only one amino acid-leucine.

purines of known nucleotides. For this valuable contribution he was awarded Nobel Prize in 1970.

By using synthetic DNA, Khorana and his co-workers prepared chains of polyribonucleotides with known repeating sequences of two or three nucleotides as follows:

(i) Poly UCUCUCUCUCUCU...
(ii) Poly CUA CUA CUA CUA CUA...

In first case CUC and UCU are two codons arranged alternately in the polynucleotide chain. This dictates the formation of a polypeptide chain having two amino acids, leucine and serine arranged alternatively. The second one is an example of a homopolymer chain. The polynucleotide chain is formed by repeated linkage of codon CUA. This dictates the formation of a polypeptide chain consisting of only one amino acid leucine.

Evolution

1

ORIGIN OF LIFE

The origin of life on the earth has been the most attracting and complicated problem for the biologists. Different views have been put forwarded concerning the origin of life by biologists of different ages. Among these some theories are *mechanistic* based on the belief that life has arisen from inorganic substances controlled by some natural laws, other theories are *materialistic* based on the belief that life has arisen from organic compounds. The mechanistic theories are quite bizarre and mearly having a historical significance.

Some of the most important hypothesis and theories concerning the phenomenon of origin of life are as follow :

1. SPECIAL CREATION THEORY

One of the foremost advocates of the special doctrine during Christian times was *Father Suarez,* (1548-1617). According to him, "The world has made in Six natural days. On the first two days the *Media Prima* was made, out of nothing, to receive afterwards those *'substantial forms'* which moulded it into the universe of things. On the third day, the ancestors of all living plants came into beings, fully grown, perfect and possessed of all the properties which now distinguish them. On the fourth and fifth days, the ancestors of all existing animals, similarly, came into existence, in their complete and perfect state, by the infusion of their appropriate material substantial forms into the matter which has already been created. Finally on the sixth day, the *anima rationales*—that rational and immortal substantial form which is peculiar to man—was created out of nothing and 'breathed' into a mass of matter which till then was mere dust of the earth, and so arose the man. But the species man, was represented by a solitary male (*Adam*) individual until the creator took out one of his twelfth ribs and fashioned into a female".

This theory was believed until the 19th century but later it has been left out.

2. THEORY OF SPONTANEOUS GENERATION OR ABIOGENESIS

According to this theory, life has originated from non-living organic matter *abiogenetically* (*Gr. A.* not; *bios*, life; *genesis*, origin) from time to time. Greek philosophers of prechristian era, like *Thales, Anaximander, Anaximenes, Xenophanes, Empedocles, Plato, Aristotle* etc. are the followers of this theory.

According to *Epicurus* (342-271-B.C.) worms and numerous other animals were generated from the soil or manure by the action of moist warmth of sun and air. *Anaxagoras* (510-428 B.C.) thought that life come in tiny seeds (spermeia) with the rain water to fructifly the earth. According to *Aristotle* (384-322 B.C.) living creatures are born from like species no doubt, but they also arise spontaneously.

Thus, it was regarded a normal thing for worms, larvae of bees, wasps, mites, glow-worms and other insects to be formed from due, rotting dung and mud, from dry wood, from sweat from meat files, moths, butterflies, midges, dungbeetles, fleas, bugs and lice arise from field humus, from moulds and dung, from decaying wood and fruits, (impurities)) of vinegar and from old wool. *Aristotle* was of the opinion that not only insects and worms but also other highly organized creatures could be spontaneously formed, for example, crabs and various molluscs from foul earth and mud; eels and many other fish from the mud of lakes, from sand and from decaying water, plants; even frogs and salamanders could arise from moist earth.

Belief in abilogenesis was so strong that *Van Helmont* (1652) claimed the formation of mice in 21 days from dirty, sweat-soaked shirt put in wheat barn in the dark.

Till the middle of the 17th century, the theory of sontaneous generation was widely accepted. But later on several scholars viz., *Francesco Redi* in 17th century and *Abbe Spallanzani* in 18th century disproved the idea of spontaneous generation.

Redi (1621-1691) described a series of experiments in which he placed meat or fish (eel) under clean muslin coverings and demonstrated that while flies laid eggs on muslin, maggots or larvae appeared only when those eggs were transferred to the meat and allowed to hatch. He concluded that maggots come only from pre-existing flies and were not spontaneously generated by any other form of material. The discovery of micro-organisms by *Leeuwenhock* (1632-1723) brought the question into the forefront of biological thoughts once again.

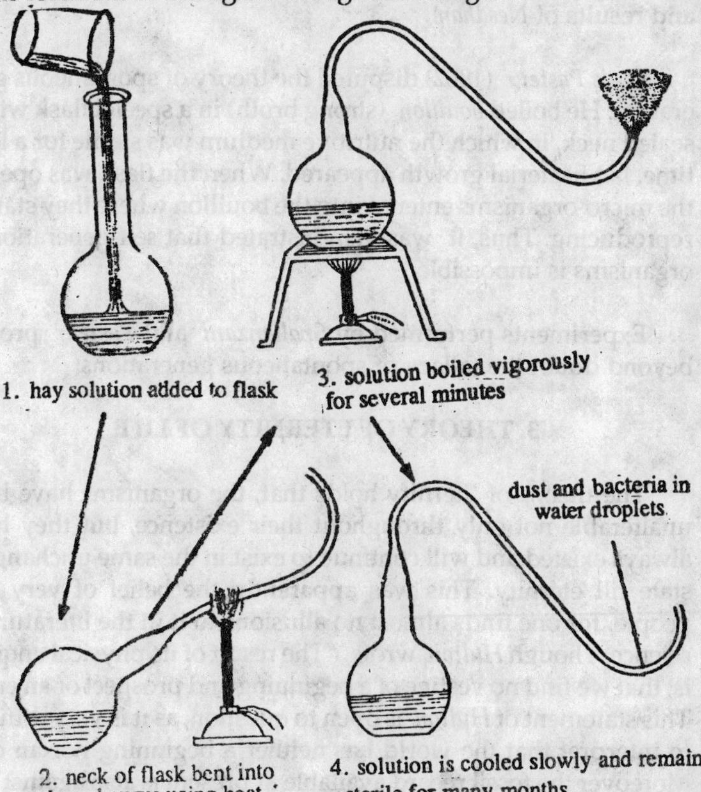

Fig. 1.1. Pasteur's experiment with bend-necked flask to disprove Theory of Spontaneous Generation.

Spallanzani (1729-1799) in his experiment sealed the necks of the flasks containing infusion so that even air could not enter inside after boiling the infusion for four hours. Some of the flasks kept open or loosely-corked. Micro-organisms appeared in those flasks which were open or loosely-corked while the sealed flasks remained sterile. According to him air carried microorganisms which germinate when get moisture and food. They were not formed abiogenetically.

In the beginning of the 17th century, spontaneous generation of more highly developed animals such as reptiles, insects, worms was proved to be impossible. *Needham* in 1745 described experiments in which sealed vessels having meat extracts were swarmed with micro-organisms. *Spallanzani* (1765) challenged the views and results of *Needham*.

Louis Pasteur (1862) disputed the theory of spontaneous generation. He boiled *bouillon* (strong broth) in a special flask with a sealed neck, in which the nutritive medium was sterile for a long time. No bacterial growth appeared. When the flask was opened the micro-organisms entered into the bouillon where they started reproducing. Thus, it was demonstrated that self-generation of organisms is impossible.

Experiments performed by *Spallanzani* and *Pasteur* proved beyond doubt the fallacy of spontaneous generations.

3. THEORY OF ETERNITY OF LIFE

The theory of Eternity holds that, the organisms have been unalterable not only throughout their existence, but they have always existed and will continue to exist in the same unchanging state till eternity. This was apparently the belief of very few people, for one finds almost no allusions to it in the literature of science. Though *Hulton* wrote, "The result of its physical enquiry is, that we find no vestige of a beginning and prospect of an end". This statement of *Hulton* is open to question, as it is very difficult to interpret that the world has neither a beginning nor an end. Moreover the fossil record available at present is also against this concept. This theory is supported by *Richter, Preyer, Helmholtz, Arrehenius, Hoyle, Bondi* etc.

4. COSMOZOIC THEORY OR THEORY OF PANSPERMIA

According to *Richter*, the protoplasm reached the earth in the form of spores or germ or other simple particle with cosmic dust from other planet.

Arrehenius proposed *cosmic panspermia theory*, according to him the life existed throughout the Universe and their spores etc. could freely travel through the space from one planet to other.

According to *Helmoholtz*, the life was brought on the earth with falling meteorites.

However this theory has been rejected due to two reasons. First, due to intense cold, extreme dryness and intense radiation of interstellar space. Even the most resistant living spores cannot withstand exposure to interstellar space. Moreover, this theory does not answer the basic question of 'origin of life' upon earth.

5. THEORY OF CATASTROPHISM

A number of biologists marked different degrees of resemblances in various types of animals and plants, showing certain relationship. This connection is evident by the fossil records. They did not accept the above theories and put forward a new idea. According to them the earth was periodically visited by catastrophes which destroyed all plants and animals from time to time and created new and special forms of lives. But this theory also has many drawbacks. A large number of fossils of plants and animals are known today. According to this theory the number of different types of fossils will correspond to the number of catastrophes which visited the earth. The number is remarkably high and appears to be impossible. *Cuvier* (1769-'83), "The father of Modern Paleontology", was the greatest advocate of this theory.

6. MODERN CONCEPTS ON THE ORIGIN OF LIFE OR CHEMICAL ORIGIN OF LIFE

Scientists are now of the opinion that spontaneous generation is not possible at present on Earth and that specific conditions are necessary for the appearance of life.

T.H. Huxley (1869) and *John Tyndall* (1874) asserted that life could be generated from inorganic chemicals. But their ideas were vague as the knowledge of biochemistry was not available at that time.

In 1920s, a new interest in the origin of life arose from independent speculation of two biologists, *A.I. Oparin* and *J.B.S. Haldane.* Both these scientists got the ideas from the new biochemistry that was founded by *Sir F.G. Hopkins.* They were of the opinion that the evolution is purely chemical—the gradual transmutation of inorganic compounds into organic ones.

After 1920s, the subject of the origin of life attracted ever increasing interest, *Pirie* coined the term *Biopoiesis* for the study of the origin of life.

Oparin first of all gave the scientific account of the origin of life in his book entitled. *"The Origin of Life"*, which was published in 1936. His main postulates were as follows :

(a) Origin of earth

The earth is presumed to have originated about 5-6 billion years ago. There are two hypothesis for its origin (i) *Planetesimal hypothesis* believes that earth is originated as a part broken off from the molten mass of sun. (ii) *Nebular hypothesis.* According to this hypothesis the earth is originated by gradual condensation of interstellar dust from which entire solar system is supposed to be formed. At that time temperature was extremely high which served as basis of primary origin of organic compound on the earth.

(b) Presence of elements on earth

In the beginning, the earth was fiery spinning ball of hot gases and vapours of elements. Gradually, through hundreds of millions of years, the gases condensed into a molten core and different elements got stratified according to their density. The original temperature of the earth was very high, about 5000-

6000°C. Due to this high temperature carbon elements existed in major forms, dicarbon (C_2), cynogen (CN), methane (CH_4), metal carbides, carbon dioxide etc. Oxygen was not existed in free state but oxides of aluminium, boron, hydrogen etc. were present. Nitrogen existed in combination with metals to form nitrides.

The earth cooled gradually and some of the gases liquefied and some solidified. Steam condensed into water and resulted in rain. The water again returned to atmosphere because of superheated earth. This cycle continued for millions of years and resulted in the cooling of earth. Due to cooling down of earth first ocean came in existence. The oceanic water contained methane, ammonia from atmosphere in dissolved condition.

(c) Inter-reaction of elements

The metallic nitrides reacted with super heated steam at that high temperature to form ammonia.

$MeN + 3H_2O \longrightarrow Me(OH_2 + NH_3$

Ammonia was also formed as follows :

$3H_2 + N_2 \longrightarrow 2NH_3$

$CaCN_2 + 3H_2O \longrightarrow CaCO_3 + 2NH_3$

Calcium Cyanamide

Calcium Cyanamide was formed by the action of nitrogen on carbides.

$CaC_2 + N_2 \longrightarrow CaCN_2 + C$

(d) Origin of organic compounds

According to *Oparin*, under the influence of electric changes, from these simple compounds more and more complex compounds were formed gradually. When the temperature of earth surface reduced to 1000°C or even lower, a number of saturated as well as unsaturated *hydrocarbons* were formed as :

$CH + CH \longrightarrow HC \equiv CH$ (Acetylene)

$CH_2 + CH_2 \longrightarrow H_2C = CH_2$ (Ethylene)

$CH_2 + CH_2 \longrightarrow C + CH_4$ (Methane)

$2CH_4 \longrightarrow CH \equiv CH$ (Acetylene) $+ 3H_2$

The metal carbides also formed the hydrocarbons with superheated steam as follows :

$$CaC_2 + H_2O \longrightarrow CaO + C_2H_2 \text{ (Acetylene)}$$
$$3Fe_4C_5 + 16H_2O \longrightarrow C_{15}H_{32} + 4Fe_3O_4$$

(e) Formation of complex organic compounds

The saturated and unsaturated hydrocarbons as previously formed combined and recombined in various ways through the process of condensation, polymerization and oxido-reduction.

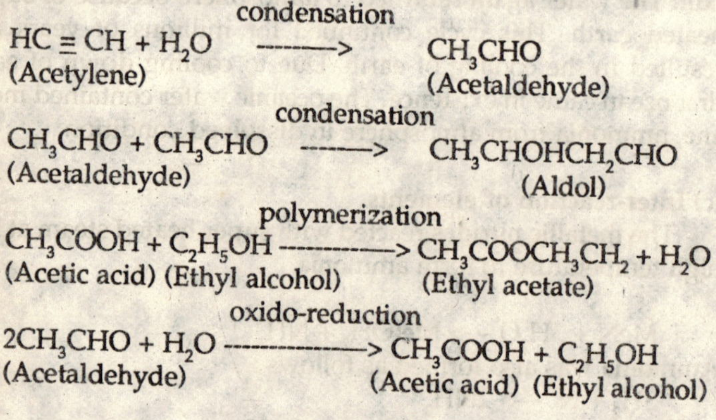

$$HC \equiv CH + H_2O \xrightarrow{\text{condensation}} CH_3CHO$$
(Acetylene) (Acetaldehyde)

$$CH_3CHO + CH_3CHO \xrightarrow{\text{condensation}} CH_3CHOHCH_2CHO$$
(Acetaldehyde) (Aldol)

$$CH_3COOH + C_2H_5OH \xrightarrow{\text{polymerization}} CH_3COOCH_3CH_2 + H_2O$$
(Acetic acid) (Ethyl alcohol) (Ethyl acetate)

$$2CH_3CHO + H_2O \xrightarrow{\text{oxido-reduction}} CH_3COOH + C_2H_5OH$$
(Acetaldehyde) (Acetic acid) (Ethyl alcohol)

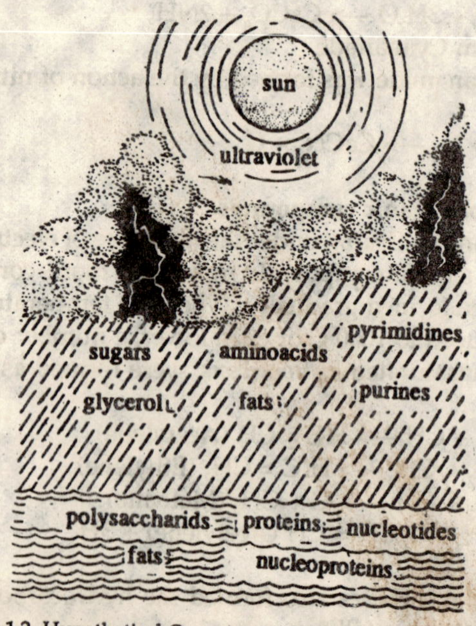

Fig. 1.2. Hypothetical Organization of Primitive Ocean

Likewise, amino acids were also produced as :

$$2HCHO \xrightarrow{\text{polymerization}} CH_2OHCHO$$
(formaldehyde) (glycol aldehyde)

$$2CH_2OHCHO + H_2O \xrightarrow{\text{oxido-reduction}} 2H_2OHCH_2OH + 2CH_2OHCOOH$$
(Glycol aldehyde) (Glycol) (Glycolic acid)

$$CH_2OHCOOH + NH_3 \longrightarrow CN_2NH_2COOH + H_2O$$
(Glycolic acid) (Ammonia) (Glycine an amino acid)

(f) Formation of Proto-Proteins, Carbohydrate, Fat etc.

Ultimately the aminc acids, sugars, glycerol and fatty acids etc. of the primitive ocean polymerized forming large macromolecules such as proteins, carbohydrates and fats. Since these complex compounds are the main constituents of the protoplasm of living cells, their synthesis established the possibilities of origin of life in the primitive ocean. As a consequence to the above chemical reactions, the oceanic water became a rich mixture of organic compound, which had been described by *J.B.S. Haldane* (1920) as *"The hot dilute Soup"*.

(g) Formation of coacervates of primary living molecules

The macromolecules of oceanic soup especially those of protein molecules having electric charges, aggregates by mutual exclusion of water, into small colloid masses, forming insoluble droplets. These droplets were surrounded by water film. These were named as *microspheres* by *Sydney Fox* (1964).

At later stages, the microspheres carrying opposite electric charges, aggregated to form larger and denser colloidal systems, named *'coacervates'* by *Oparin*.

These drops form a separate phase in a colloided system. These drops do not mix up with the surrounding medium but at the same time, the processes taking place inside them and between them and the medium, constitute the beginning of metabolism.

These coacervate drops were different in chemical composition and reaction which took place in them. They had common properties and still definite individualities and structures. These could grow in size as a result of absorbing substances dissolved in the surrounding water. These coacervate drops became more complex and created diversity among themselves. Certain combinations of compounds made them more stable, the complex molecules are more stable, therefore, they survived while the simpler ones were destroyed.

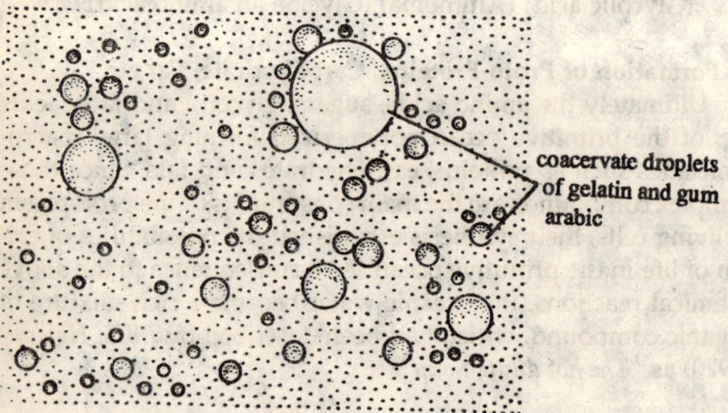

Fig. 1.3. Coacervate Droplets.

Oparin and his co-workers produced several artificial coacervates from gelatin, gum, arabic and other substances as an illustration of this theory of the origin of life.

Another important event in the origin of life was the formation of nucleic acids in the primitive ocean. Nucleic acids (DNA and RNA) are long-chain polymers of nucleotide molecules. The nucleotides were formed in the primitive ocean by combination of nitrogenous bases (purines and pyrimidines), pentose sugars and phosphoric acid. These molecules were like *naked genes*. There formation was the first step to enter the vaguely defined frontiers between life and no-life.

(h) Origin of primary organisms

Due to aggregation tendency of molecules, macromolecules of *nucleo-proteins* were formed by the union of nucleic acids and protein molecules. It is presumed that these macromolecules had certain characteristic of a *free living gene.* A number of such free genes might have aggregated to form a single large unit. That resembled the present-day *'Viruses'*, and named as *'protovirus'*.

Before the gene aggregates could develop into anything like a cell, it was necessary that they produce enzymes. Enzymes play a very important role in cellular physiology and they had to come first. With the formation of enzymes, conditions were now favourable for cells to be formed. They were very simple cells at first, without a definite nucleus (*Prokaryotes*) like bacteria.

(i) Origin of autotrophism

Nutrition was no problem at first the seas abounded in the simple soluble organic compounds which could diffuse into the cell and, by enzymatic action, be formed into cell protoplasm and growth could took place. Continued growth of cell, however, created a problem, the cells would soon have become too large for efficient functioning until cell-division intervened. Hence, a splitting of a cell into two parts must have developed early as a means of permitting continued growth.

Being anaerobic heterotrophs, the early bacteria-like prokaryotes gradually consumed all abiotically synthesized organic nutrients of the primitive sea. At this point there was danger that the life so long in developing state would perish, learning the earth once again sterile. During this course of time some of these early prokaryotes acquired enzymes which would catalyse synthesis of simple carbohydrates molecules from inorganic substances of the ocean water. This was a beginning of what is called as *autotrophic nutrition.* Energy used in the synthesis of organic molecules was solely of anaerobic break down, such a method of obtaining energy through chemical recombination with a release of a portion of the energy is known as *chaemosynthesis.* Although free oxygen was not available in the atmosphere at that time, it was possible for certain forms of chaemosynthesis to take place. Certain bacteria living today still subsist on this mode of feeding.

(ii) Phtosynthesis

The above process of chaemosynthesis could not become a

popular method on account of limited resources. Later certain autotrophic bacteria synthesized a new, green substance from a magnesium porphyrin of the ocean water. This substance, called *bacteriochlorophyll* which enabelled the organism to combine water and carbon dioxide in the presence of sunlight and obtain food. Certain changes in the bacteriochlrophyll resulted into the formation of chlorophyll.

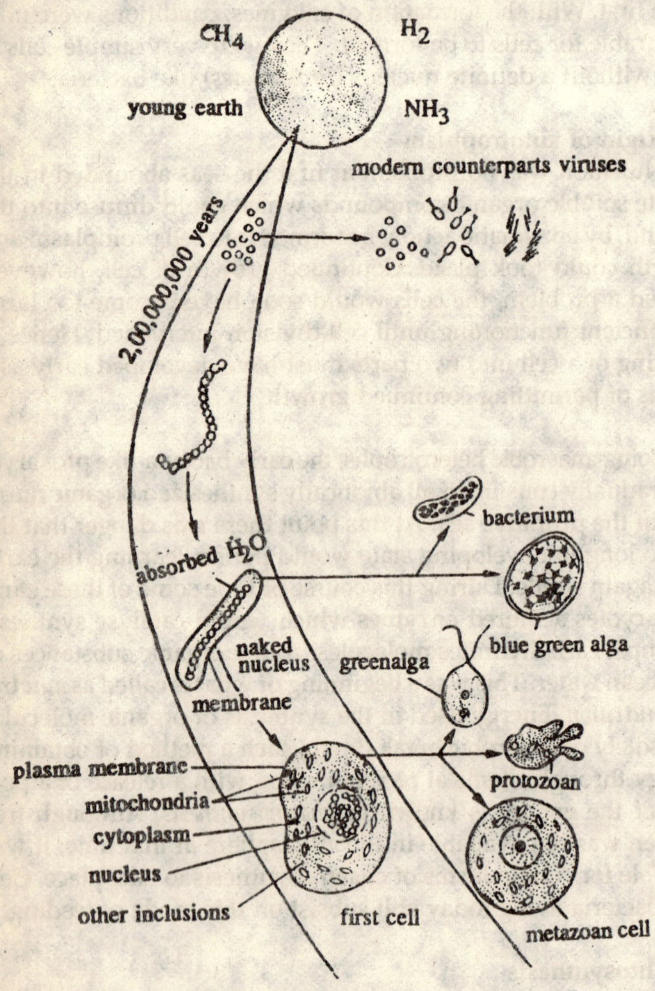

Fig. 1.4. Origin of first Organism.

$$6CO_2 + 6H_2O \xrightarrow{\text{sunlight}} \underset{\text{(glucose)}}{C_6H_{12}O_6} + 6O_2$$

Organism which developed photosynthetic activity were the first *plant-like* types and can be compared with *blue-green algae* of present day. In the phtosynthesis oxygen was liberated in atmosphere.

The entry of oxygen into the atmosphere was a major step in making possible the advanced forms of life that have developed on the earth. Not only did make possible cell respiration, but it also brought about a great change in the composition of the atmosphere. It reacted with methane and transformed into CO_2 and water.

This provided an additional source of CO_2 for photosynthesis and changed the atmosphere into a form in which animal life could exist. Oxygen also reacted with ammonia and converted it into nitrogen and water.

(iii) Environment

Oxygen in the air had another effect of great importance—— it liberated living organisms from the oceans. Much high energy radiations from the sun reached the earth, and such radiation are destructive to life, but water is a good absorber of such radiation. Thus, life could exist in the oceans, but not on the land. As oxygen was liberated, however, some of it rose and formed a layer of *Ozone* high in the atmosphere and this absorbs most of the radiation. For the first time it became possible for living organisms to leave to oceans and take up life on the land and in the air. At this time earth was cooled to a tolerable temperature; the injurious radiation was effectively blanketed ; the methane and ammonia in the air were replaced by nitrogen, oxygen, and CO_2 photosynthesis had become the dominant from the energy capture ; life was now free to develop into forms such as occur today.

Experimental evidences

The most significant experiments are those conducted by

Stanley L. Miller in 1953. A flask like the one shown in figure was used. A mixture of gases, methane, ammonia and hydrogen was kept in the flask and the flask was closed after sterilization. A high frequency spark was discharged in a constantly circulating mixture of gases for about a week. During this period a small amount of water was constantly boiled, to produce water vapour. At the end of a week a mixture of amino acids like glycine, alanine, α amino butyric acid, β-alanine, aspartic acid and glutamic acid etc., were obtained. The intermediate products of the reaction were aldehydes and HCN. In the last two decades after Miller's experiment, hundreds of such experiments, have been conducted under variety of different conditions.

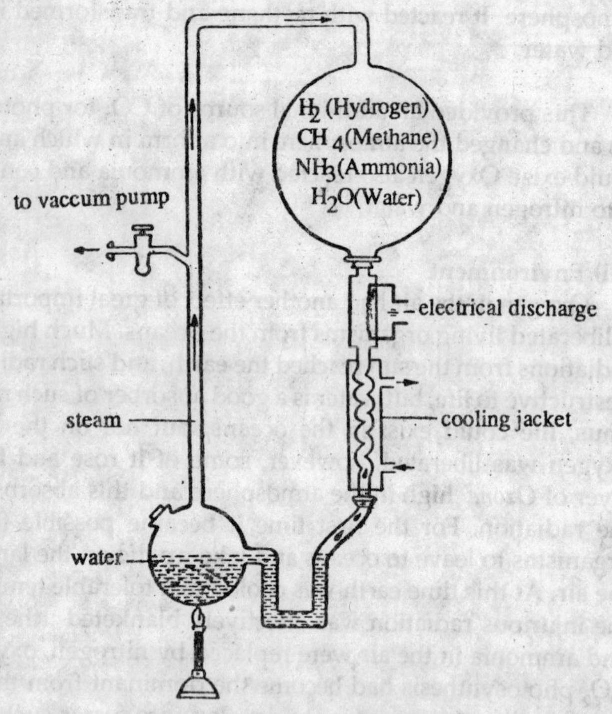

Fig. 1.5. Spark discharge apparatus.

Baly (1922)reported the synthesis of amino acids by using formaldehyde in solution. *Bahadur* (1954) obtained almost all the possible amino acids by subjecting strong sunlight to a mixture of paraformaldehyde, ammonia and ferric chloride. He concluded that this mechanism of biological synthesis of amino acids is still going on.

Purines, pyrimidines and their derivatives were also synthesized which constitute nucleoproteins essential for life. *Oro, Oro* and *Kimbell* (1960-61) obtained adenine by heating a solution of ammonium cyanide at 90ºC for 24 hrs. *Fox* and *Harade* (1961) synthesized Uracil from methane, hydrogen and water under primitive conditions.

S.W. Fox, simulating the conditions with volcanic eruptions, conducted some heating experiments and found amino acids undergoing polymerization. Since these were unlike true proteins, these were called *protenoids.* These protenoids with water may from a coacervate, were the protenoids are contained in which *Fox* called microspheres (50-80• in diameter). These protenoid microspheres can metabolize glucose. Thus both *Oparin* and *Fox* considered the protein coacervated to be the first structures in the ancestory of living systems. These protein coacervates are believed to have given rise to the first living organisms.

In 1967, *J. William Schopf* detected evidence of 22 amino acids in a rock formation which was about 3,000 million years old. These occurrence of amino acids are proof of chemical evolution of life.

Recently, *Crick* (1982) in his book *"Life Itself : Its Origin and Nature"* discussed the problem of origin of life. According to him the age of the earth does not provide enough time for the origin of life. He believed that the life on earth could have originated elsewhere in our Galaxy, the Milky Way. Thus there was enough time for intelligent being to evolve elsewhere in a suitable environment. This life elsewhere could have dispatched, by rocket to the earth, the prokaryotic and eukaryotic microbes and the sperms of primeval life. This theory of origin of life on earth by heavenly insemination is called *"Theory of Directed Panspermia"*. *Crick* admits that no evidence for this theory can be easily available and, therefore, concludes "I can not myself see just how we shall ever decide how life originated". He thinks that origin of life on earth will be an extremely rare event and that if it occurred, it must be a miracle.

LIFE ON OTHER PLANETS

It is quite obvious that life could have originated upon other planets and stars having conditions approximately similar to those of primitive earth.

Moon cannot hold even water and as such it is dry and lifeless. *Earth* is situated at the right distance from the sun so that water remains as liquid between freezing and boiling points. On *Venus* the temperature is believed to be always above the boiling point. On *Mars* the night temperature drops below freezing point but much evidence points to life present there. *Mercury* is extremely hot and is nearer to sun. *Jupiter, Saturn, Uranus* and *Neptune* have dense atmosphere made up of thick clouds of hydrogen, helium, ammonia and methane which are similar to primitive atmosphere of early earth. But these planets are supposed to be too cool. It has also been estimated that in several million stars in our own galaxy, conditions are favourable for maintenance and evolution of life.

2

EVIDENCES IN FAVOUR OF EVOLUTION

Now-a-days we firmly believe in the doctrine of *organic evolution.* According to this doctrine all the organisms (plants and animals) which are existing today have descended form simpler pre-existing forms.

The term evolution means unrolling or unfolding of events and was used by *Hebert Spencer* for the first time. *Charles Darwin* described evolution as "descent with modification". In other words, evolution may be described as derivation of new species of plants and animals from those existed in the past. A host of evidences that evolution has actually taken place have now been accumulated. A short account of these evidences is given below.

I. EVIDENCE FROM TAXONOMY

There are about 1,00,000 species of animals and about 2,50,000 species of plants in the world, many species are yet to be described. Therefore, it is evident that the study of living organisms is not at all possible if we do not categorise or classify them.

The credit of modern classification goes to the work of *Carolus Linnaeus* (a Swedish botanist 1707-1778) who undertook the work of classification of the entire living world. *Linnaeus,* in the tenth edition of his *Systema Naturae* (1750), introduced the binomial nomenclature of each animal with first part as the generic name and the second part as the specific name.

Earlier systematicists use superficial character to differentiate and classify organisms and the classification suggested was more or less *artificial*. In the classification the basic unit is the *species*, a population of closely similar individuals. *Herst* defined species as "group of individuals of common descent with certain constant specific characters in common, which are represented in the nucleus of cell by constant and characteristic set of chromosomes carrying homologous specific genes causing infrafertility and inter-sterility.

Several species have so many common characters that they can be placed together as a same *genus*. Therefore, the various species-clusters are named as various genera. The genera also naturally fall into larger groups on the basis of similarities in their fundamental characters. *Linnaeus* called these groups as *orders*. Finally these orders were grouped in classes, the diverse members of which share only the very fundamental characteristics. *Linnaeus* grouped these classes into two kingdoms-*Plantae* and *Animalia*. *E. Haeckel* introduced the term *phylum* to describe the related classes. However, various other workers before *Haeckel*, used various terms such as *sub-kingdom*, *circle* and *types* in between the class and kingdom. Etymologically the term phylum stands for a line of descent and is more appropriate to the new studies of evolution. Similarly *Haeckel* also introduced the term *family* as a category intermediate between genus and order.

Kingdom
Phylum
Class
Order
Family
Genus
Species.

The generic name is written with a capital letter, the specific and sub-specific name without capital letter. For example, *Homo sapiens*.

The above taxonomic categories represent degrees of blood relationship. For instance, all chordates have common ancestors but now only most fundamental characters are found to be common. the degree of similarity or closeness will become higher as we reach the lower scale of taxonomic categories.

The above stated facts cannot be explained by the theory of special creation. Had the species been created independently of one another, the question of grouping them would not have arisen. The ready explanation of grouping of plants and animals lied only in the concept of organic evolution which suggests an evolutionary tree or geological tree (since each taxonomic group includes the members of a common origin, all its members can be shown as off shoots, of a common trunk in the form of a tree called *evolutionary tree* where the species, genera and families etc. are comparable to the leaves, branches and large branches, all ultimately sprourting out from common stock.

II. EVIDENCES FROM COMPARATIVE ANATOMY

Study of functional anatomy is called *tectology*. The comparative anatomy provides us good evidences for evolution. All the homologous organs in animals and plants are formed on the same basic plan, though they may be modified variously. This relationship in the organisms in their anatomy shows that they have evolved from common ancestor and modifications are secondary development, according to their needs.

Some of the interesting examples are as given below :

A. Homology and Analogy

When we make a general survey of the animals or plants for structural evidences of evolution, we come across two types of characters, firstly those which are of common origin are known as *homology* and secondly, the adaptive features which are of unlike origin but are of similar functions, such are called *analogy*.

Those organs which are fundamentally unlike i.e. they have different origins but have the same function are called *analogous organs*. But the organs which are fundamentally the same in structure and have the same origin, irrespective of how greatly they may be modified to perform widely different functions, are called *homologous organs*.

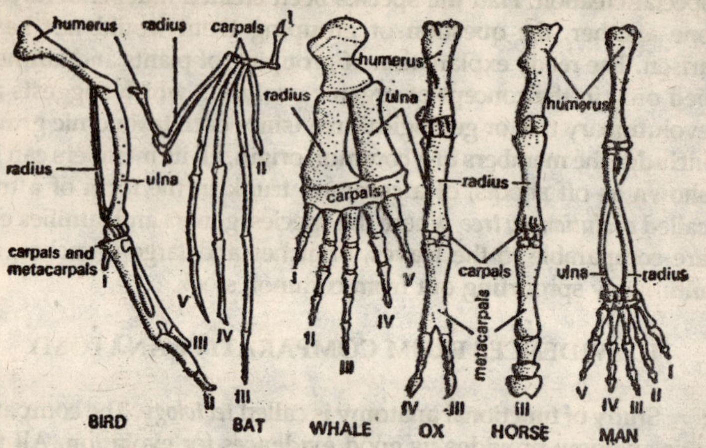

Fig. 2.1. Homology of Vertebrate fore-limbs.

Following examples illustrate homology :

1. Homology in limb structure of vertebrates

The fore-limbs of a mole, wing of bat, fore-limb of man and terrestrial horse which look so much different and perform different functions are homologous structures because developmentally all of them possess a pentadactyle plan. This structural divergence or modification from a fundamental plan of structure can be explained only on the basis of adaptation to different enviromental conditions. Thus biologists are convinced that animals have inherited homologous structures from an ancestor which they shared in common in the remote past.

2. Homology in eye structure of vertebrates

The eyes of different vertebrates, though may differ in their muscles and lenses and required by different degrees of accommodation, but they are all homologous. The eyes of vertebrate from cyclostomes to mammals, are constructed of similar parts like sclerotic, choroid, retina and lens.

3. Homology in brain structure

The brain of vertebrates ranging from fishes to mammals consists of similar series of parts, viz. olfactory lobes, cerebral

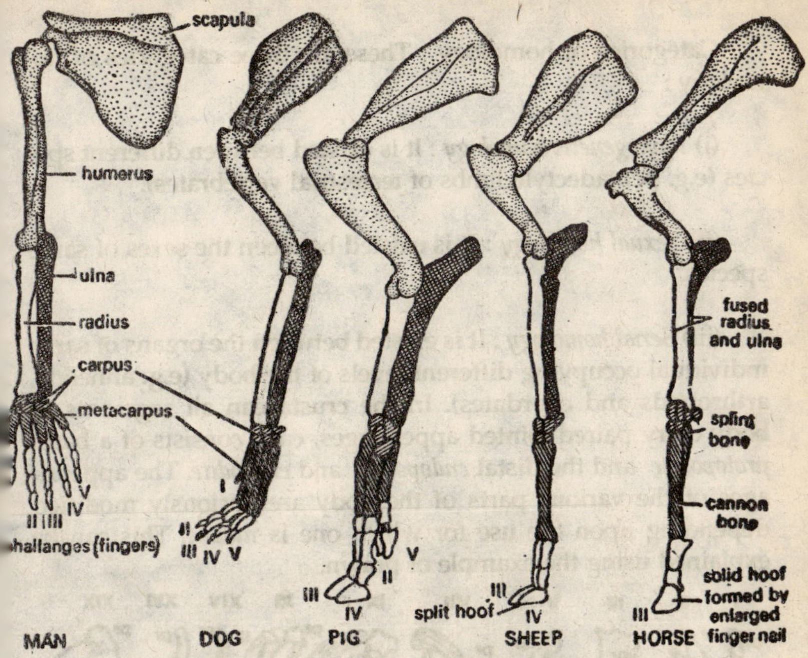

Fig. 2.2. Fore-limbs of few mammals showing serial homology.

hemispheres, optic lobes, cerebellum and medulla oblongata and other less prominent structures. As we progress through the series from fishes to mammals some lobes become more prominent than other like cerebral hemispheres which are smaller in fishes but highly developed in mammals. It is due to adaptations and evolutionary changes.

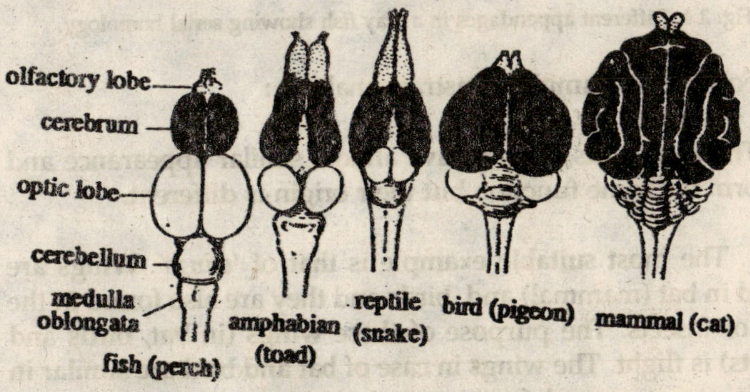

Fig. 2.3. Brains of vertebrates (Dorsal View)

Categories of homology : These are three categories of homology :

(i) *Phylogenetic homology* : It is existed between different species (e.g. pentadectyle limbs of terrestrial vertebrates).

(ii) *Sexual homology* : It is existed between the sexes of same species.

(iii) *Serial homology* : It is existed between the organs of same individual occupying different levels of the body (e.g. annelids, arthropods and chordates). In the crustacean all segments of body carry paired jointed appendages, each consists of a basal *protopodite* and the distal *endopodite* and *exopodite*. The appendages of the various parts of the body are variously modified depending upon the use for which one is meant. This can be explained using the example of prawn.

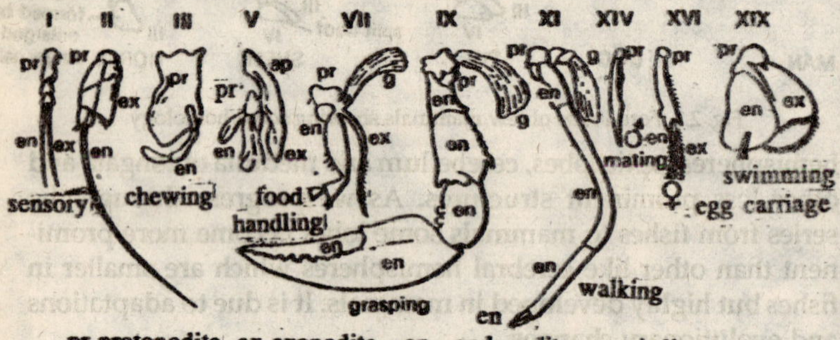

pr-protopodite, ex-exopodite, en - endopodite, ep-epiodite, g-gill

Fig. 2.4. Different appendages in a cray fish showing serial homology.

Following examples illustrate analogy :

The analogous organs have almost similar appearance and perform the same function but their origin is different.

1. The most suitable example is that of *'wings'*. Wings are found in bat (mammal) and birds and they are also found in the case of insects. The purpose of these wings (in bat, birds and insects) is flight. The wings in case of bat and bird are similar in origin, structure and function and are thus considered as ho-

mologous organs. But an insect's wing is not similar in origin and structure though it performs the same function. Therefore, it is considered as analogous organ.

2. The other example is furnished by the fins of the fishes and flappers of aquatic mammals like whale and seals. These structure have similar appearance and function but their structure found distinctly different and therefore, are analogous. The fins have very simple skeleton while the flappers resembles a pentadactyle limb.

3. The stings of honeybee and scorpion perform similar function and similar in their structure. But their origin is different, in honeybee it is a modification of ovipositor while in scorpion it is the modification of last abdominal segment. Hence these are analogous.

B. Vestigial Organs

Among animals and plants are met with reduced and functionless organs which in other allied forms are functional and of large size. Such organs which are functionless and atrophied are called *vestigial organs*. The occurrence of vestigeal organs suggest that these organs were well developed and functional in the ancestors but have become atrophied due to alteranate development in the organism and change of environment.

Following are few examples of such organs :

1. *Vermiform appendix in man* : The vermiform appendix in man is the common example. The appendix attaches to a short section of the large intestine called the caecum and the latter located at the point where the large intestine is joined with the small intestine. The caecum is a short pouch, ending blindly except for the small opening into its extension the appendix. Appendix is a small structure without any known function. However, in some other mammals specially which live on coarse diet rich in cellulose, the appendix is functional. The presence of appendix in man shows that at one time he was purely herbivorous.

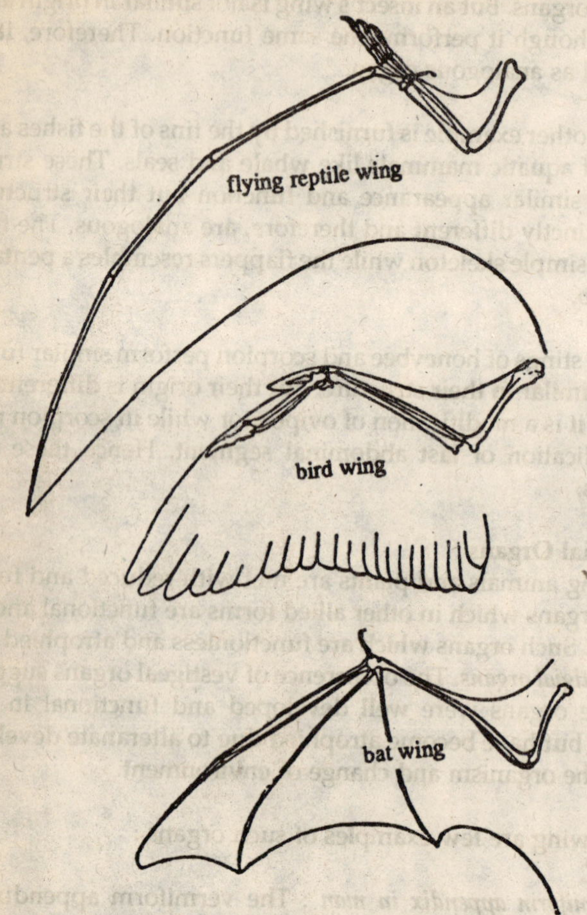

Fig. 2.5. Comparison of Vertebrate Wings.

Fig. 2.6. Appendix vermiform A=Orang utam, B=Man.

2. *Vestigial hind limbs and pelvic girdle of python* and related snakes which externally are mere spurs on either side of the vent, internally have the structure of full formed limb, made of several bones i.e. ilium, femer, tibia, claw etc.

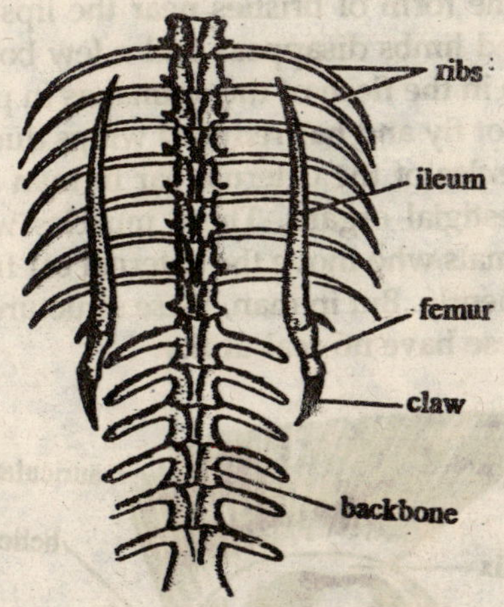

Fig. 2.7. Vestigial hind-limbs of Python

3. A protective covering, *the nictitating membrane* is found in birds on the surface of eye to keep the eyes moistened. This membrane is also found in reptiles. In human beings a functionless trade of this membrane called semilunar fold or plica semilurnaris is present in the inner angle of the eye. This shows relationship of reptiles, birds and mammals.
4. Majority of mammals have well developed tails but it is absent in man. It is represented by a caudal vertebrae even now.

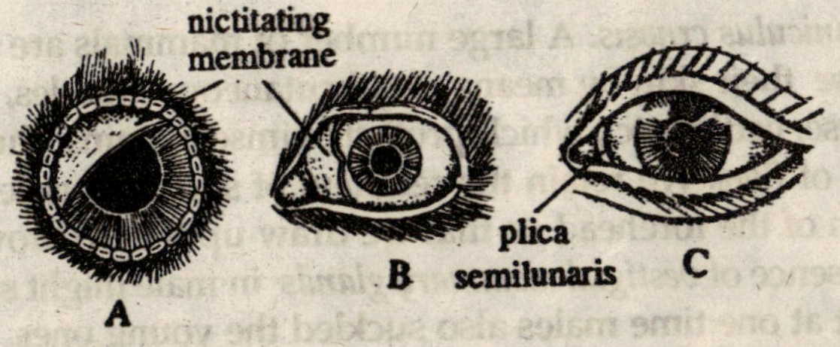

Fig. 2.8. Nictitating membranes in the eyes of various animals.
A=Owl, B=Horse, C=Man.

5. In the embryo of whales a coat of hair is generally present which was present in their vanished fore-bears. The relics of hind limbs were also present as well-developed buds. At the time of birth all the hairs are shed and only a few are present in the form of bristles near the lips. The external traces of hind limbs disappear and a few bones are found buried deep in the flesh of the animal as in python.
6. Kiwi does not fly and has reduced wings due to its disuse.
7. The ear muscles of the external ear in man is another example of vestigial organs. These muscles were useful in many mammals who move the external ear freely to detect sounds efficiently. But in man, these structures still persist, although these have no real utility.

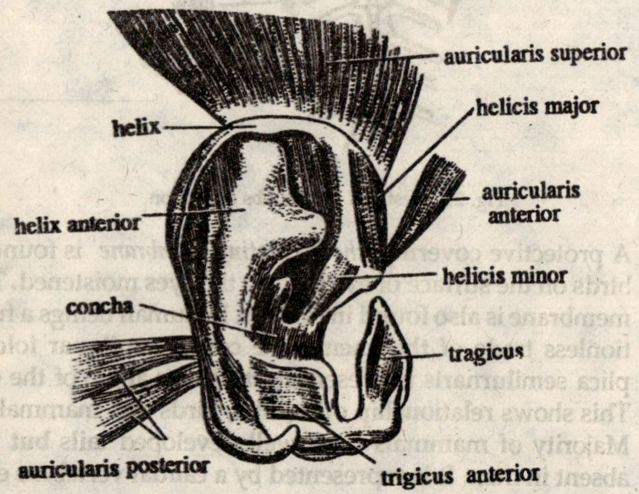

Fig. 2.9. Human ear showing vestigial ear muscles

8. *Panniculus crnosis.* A large number of mammals are able to *move* their skin by means of subcutaneous muscles, as in a horse, cattles etc., which protects himself against the sucking of flies. We retain the remnant of such a muscle in the skin of the forehead so that we draw up the eyebrows.
9. Presence of *vestigial mammary glands* in male might suggest that at one time males also suckled the young ones.
10. *Wisdom teeth.* It appears as third pair of molars are vestigial

in the more civilized races of man.

11. Cave-dwellers like salamanders, Proteus etc. live in perpetual darkness, they have lost their eyes during the course of evolution.
12. In horses and cursorial animals the third metacarpal (splint bone) in feet is reduced.
13. Presence of *coccyx* at the end of the vertebral column which is a remnant of the ancestral tail of quadrupeds. The coccyx is formed by the fusion of 3-5 tail vertebrae.

Besides few above examples in man, according to *Wiedersheim* there are about 100 vestigial structures.

C. Connecting links

There are certain animals living or extinct which possess characters intermediate between two major groups of animals. Thus, lung fishes (living) connect fish with amphibians, *Seymouria* (extinct) connects amphibians with reptiles. *Archaeopteryx* (extinct) connects reptiles with birds and Prototheria (egg laying

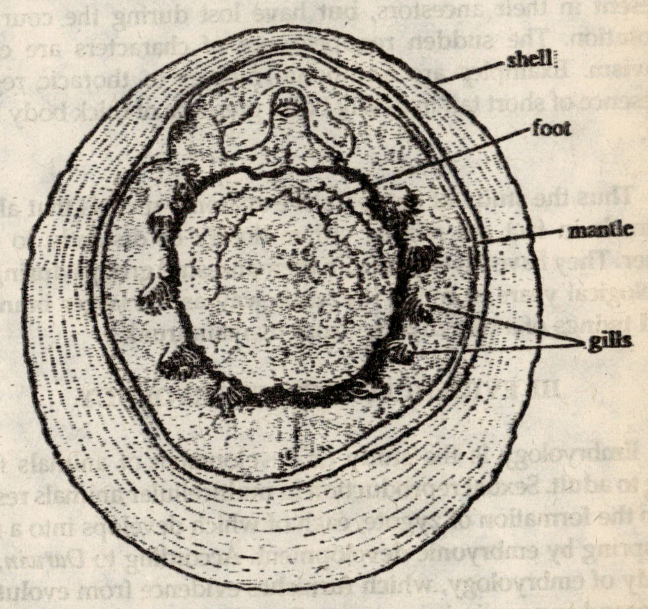

Fig 2.10. Neoplina

mammals-living) connect reptiles with mammals. *Neoplina* forms a connecting link between annelids and molluscs. *Peripatus* connects annelids and arthropods. These connecting links may not be direct ancestors of the next higher group but they do show that evolution has taken place. The lower animals during the course of time have changed into higher animals through the bridge of animals which possessed intermediate characters.

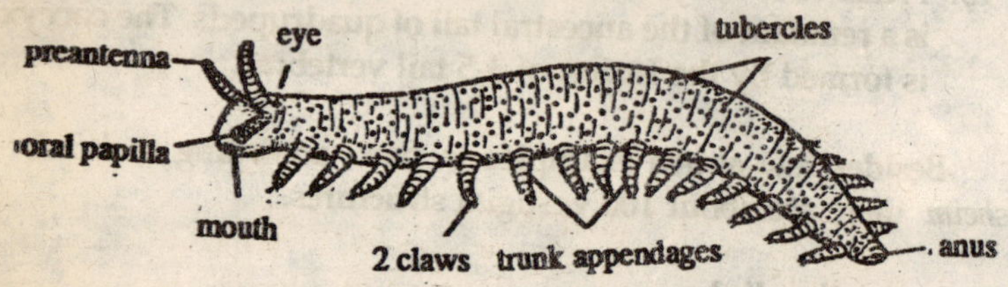

Fig. 2.11. Peripatus

D. Atavism or reversion

It has been observed that some individuals are born with some such abnormal features which are supposed to have been present in their ancestors, but have lost during the course of evolution. The sudden reappearance of characters are called atavism. Examples are additional nipples in thoracic region, presence of short tail in newly born, presence of thick body hairs etc.

Thus the study of comparative anatomy reveals that all the animals in fact are related either closely or distantly to each other. They have diverged from their ancestral groups during the geological years in much the same way as the larger branches and twings of a tree diverge from its main trunk.

III. EVIDENCES FROM EMBRYOLOGY

Embryology is the study of development of animals from egg to adult. Sexual reproduction in multicellular animals results into the formation of zygote, each of which develops into a new offspring by embryonic development. According to *Darwin*, the study of embryology, which furnishes evidence from evolution, is second to none in importance. *Ernst Haeckel* brought this into prominence through his *Biogenetic Law* which states that "Ontogeny recapitulates phylogeny". *Ontogeny* is the development of the individual from egg to adulthood while *phylogeny* is the series of the stages through which that particular species passed in its evolution. *Haeckel* in his theory believed that embryonic stages corresponded to ancestral adults, thus providing evidence for the possible line of organic evolution. The idea of *Haeckel* though is wrong in the eyes of modern embryologists yet, it has stimulated research in embryology and focused attention on the general resemblance between embryonic development and evolutionary process.

In formulating his recapitulation theory, *Haeckel* based his observations on *Von Baer's* principles of embryonic differentiation. These *Von Baer's* principles can be stated as follows—(i) General characters appear in development before special characters. (ii) After the more general characters, the less general characters and finally the special characters would appear. (iii) An animal during development only progressively departs from the development of other animals. (iv) Young stages of an animal are like the young of embryonic stages of lower animals but not like the adults.

A comparative study of the ontogeny of varied forms of animals reveals their phylogenetic relationship and, thus, confirms evolution.

In the animal kingdom there are a number of interesting examples which provides evidences for common ancestory and evolution.

(i) The zygotes from which the development of all metazoans starts are single-celled and can be compared to the simple protozoan. This indicates origin of metazoans from protozoan ancestors.

(ii) The zygote soon becomes multicellular forming morula, *blatula* and later gastrula. The blastula can be compared to a colonial protozoan or to some hypothetical blastula-like animal which has been postulated to be the ancestor of all metazoan.

Upon gastrulation, the embryo is coelenterate like, but it soon acquires triploblastic grade of construction resembling to the playtyhelminthes or to the Namertina. This indicates a monophylatic origin.

(iii) In the later stages the fundamental chordate characters are developed viz. dorsal nerve cord, notohord and pharyngeal gill-slits. The tadpole larva of amphibians is like fishes in structure and habit. Its gills are like that of fishes and tail helps in swimming. Tadpole become frog after *metamorphosis*. It is concluded that the frog has evolved from some fish-like ancestor.

(iv) The early stages of development of the embryos of fishes, salamander, tortoise, chick, rabbit and man show a peculiar similarly.

Each sequence begins with a single fertilized egg (zygote). To facilitate the comparison, the structure of different stages of different animals is drawn about the same size, although they vary in their size measurements.

In the third stage as shown in figure all of the embryos look very much alike. They all have similar segmentally arranged somites and similar gill arches and gill clefts. In the next stage in the figure, the limb primordia are forming on all of them in a similar way and they all have embryonic tails. The embryos of tortoise, chick, rabbit and man are indistinguishable upto the fourth stage while those of fish and salamander are beginning to assume recognizable forms. At this stage, gills have formed from the tissue lining the gill clefts of both the fish and salamander. However in the last stage of figure, each embryo has developed features that indicate fairly clearly its definitive nature. It may be asked as to why do the embryos of all vertebrates develop in the same way or as to why embryonic gill clefts develop in tortoise, chicken, rabbit and man where they degenerate and are never functional. These facts can only be explained on the basis of doctrine of organic evolution. All these animals have developed from a common ancestor and they possess a common heredity for the manifestation of these characters.

This development can be traced in the various systems also. When the heart first develops in the embryos of fishes, amphibians, reptiles, birds and mammals, it is two-chambered (auricle and ventricle) which is retained as such in fishes. In later stages of embryonic development of amphibians, reptiles, birds and mammals the heart becomes three-chambered and finally in birds and mammals it comes four-chambered.

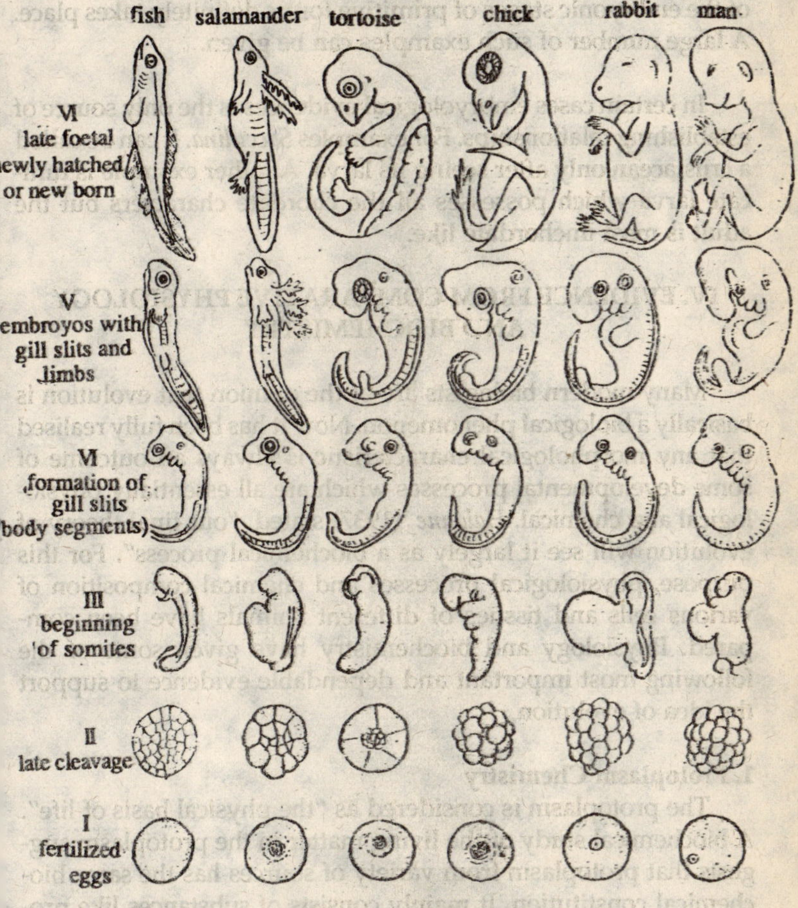

Fig. 2.12. Comparison of Vertebrate Embroys.

In vertebrates there occur three distinct types of kidneys, all of which have developed from the nephrostome. *Protonephros* is characteristic of lower vertebrates. In adult hagfish this type of kidney is present. In fishes and amphibians it is replaced by *mesonephros* while in reptiles birds and mammals the metanephros—most evolved type—is present.

The above two examples of the development of heart and the kidneys show that during the ontogenetic stages recapitulation of the embryonic stages of primitive forms definitely takes place. A large number of such examples can be given.

In certain cases embryological evidences is the only source of establishing relationships. For examples *Sacculina*. It can be called a crustacean only after seeing its larva. Another example is tunicate larva which possesses all the chordate characters but the adult is most unchordate like.

IV. EVIDENCE FROM COMPARATIVE PHYSIOLOGY AND BIOCHEMISTRY

Many modern biologists are of the opinion that evolution is basically a biological phenomenon. Now it has been fully realised that any morphological characteristic is always an outcome of some developmental processes which are all essentially physiological and chemical. *Haldane* (1937) stated, "our final theory of evolution will see it largely as a biochemical process". For this purpose, physiological processes and chemical composition of various cells and tissues of different animals have been compared. Physiology and biochemistry have given some of the following most important and dependable evidence to support the idea of evolution.

1. Protoplasm Chemistry

The protoplasm is considered as "the physical basis of life". A biochemical study of the living matter in the protoplasm suggests that protoplasm from variety of sources has the same biochemical constitution. It mainly consists of substances like proteins, carbohydrates, fats, water etc. This would suggest that during evolution the most fundamental property of living things has remained intact, while variations in essential respects produced the variability according to the needs of varied forms.

2. Chromosome Chemistry

Like protoplasm, another remarkable similarity at the bio-chemical level is found in the chemistry of chromosomes. The chromosomes of all living organism basically consist of nucleic acids (DNA , and RNA) and proteins (histones and protamines). The molecules of these chemical substances remain arranged in all chromosomes in, a almost identical fashion,. Such a uniformity in the composition of chromosomes again suggests a common origin of most living beings.

3. Enzymes

A large number of enzymes (bio-catalysts) are same in all the animals. For example *Trypsin*, a protein splitting enzyme is present from protozoans to mammals and hence called an *ancient enzyme*. Similarly *amylase* is found from sponges to mammals.

4. Hormones

There are a number of hormones which throw light on the organic evolution. For example *thyroid hormone* is common in all vertebrates and this hormone from one class of organisms can be substituted for that in another class of organisms. For the treatment of human thyroid deficiency, beef thyroid has been successfully used. Also in case thyroid gland of frog is surgically removed at a young stage, frog will not metamorphose, but if it is again fed with thyroid tissue from mammals, the metamorphosis can be easily brought about.

Another example is that of M.S.H. or *melanophore stimulating hormone* of amphibians. This hormone is found in mammals also, but has no known effect there. If the hormone, extracted from mammalian pituitary glands, is supplied to amphibians, it is as effective as the amphibian hormone itself. It suggests that this enzyme in mammals does not have any known function and is only found as a vestigial of the amphibian ancestory.

5. Excretion

In most of the aquatic animals, the nitrogenous waste is ammonia, in terrestrial forms it is urea, but in insects, reptiles and birds, it is the semi solid uric acid. This is due to economy in the supply and intake of water. Ammonia being toxic is eliminated soon in aquatic forms which have ample supply of water while in other forms it is converted into harmless urea or uric acid. An interesting example is that of embryo of birds. In birds, in the embryo for the first five days the nitrogenous wastes are in the form of ammonia, for the next few days (till 9th day) urea, and finally uric acid.

6. Haemoglobin

Haemoglobin, a respiratory pigment, when treated with glacial acetic acid precipitates in crystals call *haemin* crystals. The shape, size and structure of these crystals is similar in all the member of a species. They are different from those of other species. The dcgree of differences agrees with the classification of animals.

7. Blood Plasma

The similarity in the composition of blood plasma of different animals is very characteristic. Plasma contains proteins in the solute form. Besides, it also contains salts of sodium, potassium, calcium and magnesium.

8. Comparative Serology

If small amount of blood serum from an animal is injected into the blood of guinea pig or any other animal, *antibodies* against the *antigens* of the injected blood will be produced. These antigens will be destroyed now by antibodies thus produced in the blood stream as well as in a test tube. The strength of precipitate depends upon the concentration of *antigen.* The precipitate is the *precipitint* and the test is *precipitation test. Dr. George H.F. Nuttal* employed the precipitation method for finding out the interrelationship among different animals. Some blood of man is taken and allowed to clot. The clot is removed and the remaining yellowish fluid is left called *serum.* It is now injected in a small dose into the rabbit. The proteins of this serum act as *antigens* in the body of rabbit. Due to it *antibodies* are formed in the blood of rabbit. These antibodies clump and destroy the human blood. After the last injection of heavy dose, the rabbit is allowed to live for some days and then its blood is drained away and allowed to clot, its clots is removed and the left serum is collected called *anti-human serum.* If the serum of man is mixed with this antise rum, a white precipitate is formed. When it is mixed with the blood of dogs, cats, primates etc. With the blood of dogs and cats precipitation does not take place but precipitation occurs very frequently with blood of primates (monkeys, apes, gorilla etc.). This test shows the relationship between man and the other primates and not with the dogs and cats.

Different types of serum can be prepared in this manner and relationship can be tested *Nuttal* and *Graham Smith* concluded the following observation after conducting thousands of such tests.

(i) *Anticarnivora serum* give maximum reactions among the bloods of carnivora than others.

(ii) *Antipig serum.* It gives maximum reactions only with blood of species belonging to pig family, moderate reactions with ruminants and camel. *Anti-Llama serum* give moderate reaction with the blood of camel.

(iii) *Anti-whale serum.* It gives maximum reactions only with bloods of other whales and slight reactions with that of pigs and ruminants.

(iv) *Anti-turtle serum.* It gives maximum reactions with the bloods of turtles and crocodiles and negative with lizards and snakes.

(v) *Anti-lizard serum.* It reacts with the blood of lizards and snakes.

(vi) *Anti-mammalian serum.* It gives positive test of interrelationship with all the mammals, but degree and time taken varies in every case.

Thus the serological tests prove the relationship between different animals. In general the species of a single genus exhibits very close serological similarity, genera of the same family show moderate reaction and families of the same order show slight similarity.

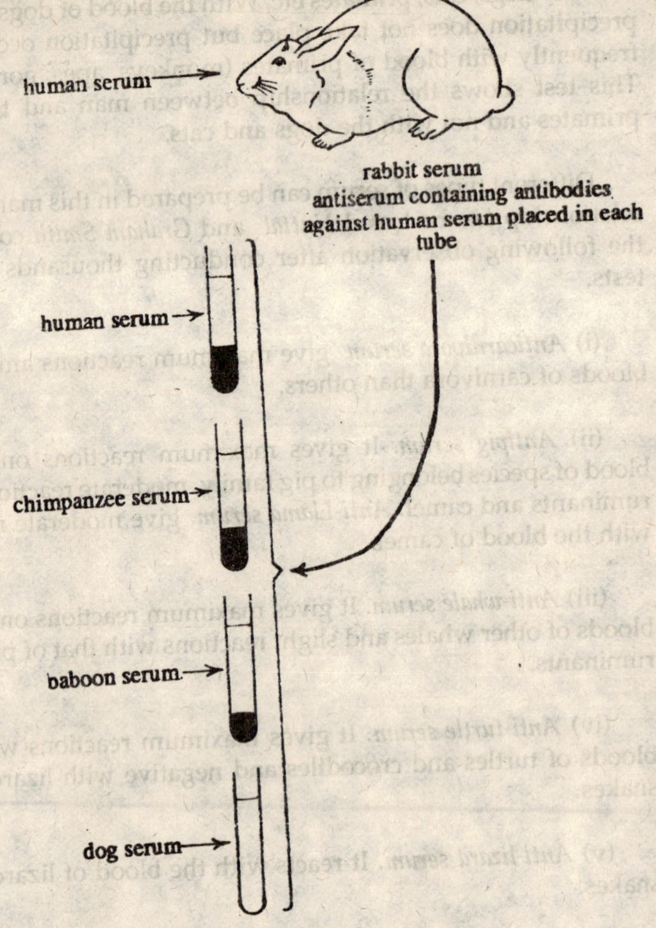

Fig. 2.13. Diagram to show precipitation test

9. Phosphagens

The phosphagens play a key role in muscle contraction and are the sources of energy for the resynthesis of ATP, once they are broken-down. In the muscles of most vertebrates, phosphagen is always a specific compound called *creatine phosphate* while in most invertebrates it is *arginine phosphate*. Hemichordates, the most primitive chordates, have both the phosphagens the creatine phosphate as well as *arginine phosphate*, such a situation is also found in echinoderms and on morphological grounds echinoderms have been considered close to the ancestor of chordates.

10. Cytochrome 'C'

It is a respiratory enzyme present in the mitochodria. It is made up of 104-112 amino acid monomers. The sequence of amino acid in its molecules has been determined by *Dickerson* (1972) and other workers in diverse forms such as man, rabbit, fishes, snakes etc. Variations found in the sequences are in agreement with accepted phylogenetic relationship.

V. EVIDENCES FROM PALAENTOLOGY

The study of past life with the help of fossils (Latin : *fosilium;* something dug up) is known as science of *palaentology*. The geological record is written in the language of fossils which may be the actual remains of the animal burried underground or may be their casts, moulds or impression in the rocks or earth's crust. There are records of fossils which animals and plants left in the rocks. These fossils found at various places in different geological periods, provide evidence for the evolution of different groups of plants and animals.

Rocks

A rock is formed by the aggregation of minerals. The rocks are found in abundance beneath the earth surface in the form of beds at various depths. Sometimes it may be found exposed on the slopes of mountains, along the stream banks etc. The rock may be formed by single mineral (rock salt) or may be composed by more than one minerals like a granite—which is formed by felspar, quartz and mica.

The nature of Rocks

The rocks, according to their origin, are of three types, *igneous, stratified* or *sedimentary* and *metamorphic*. Igneous rock were formed when the molten earth cooled down and solidified. They are the oldest rocks and contain no fossils. The fossils are found only in the stratified rocks, which have been formed by slow deposition in water of sand, clay, mud or lime formed by the weathering of igneous rocks as a result of the action of heat, cold, wind and rains. During the process of this type of rock formation at the beds of great seas countless marine animals and plants after death, have been sinking to the bottom becoming embedded in the sediments. Some land plants and animals also, after death were carried by rivers to lakes or ocean, and got embedded in sediments. They were changed to fossils. The metamorphic rocks are formed from the above two groups by changing their texture and composition. This change is caused by weight, pressure, heat and movement. The common examples are anthracite coal from soft coal, quartzite from sandlime, marble from limestone and slate from clay.

The process of rock formation is as old as the earth. The age of rock may be calculated by different methods. The deepest bed is the last in case of sedimentary rocks and most superficial one is the recent. But this does not tell us the age of earth in years. The age of fossil is determined by following way :

The element uranium changes to lead by a long process of transformation. When uranium and lead occur together in the form of small nodule in a fragment of sedimentary rock, it may be assumed that rate at which uranium changes to lead is independent of the conditions under which it occurred. It has been calculated that 7,400,000,000 gms. of uranium yield one gm. of lead per year. In this way the age of a piece or rock containing uranium and lead can be determined from the following formula:

$$\text{Age of the rock} = \frac{\text{wt. of lead}}{\text{wt. of uranium}} \times 7{,}400 \text{ million years}$$

By this method the age of earth has been calculated to be 3,000,000,000 years and rocks bearing first sign of life is about 2,000,000,000 years.

Fossilization

Usually the animals and plants, after their death are destroyed and decomposed by bacteria, fungi and predators. Besides this there are also the cases where the dead bodies of plant and animals are not destroyed but are preserved as fossils. These fossils are of various types :

(i) *Petrified fossils*

In this type of fossils, as a result of petrification the organic matter a dead animal or plant is replaced particle by mineral matter. In petrification, quartz, limestone or iron pyrites are used.

(ii) *Dead and preserved bodies*

The actual dead and preserved bodies, or parts of bodies, of animals and plant, with the original tissues intact ; and enclosed either in ice or in amber or else mummified in various ways, form one class of fossils. From the arctic ice, almost fresh bodies of mammoths, dead thousands of years ago, have been recovered. Several species of ants and insects have been preserved in amber especially found on the shallow coats of the Baltic sea. Several mollusc-shells, teeth of sharks, bones of animals have been found in well preserved condition.

(iii) *Casts and impressions*

Sometimes an animals or plant that has laid in mud or clay long enough to have left its impression ; the mud hardens about the body and forms a mold ; the organic matter disintegrates and the mold is filled with hard mineral matter ; and the matrix may then be removed so as to leave the perfect cast.

(iv) *Trails and footprints*

Fossils are also found in the form of trails and footprints. Animals when they move from one place to another leave impressions, which are preserved when sand and mud become stone. Such fossils have been found of organisms such as worms, molluscs, arthropods and vertebrates.

(v) *Cropolites*

These are the structures, which represent fossil casting or excreta.

(vi) *Gastroliths*

These are present in the body cavity of certain reptiles. These structures are believed to have been of some use of grinding the stomach contents of the extinct reptiles.

(vii) *Pseudofossils*

Many objects of inorganic origin closely resembles the forms of organic origin, and are found in the sedimentary rocks. These are called pseudofossils.

Conditions for fossilization

There are two important conditions for fossilization (i) hard parts and (ii) immediate burrial.

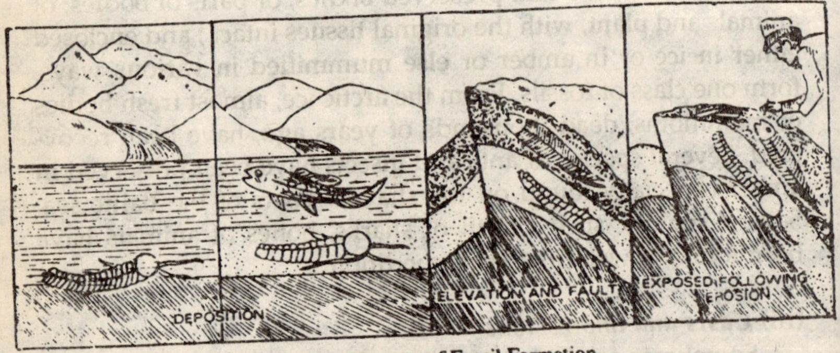

Fig. 2.14. Process of Fossil Formation.

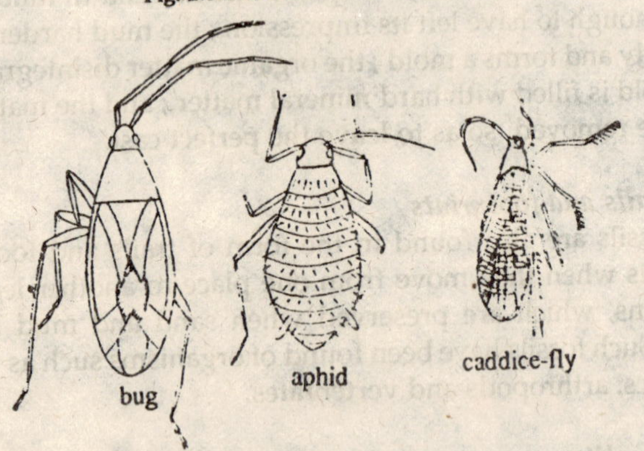

Fig. 2.15. Insects preserved in Amber

The Geological record

On the basis of their studies palaentologists have divided the geological history of earth into five major *eras* ; these are in turn divided into *periods* and periods into *epoches*.

Importance of fossil record

1. Most primitive forms of life are present in the oldest rocks.
2. From older to recent strata or layers, there is a succession of higher and more complex forms.
3. In many cases, a group arose in one era or period and remained scare. However, in the next period or era it became dominant due to adaptive radiation.
4. Large groups became extinct but after establishment of all the major phyla, some species of each phylum remained upto the present.
5. The past forms of life are not exactly similar to any of the living forms.
6. The main trend in evolution has been a gradual progression from simpler and more generalised types towards more complex and specialized forms, as one proceeds from the lower towards the upper strata.
7. It is seen that a new group arises near the close of a geological period during which great climatic changes were taking place. Such a incipient group become dominant and characteristic group of next period.
8. Many complete fossil pedegrees have been worked out which establish the most convincing evidence at our disposal that evolution has taken place.

Transitional or intermediate fossil forms

Transitional fossil forms are known between different existing group from fishes to amphibia, from amphibia to reptiles, from reptiles to birds and from reptiles to mammals. For example :

Stegocaphalus is a form linking fishes and amphibians. *Archaeopteryx* and *Archaeornis* are the toothed birds connecting reptiles and birds. *Inostracevia* was a intermediate form between reptiles and mammals. *Manchurosaurus* was also a link between reptiles and mammals.

Incompleteness of the Geological Record

Unfortunately the geological record does not give a complete picture of all the plants and animals which existed in the past. If it had been complete no further proof of organic evolution, would have been required.

The incompleteness of the geological record is due to various reasons, some of which are listed below.

1. In the earlier time plants and animals were soft and usually not fossilized. Most of them, after the death, were destroyed by micro-organisms, predators, etc. In some cases some part fossilised and some not, as in the case of plants where wood is preserved and flowers, leaves etc. are destroyed. In this way we find that most plants and animals are poorly fossilised.
2. Several examples of the cracking of rocks have been found. The cracking may be caused by tension. Many such rocks containing fossils have been destroyed in the world's history.
3. Fossil formation generally takes place at the bottom of sea. Many land animals and plants could find no chance to reach the sea.
4. Sometimes the superficial rocks are flown away with the moving glaciers due to which the deeper strata are exposed and these exposed strata are eroded by wind and water destroying the fossils preserved there. This incompleteness of fossils record does not give a complete picture of progressive evolution.
5. Fossils lying at great depths have been destroyed by pressure of the overlying rock layers and heat.

Evolution of horse

This history of horse dates back to about 60 million years in the eocene period, involving about 20 genera. The horse phylogeny starts with *Hyracotherium* (including *Eohippus*) a member of Equidae. This animal was a little less than a foot high, the teeth were 44 and the check teeth were only moderately specialised for grinding. The front foot had four toes and a splint and hind foot with three toes and two splints. The line of a descent perhaps passed from *Hyracotherium* through *Mesohippus, Miohippus, Parahippus, Merychippus* and *Pliohippus* to *Equus*, which represents the modern horse and its allies.

In the above transition, changes were brought about from the size of fox to that of horse. The teeth became specialised for grinding coarse siliceous grasses. These changes were associated with elongation of jaws. The limbs were elongated and the toes were lost. The metacarpels and metatarsals were fused. The neck became much longer and mobile.

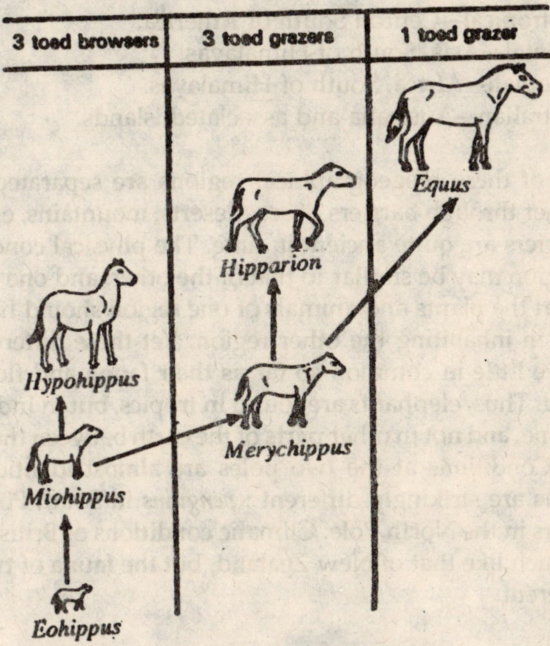

Fig. 2.16. Evolution of horse.

VI. EVIDENCES FROM GEOGRAPHICAL DISTRIBUTION

The geographical distribution or *biography* of animals and plants on the earth give a clear understanding of the organic evolution theory (*Wallace*). Geographical distribution may also be called a study of the *horizontal distribution* of organisms known as *spatical distribution* of the earth's surface at a given time. The distribution of animals is governed by many factors such as environment, temperature, availability of required type and amount of food, salinity, enemies, topography and barriers.

On the basis of similarity and differences of fauna and flora in different regions, the world has been divided into following six biogeographical regions.

(a) Nearctic—North America down to the Mexican Plateau.
(b) Palearctic—Asia North of the Himalayas, Europe and Africa, North of Sahara Desert.
(c) Neotropical—Central South of America.
(d) Oriental—Asia, South of Himalayas.
(e) Ethiopian—Africa, South of Himalayas.
(f) Australian—Australia and associated islands.

Most of these biogeographical regions are separated from one another through barriers of sea, deserts, mountains, etc. and these barriers are quite ancient in time. The physical conditions of one region may be similar to that of the other, and one would expect that the plants and animals of one region should have no difficulty in inhabiting the other region. Yet these different regions have little in common so far as their fauna and flora are concerned. Thus, elephants are found in tropics, but in India and Africa alone, and not in other parts of the earth between the same latitude. Conditions at the two poles are almost identical but their fauna are strikingly different : *penguins* in South Pole and polar bears in the North Pole. Climatic conditions of British Isles is very much like that of New Zealand, but the fauna of two are very different.

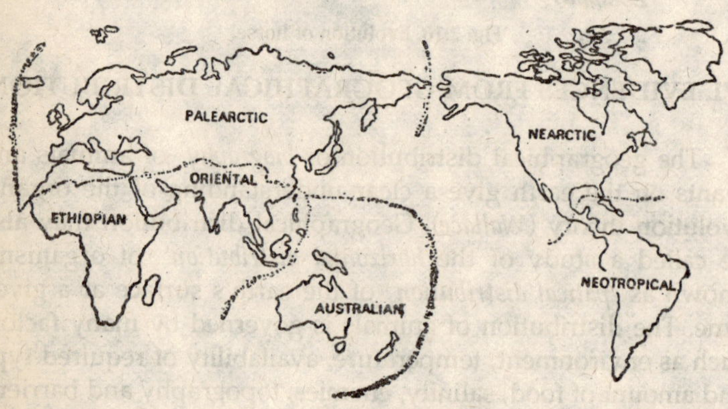

Fig. 2.17. Geographical Regions.

Marsupials are restricted to Australia and South America (with the exception of North American *Opossums*). *Anthropoid apes* occur in isolated areas in West Africa and South East Asia. On the other hand, dogs, mice among mammals, thrushes, swallows and plovers among birds and many families of insects are examples of almost universal distribution. The fauna of West of Africa (elephant, antelopes and gorilla) is entirely different from that of Brazil (tapirs, sloths and monkeys with prehensile tails). Distances also do not destribution. The fauna of West of Africa (elephant, antelopes and gorilla) is entirely different from that of Brazl (tapirs, sloths and monkeys with prehensile tails). Distances also do not determine determine distribution. Great Britain and Japan separated by long distances possess similar fauna while the islands of Bali and Lombock separated by only a sea of 15 miles distance contain entirely different faunas.

The above facts cannot be explained by the theory of special creation ; but the explanation lies in the doctrine of organic evolution. The dissimilarities in the fauna and flora of regions having identical environmental conditions, can be interpreted as under :

1. Each species has originated only once. They originate in all habitats at all times.
2. Each species tends to expand from its centre of origin and this migration is blocked by physical or climatic barriers.
3. New species can arise only in isolation and hence related species tend to found in adjacent areas.
4. Due to geological changes or action of enemies in the course of time, extension took place in large areas. This resulted in *Discontinuous distribution.*

VII. EVIDENCES FROM CYTOLOGY

Animals are made up of the aggregates of cells. The fundamental structure of a cell is similar throughout the animals kingdom. It consists of nucleus, cytoplasm and the surrounding cell membrane. Process of cell division (mitosis and meiosis) are also the same throughout the animal kingdom. The only explanation is that all the animals had a common origin.

VIII. EVIDENCES FROM GENETICS

The final line of evidence for evolution is drawn from Genetics, the science of heredity and variations. Hereditary variations on which the whole idea of organic evolution is based will result only through the application of certain basic principles of genetics. There are mainly two sources of hereditary variations namely, recombination and mutation. While recombinations after hybridization will yield new combinations, mutations will create new genetic material which never existed earlier.

Examples of hybridization and mutations are available which show that evolution has taken place. Man has tried to cross different species of animals to give rise hybrid. Besides artificial hybrids, there are some naturally occurring hybrids in plants.

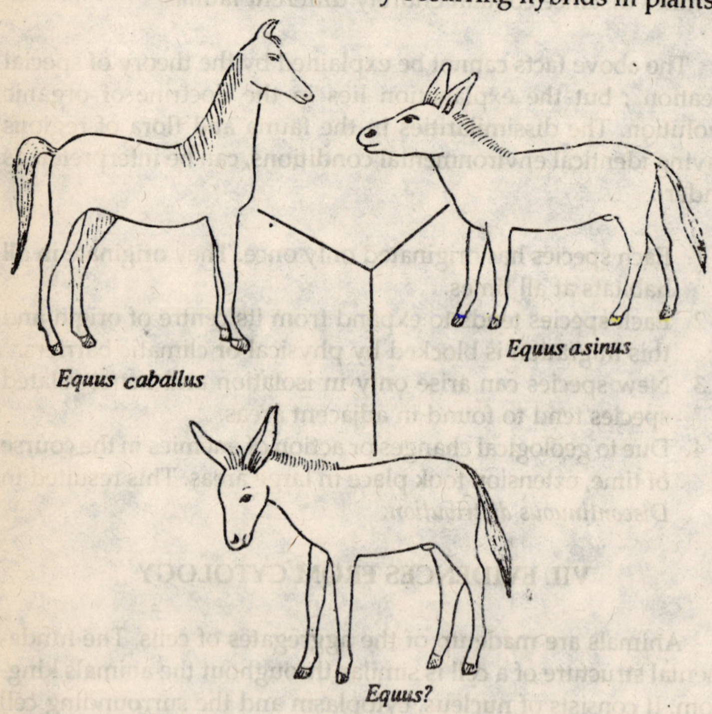

Fig. 2.18 Mule, an offspring of mare and jackass

A *mule* is the offspring of a jackass (*Equus asinus*) and a mase (*Equus calabus*) is sterile hybrid. Natural hybrids in animals are among butterflies, moths, crickets, fresh water fishes, toads and ducks. Hybridization is uncommon in reptiles and birds. Changes in the basic number of chromosome can occur due to breakage and reunion of chromosomes.

Different kinds of mutations-namely gross mutation due to variation in chromosome number (polyploidy and aneuploidy), and point mutations (see chapter of mutation) introduce different kinds of variations in plant and animals are consequently result in *speciation*. Plant breeders have employed induced polyploidy methods in producing numerous economically important varieties of plants. Geneticists have produced many new strains of micro-organisms, plants and animals (*Drosophila*) by artificially inducing point mutations in them.

Mutations form the raw materials for evolution. Experimental data with induced mutations proves beyond any doubt "descent with modification". The cross breeding in animals and plants has frequently resulted in the production of sudden and unpredictable new types from older parent types.

3

LAMARCKISM

Until the middle of the 18th century, there was a firm and widespread belief in spontaneous creation and the fixity of species. The idea that living organisms are subject to constant change in structure and habit was first developed by a French biologist, Buffon in his *Histoire Naturelle* (1749-67) and later elaborated slightly by *Erasmus Darwin* in long paper entitled *Zoonomia* (1749). Although they accepted the idea of evolution, they did not propose any hypothesis to explain the means by which it might come about.

LAMARCKISM

The first extensive and coherent theory of evolution was put forward by *Jean Baptiste Lamarck* (French) in his *Philosophic Zoologique* in 1816.

Lamarck was very much impressed by the effect of environment on plants and animals. His conclusions are summarized as follows :

(1) The internal forces of life tend to increase the size of an organism i.e. the whole body and also the different parts upto a limit which it brings about itself. (There is gradual increase in size).

(2) The production of a new organ in an animal body results from the arisal and continuance of a new need, and from the new movement which, this need brings into being and sustains. (New need produces new organ).

(3) The degree of development and their forces of action are directly proportional to their use, continuous use strengthening the organ while disuse have reverse effect.

(4) All that has been acquired, imprinted or changed in the organization of the individual during the course of its life is preserved by generation and transmitted to the new individuals that descend from the individual so modified. (Acquired characters are inherited).

The fourth principle, that is, acquired characters are inherited is the most attractive and controversial law, now known as *'Lamarckism'* or *'Lamarckian doctrine'*.

Analysis of Lamarck's Theory

(I) The first of his law is the statement of a supposed fact, which is regarded to be universally far from truth. While the evolutionary trend in certain groups may be associated with increase of size, there are a number of cases, where evolution proceeded not only without any increase in size but rather through a reduction in size. In several groups of plants such a reduction in size can be seen.

(II) According to 2nd law of *Lamarck*, the development and efficiency of an organ is in proportion to the use of that organ. If an organ is used constantly, it will tend to become highly developed and if it is not used by the organism, then it would atrophy or may disappear altogether in the course of future generations.

(III) The law of use and disuse of organ appears satisfactory and is supported by the following evidences :

1. Giraffe is found in forest of Africa. In an attempt to catch the leaves of the branches, high above the ground, its neck went on elongating and attained the present day form. In this effort, his front legs were also used alongwith the neck, as a result of which the legs were lengthened with the stretching of neck. This change was inherited to the offsprings gradually and caused the evolution of present giraffe.
2. The snakes live in bushy places and therefore they have got a long body. *Lamarck* explained that the ancestors of the snakes were 4 limbed and tried to conceal themselves in the bushes. This required creeping habit and elongated body. These efforts resulted into aborted limbs and elongated body of snake. The locomotion was carried by the abdomen.

3. The flat fishes (flounder) have their both eyes on one side of the body. It is assumed that the ancestors of these fishes used to turnover to one side of the body in order to swim over in shallow water. They, therefore, made efforts to bring both the eyes on the upper side. This adaptation was inherited and all the flat fishes now have their eyes on one side.
4. Ducks and allied birds, when did not get enough food on land, they were forced to search it in water. Here they spread their toes and stretched their legs for wading purpose, resulting into webbed feet and long legs.
5. An athelete or a wrestler has at the peak of his training more powerful muscles than a bed ridden individual who has powerless leg muscles due to his protected illness. A black-smith develops a large and strong *biceps* muscle due to his constantly pounding on his anvil.
6. The forelimbs in birds have developed into wings with which they fly, but then continuous disuse in Ostrich and Kiwi has resulted in their reduction and weakness.

The third law of *use* and *disuse* of organs is true but it does not form a principle of evolution except in conjunction with the fourth law of *inheritance of acquired characters.*

(IV) The inheritance of the characters acquired during the life time of an individual is the fourth postulate and is an essential requirement, if the modifications produced due to changes in environment, have to have an evolutionary significance.

Lamarck recognized that such structural changes, irrespective of whether they are progressive or retrogressive, acquired by the individual during its life span are inherited or transmitted to the offspring.

Origin of New Species. Lamarck considered that existing individual is the sum total of characters acquired by its ancestors in the preceding several generations, so that the present form is so markedly different from is ancestors, that it has become a new species.

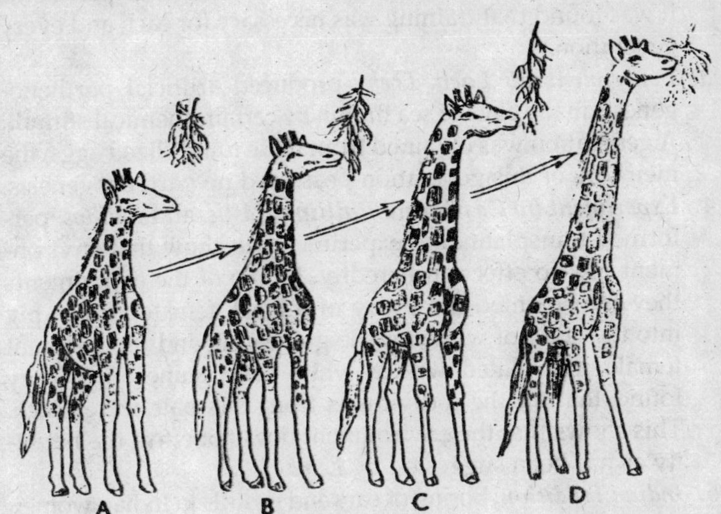

Fig. 3.1. A=Original short necked ancestor of Giraffe,
B=Keep stretching the neck,
C=and stretching, D=Until neck becomes progressively longer.

The evolutionary theory of *Lamarck* was strongly supported by *E. Geoffroy* (1772-1844).

CRITICISM OF LAMARCKISM. All experiments performed to test this postulate gave negative results with the possible exception of McDougall's experiments on rats. Following are some objections to Lamarckism.

1. ***Experiment by Weismann. August Weismann*** was the first who for the first time made a definite distinction between heritable changes and those which cannot be inherited. In 1890, he performed some experiments to test if characters disappear due to disuse. This he did by cutting the tails (*mutilation*) of white mice for more than 20 generations to see if this has any effect on tail length. The measuring of tail length of the offsprings of 20 successive generations, revealed that on average, the tail were not shorter. It means that acquired character (cut tail) was not inherited.
2. ***Experiment by Pavlov***. *Pavlov,* a Russian scientist, wanted to show the inheritance of learning. He trained the mice to

come for food on hearing the bell. But in later experiments it was found that training was necessary for each and every generation.

3. *Experiment by Loeb. Loeb* produced artificial parthenogenesis in the eggs of sea urchin by certain chemical stimuli. A generation was obtained from these unfertilized eggs, the members of this generation possessed no parthenogenesis.
4. *Experiment by Castle and Phillips. Castle* and *Phillips* performed transplantation experiments to show that environment has no effect on heredity. In one of the experiments they transplanted the ovary of a black female guinea pig into the body of white female guinea pig and the recipient female was mated with a white male guinea pig. They found that all the individuals from this pair were black. This shows that the environment does not effect the heredity as has been suggested by *Lamarck*.
5. *Indian Tradition*. Boring of ears and nostrils in Indian women has been continued from centuries but their female offsprings do not show any trace of holes in ears and nostrils.
6. Chinese women use iron shoes to keep their feet short but young ones at birth have normal size.
7. Muslim and Jewish boys have been circumcised for so many years, yet this has not resulted in a tendency towards the reduction of the produce in them.

Besides the above, there are evidences which support that acquired characters are inherited from generation to generation. These are as follow :

1. *Guyer and Smith's experiment. Guyer* and *Smith* crushed the crystalline lens of the eye of rabbit and inoculated it into fowl which developed antibodies. The antiserum of fowl (the fowl serum containing antibodies) was injected into pregnant rabbits. Some of the offsprings of rabbits were born with defective eyes and this character was inherited in successive generations.
2. *Experiment by McDougall. McDougall* trained the rats to escape the water tank only through the dark route as against the lighted route. This training was continued through several generations in the progency which make fewer and fewer

mistakes in succeeding generations.

Agar et at. (1954) also repeated the experiments of *Mc-Dougall* for 50 generations, covering a period of 20 years. They got clear evidence against the hypothesis that effects of training are inherited.

3. ***Experiment by Brown Sequard.*** Various diseases like *Exopthalmia, Haematoma* and *Dry gangrene* are inherited from generation to generation by injuries in the restiform body of the brain shown by *Brown sequard*.
4. ***Melanism in moth.*** *Haslop Harrison* claims to have induced the formation of melanic mutants by feeding larvae of moth (*Selenia bilunaria*) on hawthorn leaves which had absorbed small quantities of salts of magnesium and lead. This has reference to the spread of melanic forms in the industrial areas of England.
5. ***Experiment by Lindsey.*** *Lindsey* subjected certain cold-blooded animals, warm-blooded animals and plants to unusual environmental conditions and found that environment affect certain changes in these organisms and these acquired modifications were inherited upto some extent in their offsprings.
6. ***Experiment by Summer.*** *F.B. Summer* reared the white mice at 20°C to 30°C. He found that they developed longer bodies, tail and feet. When these mice were bred at lower temperatures their offsprings showed their abnormal proportions of size from generation to generation.
7. ***Kammerer's experiments on Salamander.*** The skin of *Salamandra maculosa* is black with yellow sports. He kept some of them for four years in yellow box and found that yellow sports become much larger and united together to form a yellow band on the back. These salamanders were then mated with each other and the resulting offsprings were found to be more of yellow colour.

   In another experiment the salamanders were kept in black box due to which yellow sports reduced and their offsprings were black.
8. ***Inheritance of food habit.*** *Sladden* (1934-38) produced the inheritance of the acquired ability of stick insects (*Dixippus morouns*) to subsists upon ivy (plant) instead of their normal diet privet (plant) after repeated forced feeding trials through

six generations.

9. ***Tower's experiment of potato beetles.*** *Tower* found that exposing the young stages of potato beetles to extreme conditions of temperature and moisture, produce marked changes in offsprings and these modifications were inherited from generations to generations.
10. ***Experiments by Griffith and Detlefson.*** *Griffith* and *Detlefson* reared the rats in cages placed on rotating tables for several months. The rats were adapted to rotating conditions to such an extend that when the rotation was stopped, they showed signs of dizziness (*nystagmus*). This condition was inherited for several generations.

NEO LAMARCKISM

In the present century, the scientists have again started thinking on Lamarckism and supporting it on the basis of many evidences. They are trying to fit it in modern science. These scientists are call *Neo Lamarckians* and the modernised theory of *Lamarck* is known as *Neo Lamarckism*. Among the neo-Lamarckians notable supporters are *Herbert Spencer, Eimer, Cope, Hyatt, Naegeli, Dall, Haeckel* and *Gadow.*

At present the concept of Neo-Lamarckism is :

(i) Developed characters (whether acquired or not) are never transmitted by heredity and the hereditary constitution of the germ is not changed by changes in such character.
(ii) Possibly the environmental stimuli act upon germ cells at an early stage in their development. This may rarely cause changes in hereditary constitution ; but changes produced in somatic cells, by environment, do not cause corresponding changes in the hereditary constitution of germ cells.
(iii) Germ cells may undergo modifications which are not hereditary. Such influence may be carried over to next generation without becoming hereditary. All such cases are called *induction.* And many instances of supposed inheritance of acquired characters come under this category.
(iv) Environment may profoundly modify individual development but it does not generally modify heredity.

Thus neo-Lamarckism is neither a complete denial nor the complete acceptance of the old Lamarckism. It is merely, a slight modification of inheritance of acquired character and it explains the appearance of acquired characters in a few succeeding generations by after effect or induction.

4

THEORY OF NATURAL SELECTION

Charles Darwin was an English Naturalist. He was born on 12th February 1809 in Shrewsbury. After his school education he was send to Edinberg for medical studies but finding medicine unsuited to his taste, he entered Christ's College, Cambridge. After graduation, it was with *Dr. Henslow* that *Darwin* later had the privilege of going in voyaga to exploration on the famous *H.M.S. Beagle* (a vessel that explored *S. America*, the *Galapagos island* and other regions). Soon after his return he read an essay of *Thomas Malthus* (*Malthus on Population*) in 1838 and was greatly impressed by the alarming potential speed of multiplication of the human race. After 1854, Darwin devoted all his time to the writing of "Origin of species". In 1858 *Alfred Russel Wallace* (a young English naturalist) sent a short essay entitled, "On the tendency of varieties to depart indefinitely from the original type", for Darwin's advice. Since *Darwin* thought well of Wallace's work, Darwin's work was jointly published with Wallace's paper entitled". The Theory of Natural selection", in the Proceedings of the Linnaen Socicty". In 1859, *Darwin* published his findings full in a book, "The Origin of Species". The publication of this book was the important event in the biological history and it was regarded as the most important book of the 19th Century.

Darwin produced a large number of books, some of which are listed in the following table :

Table. 4.1 : Some publications of Charles Darwin

	Title of Book	*Year of publication*
1.	The Structure and Distribution of Coral Reefs	1842
2.	Geological Observations on Volcanic Islands.	1844

3. Geological Observations on South America. 1846
4. 'A Monograph on Cirripedia' (four volumes) 1851, 1854
5. Origin of Species. 1859
6. The Fertilization of Orchids. 1862
7. The Variation of Plants and Animals under Domestication. 1868
8. The Descent of Man. 1871
9. The Expression of the Emotions in Men and Animals. 1872
10. Insectivorous Plants. 1875
11. The Effects of Cross and Self-Fertilization in the Vegetable Kingdom. 1876
12. Different Forms of Flowers on Plants of the same Species. 1877
13. The Power of Movement in Plants. 1880
14. The Formation of Vegetable Mould Through the Action of Worms. 1881

Darwin died on 19th April 1882, when he was 73 years old.

Natural selection is one of the most important facts of evolution. It is a continuous and real process. The elements of this theory may be enumerated as follows :

1. Prodigality of Nature

Darwin accepted that in nature every animal and plant shows an extensive rate of multiplication. The power of reproduction, in animals, is much greater than their requirement to maintain their number. For instance, the elephant is slowest breeder among the mammals but *Darwin* concluded that a single pair is able to breed at 30 years of age and continue to do so until 100 years age. They produce on the average six children and would have in 750 years about 19 million from the same parent. Similarly a Salmon produces 28,000,000 eggs in a season.

With the invertebrates the power of production is very higher. *Huxley* estimated that the descendants of a single pair of green fly, if all survived and multiplied would at the end of summer, weight down the population of China. Similarly, an Oyster may pass as many as 114,000,000 eggs at a single spawning. A starfish lays 1,000,000 eggs in a year. *Woodrulff* after his studies on *Paramecium* found that if a race is maintained for five years, and if all the descendants of one wild individual survive and multiply their volume of protoplasm will approximately be equal to thousand times the volume of the earth. Not the animals, the same condition is with plants. For example : a single plant of *Amaranthus* may produce 2,000,000 seeds; a single orchid flower may yield more than a million seeds; a fern may scatter more than 2,000,000 spores during its life cycle.

It is therefore evident, that the number of a species would soon become enormous if all the offsprings survived and reproduced because the rate of increase is geometric. But, on the other hand, it is an observed fact that the number of a species remain constant to a fair degree. The number never approaches the size calculated from the reproductive rate. It is clear therefore that the difference between the calculated rate and the observed number must be due to the severe struggle for existence.

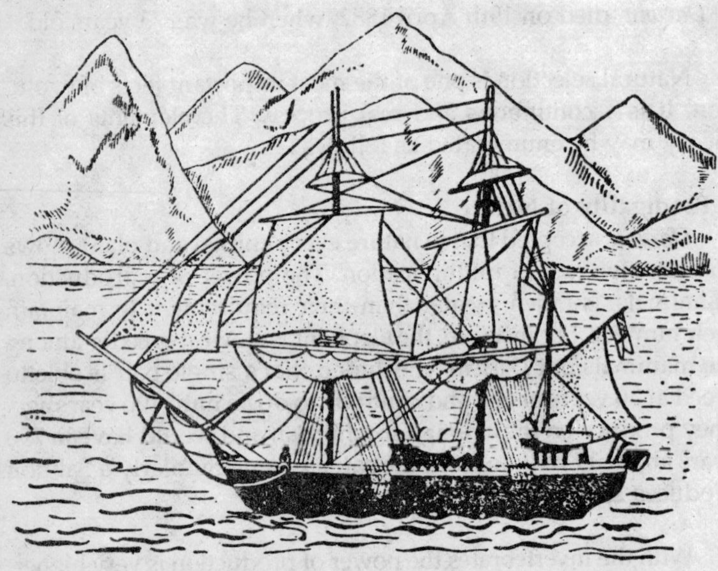

Fig. 4.1. Diagram of The Beagle in which Darwin sailed around the world.

2. Struggle for Existence

The struggle for existence is the competition between all the organisms and between each individual and the physical environment. This competition or struggle is for the survival and may be classified as :

a. *Instraspecific struggle*

This type of struggle is found within the species i.e. similar kind of organisms. In most cases it is most severe check up of the rate of reproduction. In forests young and smaller trees often die due to lack of sufficient food, moisture, light and mineral etc. In animals also when a number of offsprings are produced and if they do not get sufficient accommodations, they struggle for life. Cannibulistic selection is most severe one. It is found that in artificial lobster culture the braver ones feed their brother and sisters.

b. *Interspecific struggle*

This type of struggle is found between different groups of animals. The total number of persons killed by animals (tigers, leopards, elephants etc.) recorded in 1925, in India, was 2,585. The number of deaths from snake bite was 19,258. In plant kingdom a number of plants are destroyed by man, animals, insects and other predators.

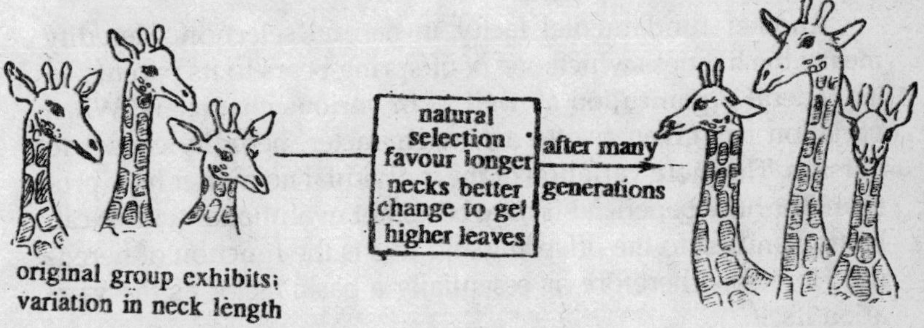

Fig. 4.2. Giraffes to show Darwin's idea about their elongation of neck.

c. *Environmental struggle*

Animals and plants also struggle with the adverse environmental conditions, e.g., excess of moisture, drought, heat, cold, and also the lightening, earthquake, volcanic eruptions etc. In 1908 in Japanese earthquake, 4,63,000 souls were destroyed. Several other cases of such type of struggle are found throughout the world.

The struggle may occur at any stage of the life cycle. Obviously this results in an equilibrium among the species growing in a particular region. Such an equilibrium persists so long so factors tending to disturb this equilibrium do not arise.

3. Variation

It is a progressive factor in evolution for without variation no change would occur and evolution would be impossible. It is also evident after observation that no two individuals are alike and the requirements of any two individuals are not exactly the same.

Darwin recognized two principal kinds of variations (a) *continuous variations* showing the whole range of variation in a particular character, and (b) *discontinuous variations* which appear all of a sudden and show no gradation. This second class of variations were called as *sports*, which were later called "mutations" by *de Vries, Darwin* though that only the continuous variations are important for evolution.

4. Heredity

Another fundamental factor in natural selection. Heredity means the likeness which one of offspring bears to its parents, in its general organization as well as in various characters. When variation has given rise to a new character, heredity causes to persists. The mere variation of the individual no matter how profound or how beneficial it may be, is not evolutional until it can be transmitted to the offspring and this is the function of heredity. Heredity, therefore, is essentially a basic factor as the variation itself.

5. Natural Selection or Survival of Fittest

Darwin regarded that in the struggle for existence those individuals, which are provided with favourable variations, will lead a more successful life and would survive and propagate their offsprings. It is called *Natural Selection* by *Darwin* and *Survival of Fittest* by *Herbert Spencer*.

According to *Darwin* several variations take part in the process of natural selection and these small variations gradually lead to the formation of species and sub species.

An interesting aspect of the problem was, that *Darwin* was not aware of the cause of variation and also knew nothing about heredity, for he never came across Mendel's work ; yet he was conscious of it. To explain his hypothesis of inheritance of acquired character *Darwin* proposed his *theory of pangenesis.* According to this theory all organs of an individual produce *Pangenes,* which are minute particles carrying information about the organs. The pangenes travelling through the blood stream will ultimately reach the gametes, so that each gamete will have panagenes from each of the different organism. After zygote formation, the pangenes tend to form the same organs from which these pangenes were produced. In 1875, *Galton* made pangenesis hypothesis untenable by presenting several experimental proofs.

ORIGIN OF NEW SPECIES

Darwin believed that inheritance of useful variations into the offsprings continued through many generations resulting in slow but increasing modification of the species towards their better adaptation for survival in the environment. Due to the cumulative effect of all these variations, gathered through many generations, individuals with character markedly different from those of their original ancestors, were formed which are termed as new species.

A species is a group of similar individuals, which breed freely into one another but not into members of other such groups.

The theory of *Darwin* can be summarised according to *Wallace* in the following way :

S.No.	*Proved fact*	*Consequences*
1.	Geometric ratio of increase	
2.	Total number of survivors roughly stationary	Struggle for existence
3.	Struggle for existence	
4.	Variation and heredity transmission	Survival of fittest or Natural selection
5.	Survival of fittest	Origin of new species or
6.	Environmental changes	Structural modification

CRITICISM AND OBJECTIONS TO DARWINISM

There are several objections against Darwin's theory of natural selection.

1. *Lack of experimental proof.* He believed in the effectiveness of natural selection was a logical detection from the facts of life of the organisms in nature as *Darwin* knew them, but he had no experimental evidence in the favour of it. It was an unavoidable conclusion from the condition of life.
2. *Johannsen* made experiments to increase the size of *Paramecium* by selecting the largest ones but no improvement could be made *Locke* tried to improve the quality of sugarcane. First there was increase in the content of sugar but very soon it became constant. When the strain became genetically pure, no difference could be made. Similarly *Agar* tried to increase the size of the carapace (a hard covering on body) of water flea (a beetle), but slight or no variation he could get.
3. It does not explain the causes of variations.
4. *Darwin* based his theory upon the idea that minute fluctuating variations, which are to a large extent non-heritable, were the principal if not the sole material for natural selection to work upon.
5. *Darwin* in fact considered all variations as heritable. Today we know that only those variations are inherited which are germinal not the somatic.
6. The theory dwells upon the inheritance of acquired characters, which is not correct.
7. Natural selection is said to be incapable to explain the origin of co-ordinated structures and highly complex organs whose effectiveness depends upon the perfection. For example electric organs of fishes.
8. The theory of natural selection does not give an adequate explanation of the occurrence of vestigial organs generation after generation.
9. The theory of natural selection does not give explanation of mimicry.
10. Sometimes certain characters in an animals develop upto a stage that they surpass their usefulness and become harm-

ful to the possessor. Example Irish Elk. (overspecialization), mammoth etc.

11. Absence of connecting links cannot be explained on the basis of this theory.
12. Theory of Pangenesis also lacks experimental support.
13. The theory underlines the occurrence of repeated variations in the same direction, which is wrong because the variations may follow a diverse course.
14. It is objected that natural selection might explain the survival but not the arrival of the fittest.
15. Special objection was raised to the theory of sexual selection proposed by *Darwin*. The theory involves passivity on the part of male and an active choice on the part of female of a more beautiful, attractive and more powerful male.

NEO DARWINISM

Darwin's theory of Natural Selection was accepted by the biologists of the 1900. The supporter of Darwinism were, *Wallace, T.H. Huxley, Haeckel, Weismann* etc. There are several evidences which have been put forwarded to prove Darwinism. These supporters are known as *Neo Darwinians*. Some of the evidences are as follow :

1. Production of various domesticated varieties by artificial selection.
2. In Austria, Hungary there is a zone of 600 m. which is divided into eight stages. In all these eight stages a transition, from shell-less to shelled molluscs are found.
3. *Censola* performed several experiments by the selective value of mimicry. He fixed several specimens of *Mantis religosa* on the plants. He observed that those having colour markings harmonious with the background survived, whereas other were devoured by birds.
4. *Davenport* took a few chicken, which were black, white, barred and checkered colour pattern. He allowed them free in fields. It was observed that hawk killed majority of white chickens, many of black coloured but those with barred and checkered type were spared, as they were less conspicuous and difficult to detect against the surroundings.

5. *Weldon* found out that because of the variations caused by the process of natural selection and changes in environments, new changed species are formed. He conducted his experiments on the shore crabs of Plymouth sound. He placed a large break water near the mouth of plymouth sound. This slowed the rate of flow of river water and China-clay deposition was increased, results in the death of numerous crabs. The survivors, had a slightly narrow frontum and there was a progressive narrowing in succeeding generation of the species *Carsinus moenae.*

The progress of evolutionary theory in the last 30 years is a complex subject because a number of new facts have been added to the knowledge of evolution. The theory of Natural Selection has been rearranged. At the time of *Darwin* and his contemporaries, there was no knowledge of genetics and cytology. The researches on these subjects started later and the work of *Mendel* was recognized only in 1900. The Neo-Darwanian included such outstanding scholars as *Dobzhansky, Stebbins, Ernst Mayer, J. Huxley, Wright* etc. who performed many experiments which removed several defects of Darwanism. Modern Neo-Darwinian stressed the significance of mutation against Lamarck's theory of acquired characters. Mutation can be defined as "Any alteration in the chemistry of gene which is able to change its effect is known as gene mutation". Generally, new species are formed by mutations in genes. Mutations have also been produced artificially through radiation. *Ronald Fischer* and *Wright* have suggested mathematical formulae so as to deal with theoretical genetics of entire population. *Fisher* showed that dominance of useful genes over the less useful allelomorphs (alleles) is due to natural selection. Mutation occurs at a definite rate which is known as *mutation pressure.* Natural selection, mutations, and heredity all together and with other factors produce less evolved changes.

The modern concept of evolutionary theory is now more intricate and complex due to the knowledge of *gene-pools* than individual. Darwinism has become much more complex but there has been no changes in its basic form. In this way, Darwinism has been approved and has withstood the testimony of the criticism.

5

MUTATION THEORY

Hugo De Vries (1848-1935), a Dutch Botanist, on the basis of his studies on a number of plants, put forth his views on the origin of species, in 1901, confirming some of the objections to Darwin's theory of Natural Selection. He was of the opinion that the new species arise not by accumulation through natural selection of minute fluctuating variations but by sudden appearance which he called *mutations*. It is also possible that such new species may continue to live side by side with their parent species. According to *De Vries* the mutations may be advantageous or disadvantageous and are heritable. *Bateson* (1894) called these sudden changes as *discontinuous* or *salutatory variations*.

De Vries began a systematic research for species of plants in nature that were giving rise to new species. Many species were examined in their natural surroundings and were then brought into the experimental garden for more careful observation. Finally in a field near Hilversum, in the vicinity of Amsterdem. In 1887, he noticed two distinct varieties of evening primrose (*Oenothera lamarckiana*) differing in the length of stem and colour; shape of flower and colour, and form of leaves. These were *O. brevistylis* and *O.laevifolia*. *O.laevifolia* is distinguished from Lamarck's evening primrose by its smooth narrower leaves.

O. lrevistylis is characterized by its short-styled flowers. The leaves are more rounded at the top.

Further breeding of these two distinct forms, by him, showed that they bred true to their own characteristics. *De Vries* continued with the breeding of these distinct forms and in later years discovered. that these further gave rise to some more distinct forms which, otherwise would have been classified as different species, had they passed unobserved. In them, the differences were well marked in the habit of growth, colour of the stem, shape of the leaves, size of the flowers and size and distribution of the seed capsules; *De Vries* gave them the name of 'elementary species' or 'primary species'.

The other varieties produced by *O. lamarckiana* are *O. nannella, O. gigas* and *O. rubrinervis*.

O. nannella is a dwarf and most attractive plant. The leaves are broader and shorter.

O. gigas is giant event primrose consisting of stout stem often twice the diameter than that of *O. lamarckina*. The leaves are broad, of a deeper green colour and leaf bladers are sharply set off against the stalk.

O. rubrinervis or red-veined evening primrose is more slender than *O. gigas*.

Besides above varieties there occurred two weak forms that could survive only if reared under protection and would have failed to survive in nature. These are *O. albida* and *O. oblonga*.

O. lata had only pistillate flowers and therefore, could not be fertilized by pollen of the same mutant. *O. scintillans* and *O. elliptica* are fertile to their own pollen but produce progeny only partly like the parent, the rest reverting to the original type (*O. lamarckiana*).

On the basis of these sudden changes, mutation theory was proposed which can be summed up in five main points as follow:

1. New species evolve, not gradually with transitional forms, but by sudden and distinct heritable changes called *mutations*.
2. The first individual showing a mutation is called *mutant*. It is pure breedings. Obviously it transmits its variations to its offsprings and thus starts a new species.

3. Mutations are large and sudden and are totally different fluctuating variations of *Darwin*, which are small and directional. They may occur is any direction.
4. Mutations are intermediate; one or more parts of mutant may undergo abnormally better or poor growth, or may ever completely disappear or altogether new part may appear. Thus mutation may be advantageous or disadvantageous.
5. Being intermediate, different mutations may occur in different members of same species giving rise to several related new species simultaneously from the same ancestral species.

Several workers such as *McDougall* and *Shull* in America and *Gates* in England have fully supported that the views of *De Vries*. However, some suggest that the 'elementary species' of *De Vries* are simply the Mendelian crosses of hybrid *Oenothera lamarckiana*. But the different number of chromosomes in each 'elementary species' of the genus is a sufficient proof of their being true species and not merely the Mendelian combinations. For instance *Oenothera Lamarckiana* has 14 chromosomes as its diploid number and the new species resulting from mutation were found to have 15, 16, 20, 22, 24, 27, 28, 29 and 30 as their chromosome number.

CRITICISM OF MUTATION THEORY

Morgan (1909), *Muller* (1912) and other studied the occurrence of mutation in animals and plants. However, the theory of *De Vries* was widely criticized on the point that, "new species arose only by mutation".

The main objections are as follow :

1. *Davis* discredited mutation theory by claiming that *O.lamarckiana* is of hybrid nature, which could be produced by crossing two wild American species. *Jaffreys* and *Gates* also confirmed *Davis* view. *Balkeslee* studies on *Datura* and *Morgan* on *Dorosophila* have shown that origin of species (as described by *De Vries*) is by no means exceptional but is a common thing among the plants.

2. Mutations may rander the possessor so much different from other members of the species that they generally fail to complete with the others and, therefore, perish. Being random they are harmful.
3. Mutations cannot explain the presence of flightless birds on oceanic islands.
4. Though mutations are quite frequent in certain plants like *Oenothera, Datura,* Boston ferns and a few animals yet they have never been found in certain groups of animals and plants.

Very recently, with the advancement of general science, the theory of mutations has been studied in more details. In the broadest sense, the changes in the genetic material are called *mutations*. Mutations fall in two categories :

1. Gene mutations or point mutations : Gene mutations are those which are caused by chemical alteration of individual genes.
2. Chromosomal mutations or chromosomal observations : These are involved in the loss, multiplication or arrangement of genes in the chromosomes.

1. Gene mutations

A change in a very segment of DNA (deoxyribonucleic acid); usually considered to involve a single nucleotide or nucleotide pair.

Gene mutations may occur due to following types :

(a) *Deletion mutations* : It is caused due to loss or deletion of some portion in a tiplet codon of a gene.
(b) *Insertion mutation* : It is caused due to addition of one or more extra nucleotides to a gene.
(c) *Substitution mutation* : It is caused due to substitution or replacement of one nucleotide by another. It is of two types:
    (i) *Transition mutation* substitutes one purine for another or one pyrimidine for another.
    (ii) *Transversion mutation* substitutes a purine for a pyrimidine or vice versa.

2. Chromosomal mutations

Mutations due to change in the whole set of chromosomes are called chromosomal mutations. Chromosomal mutations are of two types.

(A) ***Change in the number of chromosomes***

Each species has a fixed number of chromosomes. The gametic chromosome number constitute a basic set of chromosomes called *genome*. A gamete contains single genome called *haploid*. A somatic cell contains two genomes called *diploid*. Sometimes the number in chromosomes in a haploid or diploid cell does not remain constant and may result in mutations. These variation in the numbers of chromosomes is of two types :

(i) Euploidy and (ii) Aneuploidy.

(i) *Euploidy*. An increase or decrease in the chromosomes by multiples of the haploid number is euploidy. It may be monoploid, triploid, tetraploid and so on. The increase after diploid is known as polypoidy and it is considerably phylogenetic significance in plants, although it appears to be relatively uncommon in animals. *Oenothra gigas* has been shown to tetraploid while *O. semigigas* is triploid.

(ii) *Aneuploidy*. Variation in chromosomes number may occur which do not involve whole sets of chromosomes but parts of a set. It is of following types :

(a) *Monosomic*. Loose of one of number of a pair (2n-1)
(b) *Nullisomic*. Loss of a homologous pair (2n-2)
(c) *Trisomic*. Diploids which have one extra chromosomes (2n+1)
(d) *Double trisomic*. Diploids which have two different extra chromosomes (2n+1+1)
(e) *Tetrasomic*. Diploids which have one pair of extra chromosomes (2n+2)

B. ***Changes in the chromosomes morphology***

The chromosomes are the structure with definite organization. Genes are arranged in linear fashion in them. Sometimes changes in the morphology of chromosomes have been observed resulting in mutations. These are of two types.

1. *Intrachrmosomal*. Changes occur with same or other chromosomes.

(a) *Deletion.* Results when a small piece of chromosomes becomes detached and lost.
(b) *Duplication.* Here an extra piece carrying genes may be added to a chromosome.
(c) *Inversion.* In this case, the number of genes in a chromosome is not changed but the order or sequence is changed.

2. *Inter-chromosomal*. When breaks occur in non-homologous chromosomes and resulting fragments are interchanged by both of the non-homologous chromosomes results in the inter-chromosomal aberration. It is only of one type i.e. traslocation.

Causes of Mutations

There may be several causes of mutations.

1. Cause of chromosomal aberration may be due to environmental changes such as sudden lowering of temperature during germ cell-cycle.
2. Sometimes natural or spontaneous mutations are due to chemical environment, including those chemical substances which usually come along food.
3. It has been noted that the rate of spontaneous mutations is increased with the rise of temperature.
4. Chemicals such as carcionogenic chemicals (like mustard gas) also induce mutations.
5. Mutation can also be induced by exposing the animals to X-rays (*Muller*, 1926).
6. It has recently been found out that antibodies are also capable of inducing mutations. (*Guyer* and *Smith*).

Mutagenic agents. *Muller* (1927) showed that wide variety of chemical and physical agents that can cause mutations in *Drosophila*. some of the mutagenic agents are X-rays, ultraviolet rays, radium, heát and temperature, mustard gas, hydroxylamine etc.

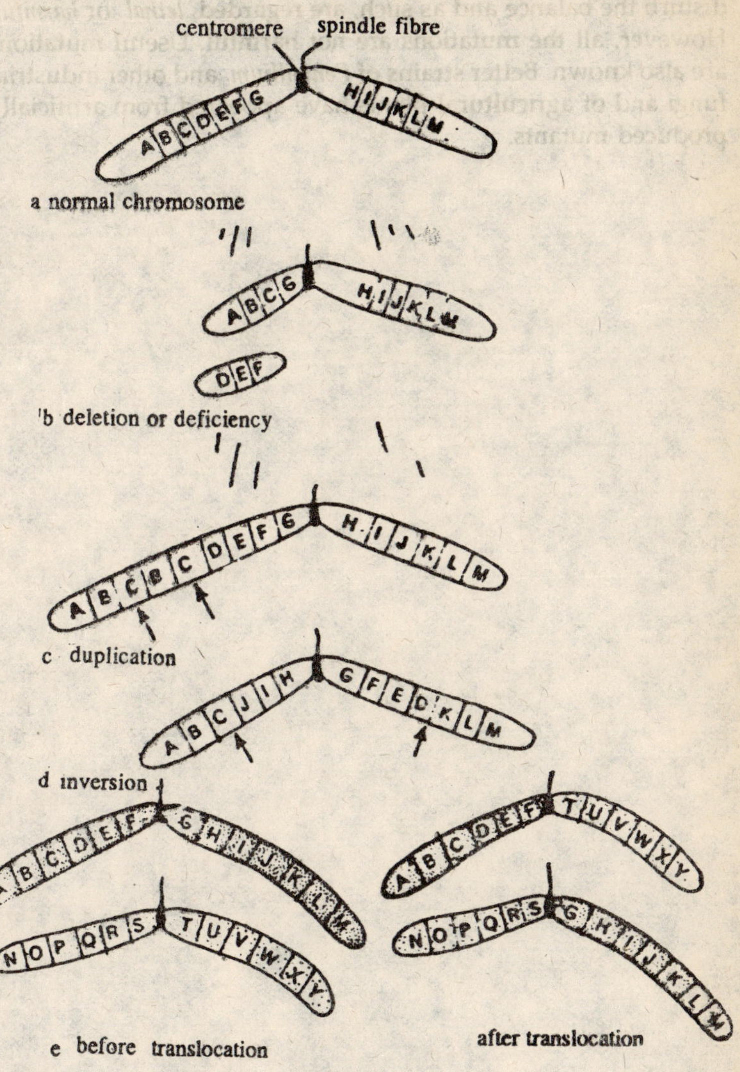

Fig. 5.1. Chromosomal abberrations.

Significance of mutations

At present mutations are considered to be raw material for evolution. Other forces of evolution like natural selection, isolation, genetic drift etc. operate on mutations to bring divergence in the naturally inbreeding populations. New mutations possibly disturb the balance and as such, are regarded, *lethal* or *harmful*. However, all the mutations are not harmful. Useful mutations are also known. Better strains of *Penicillium* and other industrial fungi and of agricultural plants have appeared from artificially produced mutants.

6

ISOLATION

According to *Metcaf*, "Anything which divides a species into groups which do not freely interferes, is said to segregate (isolate) the members of the species into these sub-divisions".

In the broadest sense, any factor may be said to play an isolating role, if it interfers with free interbreeding among all the members of a species. The new species are formed when free inter-breeding among the members of a species is checked.

The importance of isolation was first strongly insisted by *M. Wagner* (1868). *Darwin* also allowed its influence to be considerable as for instance in the production of island races. The rise of Mendelian genetics with new conception of the genotype, and population studies has only confirmed that without isolation or the preventation of inter-breeding, organic evolution is in no case possible. Like natural selection, isolation does not get to root of the problem for it does not explain the origin of variety. *Kellogg* says, "Isolation is tremendously favouring condition but not a primary cause of species disintegration, not to initiate it. It is a biological catalytic agent."

According to *Newman*, the isolation is an absolutely essential part of any complete explanation of evolution, but that it is a subsidiary factor often working in such intimate relation with natural selection and Mendelian heredity as to be almost inseparable from them. *Dobzhansky* (1937) used the term *isolating mechanism* in his book, *"Genetics of the Origin of Species."*

ISOLATING MECHANISM

The isolating mechanisms put a check on the inter-breeding amongst related species and serves as *external barriers*. There are a great many ways in which free inter-breeding may be interferred with. These are as follows :

1. Geographical isolation.
2. Spatial isolation.
3. Reproductive isolation.

1. Geographical isolation

When two populations or two parts of a population are separated by geographic barriers, it is called geographical isolation. *Wagner* (1868) was the first who mentioned that geographic isolation was a factor of condition in the formation of every species, race or tribe of animals or plants on the earth. The organisms are separated by geographical barriers, such as *land masses in seas, bodies of water over land, mountains, deserts* etc.

For example in the central Arabian desert, two races of rodent, *Meriones syrius* inhibit different stream valleys separated by only a mile of base limestone plateau. In the same way, high mountain-ranges, deserts, dense forests and extremes of temperature also act as effective barriers. Such populations are completely cut of from one another genetically. Such a type of geographic barrier is found between the fauna of an oceanic island and that of mainland. In Britain, a famous example of geographic isolation among birds has been given by *Salomosen*. The Wren, *Troglodytes troglodytes* forms distinct subspecies, on St. Kilda in the shetlands and on the other Outer Hebridean island.

S. sp.	*Locality*	*Wing length*	*Appearance*
T.t. hirtensis	St. Kilda	51-55 mm	Greyish brown above, paler under parts.
T.t. zetlandicus	Shetland Is.	50-54 mm	Darker and more bulky in appearance
T.t. hebridensis	Outer Is. Hebridean	48-53 mm	Under parts buff coloured and are less heavy.

Another interesting example of geographic isolation was given by *Gullick* as the distribution of Hawaiian land-snails. Each variety of snails occurs not only in one island but in a definite valley on the island. *Gullick's* findings were confirmed by *Crompton.*

Two species of mosquito (Genus-*Anopheles*) in Africa are separated by salinity of the water. The larvae of both can live in fresh water but one of them can endure brekish water and perhaps to avoid competition usually does live in such water.

Another example of geographical isolation is that described by *Darwin* for finches. *Darwin* found that there were 26 groups of finches among the Galapagos Islands (which lie a few hundred miles west of South America). Only five of these groups were the same as the finches found of the mainland. The other twenty-one groups interbed quite freely, while others did not. Apparently, each of the groups became isolated by migration. Each group evolved separately from the continental forms as well as from other isolated groups on the islands, forming a series of species and subspecies.

2. Spatial Isolation or Isolation due to sheer Distance

If a species ranges all over a wide extent of territory which is unbroken by barriers, there may be isolation because of great distance between extreme outlying section of the range. Its example is *wrens* (birds) of South America. Wrens are found all over the continent but the wrens of one region differ from those of the other in colour patterns, size, proportions and habits. It shows that without any barrier, sheer distance apart tends to produce local races (subspecies).

3. Reproductive isolation

The mechanisms of reproductive isolation can be varied. Most modern evolutionists such as *Mecham* (1961), *Mayr* (1948, 1970) and *Stebbins* (1966, 1971) have classified the reproductive isolation mechanism into two classes :

(a) *Prezygotic mechanism,* which either prevent contact between species at the time of active reproductive period or else the fertilization is checked even if pollination may be effectively brought about.

(b) *Postzygotic mechanisms*, where fertilization is brought about, but the hybrids are either inviable or weak, or the hybrids are sterile or in still other cases the F_1 may be fertile but F_2 progency will be sterile.

Both types of isolating mechanisms include many sub-types, all of which has been given in the table.

Table

(a) **Prezygotic isolating mechanisms.** Mechanisms that prevent interspecific crosses (i.e., fertilization and zygote formation).

1. **Habitat isolation.** The population live in the same regions, but occupy different habitats, so that potential mates do not meet.
2. **Seasonal or temporal isolation.** The population exist in the same regions, but are sexually mature at different times, so that, potential mates remain unable to mate.
3. **Ethological isolation.** The populations are isolated by (in animals only) different and incompatible behaviour before mating so that, potential mates meet but do not mate.
4. **Mechanical isolation.** Cross fertilization or pollination is prevented or restricted by differences in structure of reproductive organs (gentitalia in animals, flowers in plants), so that, copulation is attempted but no transfer of sperm takes place.

(b) **Postzygotic isolating mechanisms.** Fertilization takes place and hybrid zygotes are formed, but these are inviable, or give rise to weak or sterile hybrids.

1. **Gametic mortality.** Sperm transfer takes place but egg is not fertilized.
2. **Zygotic mortality.** Egg is fertilized but zygote dies.
3. **Hybrid inviability or weakness.** Zygote produces and F_1 hybrid of reduced viability.
4. **Hybrid sterility.** Hybrids are sterile because gonads develop abnormally, or meiosis breaks down before it is completed.

5. **F_2 breakdown.** F_1 hybrids are normal, vigorous, and fertile, but F_2 contains many weak or sterile individuals.

(A) PREZYGOTIC ISOLATING MECHANISMS

1. Habitat isolation

Population of different races or of a species may occupy different races or of a species may occupy different habitats in the same geographic region because of their preference to different ecological factors such as soil composition, soil water, attitude, etc. Such habitat isolation gives the individuals of the species little or no opportunity to meet and interbreed. Examples are : a fish and a seed-eating bird, which are environmentally isolated, although they live in the same locality. Similarly, beetles, which burrow in the ground are environmentally isolated from beetles, which live on trees. In this case, environmental conditions are not similar. *Moore* (1949) said, "The difference between geographic and habitat solution is merely quantitative." *Stebbins* (1965) mentions that ecological or environmental isolation is much more effective in plants than animals.

In some cases, evolution may be due to combined action of ecological and geographic isolation working together. This has been shown by *Camin* and *Ehrlich* for water snake, *Natrix sipedon* found in Florida. One race of it is found in fresh water and the other in salt water. They do not mate when come close to each other.

2. Seasonal isolation

Specific differences in breeding season or seasonal occurrence are extremely common in insects and are not rare in other groups. In *Cicada* of the United States there are two races, the 17-year race and the 13-year race. The numbers refer to the time in years spent as a subterranean nymph. These two main races scarcely differ in structure, but do not appear to interbreed. Similarly, in the United States *Rana clamitans, R. pipiens* and *R. sylvatica* may all breed in the same pond but they do not interbreed as individual breeding is determined by water temperature

R. syllvatica breeds when water temperature is as low as 44°F. *R. pipiens* starts breeding at 55°F, while *R. clamitans* requires 60°F.

In *Cocklebures,* the flowering time of two species have become so different that in the same area one species flowers only after the other has formed seed capsules. Thus, chances of crossing do not occur.

3. Ethological isolation

There are many instances in which behaviour differences particularly in regard to courtship, restrict copulation. The males of every species have specific courtship behaviour and females of the same species are receptive. Courtship involves an exchange of stimuli (visual, auditory, tactile, olfactory or chemical) between male and female continuing until both have reached a state of physiological readiness in which successful copulation can occur.

The visual stimuli includes colour, colour patterns on the body of organisms, the shape, size and their movements as seen in birds, insects etc. The auditory stimuli include songs, calls and other acoustic signals. The chemicals stimuli includes the scents or specific odours as seen in insects and mammals.

It appears that unless the female recognizes the male as belonging to her species she will often eat him and the peculiar dances or scent or sound of males assist the females to avoid mistakes.

4. Mechanical isolation

Mechanical isolation is provided due to differences in the genital organs of different species in animals, so that copulation may not be easily brought about. However, this mechanical isolation in animals has now been shown to be fairly ineffective. According to *L. Durfour* (1844) the genitalia in insects are developed on *'lock and key'* principle. Certain type of key can fit and open a particular lock. According to *Durfour* the male and female genitalia are so exactly fitted to each other than even slight deviation in structure of either renders, copulation impossible.

No doubt mechanical isolation was considered to be an effective barriers to mating in some species, but it is not applicable to all.

(B) POST-ZYGOTIC ISOLATING MECHANISMS

If the prezygotic isolating mechanisms fails then the postzygotic isolating mechanism prevents the successful hyberdization. They are of following types :

1. Gametic mortality

The gametic mortality is seen in forms both with external and internal fertilization. Even when mating occurs, the sperms are killed in an antigenic reaction in female genital tract before they could reach the eggs. *Patterson* found in cross-insemination between related species of *Drosophila*. The mucuous membrane of vagina swells markedly after mating. The swelling is stimulated by spermatic fluid, even without any sperm in it. If the mating has been with a male of same species the vagina returns to normal size within few hours. In an inter-specific mating, it may remains swollen for days. Eggs are destroyed in a swollen vagina.

2. Zygotic mortality

Sometimes the gametes of different species have succeeded in uniting, there still may be complete isolation of the contributory species. The development of hybrid zygote is often irregular and the zygote may died at any stage during development (between fertilization and adulthood). For example in a cross between *Datura stromonium* and *D. metel* development takes place upto 8 celled stage and then stops.

3. Hybrid inviability

Many naturally occurring hybrids have been found to leave no offsprings, even though they seen fully fertile. The weakness of hybrid is attributed to some physiological disturbance or ecological differences.

4. Hybrid sterility

Hybrids may be formed, may be vigour and appears to be normal, yet it is sterile. The mule is hybrid of jackass (*Equus asinus*) and a mare (*Equus calabus*). It is a vary vigrous animal, superior in many respects to both of its parents, but it is a sterile one.

Whether sterility is gametic or zygotic (haplontic or diplontic), basically it will either be due to genic disharmony or due to chrmosomal differences. The genic sterility may be caused due to genetically controlled spindle abnormalities, asynapsis or desynapsis and similar other abnormalities. Chromosomal sterility will be mainly due to lack of homology between chromosomes of two parents.

The chromosomes do not pair at all, thus resulting into meiotic irregularity leading to strong gametic sterility.

5. Hybrid break-down

Merrell (1962) describes that even vigorous, fertile F_1 hybrids produce hybrid breakdown in F_2 generation may be responsible for reproductive isolation. In such cases, subsequent generations may show reduced vigour or fertility or both.

An example of hybrid breakdown is provided by F_1 hybrids, *Gossypium arboreau* X G. *herbaceum* this case, F_1 progeny is either missing or is very weak.

Genetic Basis of Isolating Mechanism

Each type of isolating mechanism is based upon differences in respect to many different genes or chromosomal segments. The progency of hybrids do not sort out in clear cut Mendelian ratios meaning thereby, the action of multiple genes. The sterility of hybrids may be due to following causes :

(i) If the parent species have different chromosome numbers, the chromosomes cannot usually be arranged in homologous pairs as some of them will be left unpaired. This irregularity of chromosome number in the gamets and consequently in the zygote should be fatal.

(ii) The pairing chromosomes (Synapsis) involved pairing of homologus genes. If the two species crossed are not very much alike; synapsis may not take place in the hybrids.

(iii) Gene mutations and chromosomes aberrations such as duplications and deletions are almost fatal as they will cause difficulty in pairing of chromosomes. Inversion and translocations may not be fatal but reduce fertility of hybrids to a great extent.

(iv) Another means of producing sterility of hybrids is through combined action of certain genes. Thus, the genes S_1 (S_1 S_1) and S_2 (S_2 S_2) alone may not produce any untoward effect but when both (S_1 S_2) occur together in the same individual, they may result in abnormal development of the hybrid with reduced fertility.

ORIGIN OF REPRODUCTIVE ISOLATION

Two major theories have been proposed to explain the origin of reproductive isolation :

1. Muller's view

Muller regarded that reproductive isolation is an incidental by-product of genetic divergence, which takes place during the origin of subspecies and species in allopatric populations. (When the population of a species occupies different environments or becomes isolated into subgroups by geographical isolation, each isolated subgroup behaves as an independent population it is called allopatric population). To simplify, it can be said that evolving population adapt themselves to different environments. Therefore, a reshuffling and restructuring of the genes, chromosomes and entire genotype takes place.

2. Dobzhansky's view

Dobzhansky suggested that reproductive isolation arises as a result of natural selection. He noted that the hybrid of the spicies are often less adapted or may be even sterile or inviable. These will tend to be eliminated by natural selection. The hybrids and those genes favouring hyberdization will slowly be eleminated from the population. Thus, natural selection serves to reduce the wastage of gametes an less-fit hybrids.

ROLE OF ISOLATION IN EVOLUTION

Isolation has been recognized as one of most important factors in the process of speciation. Each species has a delicate integrated genetic system. The genetic system has been selected through many generations to fit into a particular habitat in the environment. One way to reduce the viability of progency is to limit the mating of parents to individuals more or less like themselves. If such limitation is desirable, any individual which has developed an isolating mechanism preventing its breeding with distinictly unlke organisms will furnish the unchanged type of offsprings which the unchanged environment can accommodate. These offsprings will survive, carrying with them their isolating mechanism. Hyberdization usually leads to a breakdown of this system and results in the production of disharmonious forms. Isolating mechanisim prevents the hybrid breakdown and protests the identity of genetics system of that species.

7

ADAPTATIONS

There are two primary requirements food and safety for which animals compete with each other. In the course of time the animals become adapted to all possible conditions of life on earth, water and air. These adaptations are manifested in various structural modifications which enable their possessors to survive the competition.

Adaptations can be classified under four headings :

I. Structural Adaptations
II. Physiological Adaptations
III. Protective Adaptations
IV. Animal Associated Adaptations.

I. STRUCTURAL ADAPTATIONS

Structural adaptations may be *morphological* i.e. confined to the shape, size and external features or *anatomical* in which visceral organs are adapted according to need. *Lull* (1952) classified adaptations into the following types.

1. Cursorial or terrestrial adaptations.
2. Fossoreal adaptations.
3. Aquatic adaptations.
4. Scansorial adaptations.
5. Volant adaptations.
6. Cave adaptations.

However, *Mathew,* added one more adaptation to the above i.e. Deep sea adaptations.

CURSORIAL ADAPTATIONS

Animals living on land need bodily structures enabling them to run away quickly. Thus these adaptations are also called *speed adaptations*. These adaptations can be seen in reptiles like snakes, lizards, birds like *Emu, Ostrich, Rhea, Moa* (all are flighless birds) etc. and more perfectly in mammals. They are characterized by following changes.

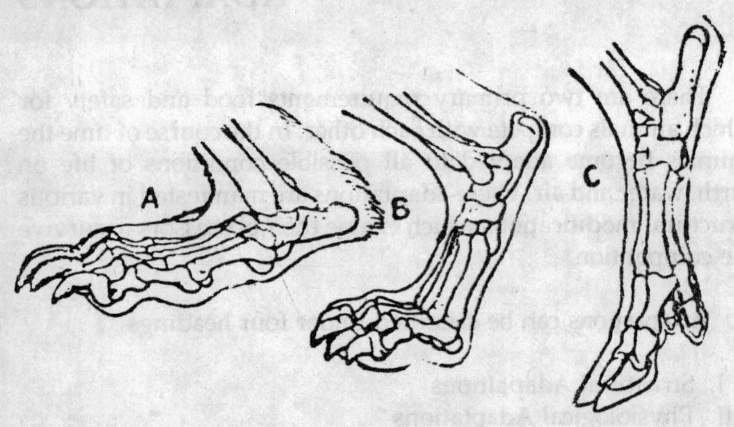

Fig. 7.1. Foot postures A = plantigrade, B = digitigrade, C = unguligrade.

1. *Body contour.* The bodies of all the speedy animals are moulded externally in such a way as to offer least resistance to the medium through which they pass. The perfectly adapted mechanism is evident in a racehorse with head and neck extended, ears thrown backwards, every tense muscle of the body working with machine-like precision exhibits the beautiful body contour.
2. *Less development of fore-limbs.* Among the propelling organs, the forelimbs are less developed as they may be concerned in food gathering. The mind-limbs are highly modified and are main divers.
3. *Changes in foot poiture.* The primitive terrestrial foot is *plantigrade* while walking, the entire palm and sole rests on the ground. Examples are : bear, racoon, baboon. Next stage is *digitigrade* i.e., walking or running upon the digits themselves. Examples : dogs, birds dinosaurs and mammals

except ungulates. The third stage is *unguligrade* i.e., walking on modified nail or hoofs. Examples : horse, and other ungulates.

4. *Loss of digits.* Plantigrade animals are those whose entire palm of sole rests on ground. The plantigrade animals are generally five toed : The digitigrade animals are four-toed. Plantigrade four-, three, two-or even one-toed. Arteodactyles have two toes while Parissodactyles have only one. Hence speed adaptation has its influence in determining digital reduction.
5. *Reduction of Fibula and Ulna.* These bcnes tend to be reduced and in exclusively locomotor limbs these bones are mere vestiges. These are well developed in slow moving forms.
6. *Loss of Universal Movement.* The entire movement of limbs is restricted to movement is only one plane. However, where universal movement is retained through the movement of ball and socket joint.
7. *Lengthening of distalia of limbs.* The lengthening of limbs is accomplished by the growth of the distal elements only. The powerful muscles are attached at the proximel end of the limbs. Moreover, the muscles are short and stout which increase their power and speed of contraction.
8. *Bipedality.* In bipedal forms (birds, marsupials and man) the cursorial adaptations include reduction of fore-limbs. Fore-limbs are also often used as efficient organs of prehension and food capturing.
9. *Importance of Tail.* Tail takes up different functions. In some, the tail may be short or heavier or it may be extremely long and selender. In Kangaroos, tail is powerful organ and serves as a third limb, when animal rests. Tail is not found in birds but features serve collectively as a balancing organ.
10. *Shortening of neck.* In bipedal mammals, there is tendency of reduction in the neck size (e.g. Jerboa) though these are seven cervical vertebrae.
11. *Mental Alterness.* Animals, which depend upon speed for safety, have alert young ones which keep up with the herd almost at once. In carnivorse and rodents, young ones are feeble and are, therefore, kept hidden until able to move independently. The newly born camel, deer, or horse with

long limbs, have more mental alertness, therefore, there is little or no period of helpless infancy.

FOSSORIAL OR SUBTERRANEAN ADAPTATIONS

These adaptations are seen in those creatures which live above ground but dig for their food. The modifications may be enhanced in animals digging for retreat. In general fossorial animals are primitive defenceless members of their respective groups. The common examples are *Caecilians* (Amphibia), *Uromastix, Sphenodon,* snakes and limbless-lizards (Reptilia); burrowing owls (Birds); monoterms, marsupials (Wombat, Kangaroo rat; moles, hedgehog, hare, squirrel, otters etc. etc. The modifications are :

1. *Body contour.* Fusiform body with greatest diameter near shoulder and with head tapering makes an efficient burrowing form. Tail is usually short, e.g. in moles. The cylindrical body is found in legless animals like snakes, lizards and caecilians.

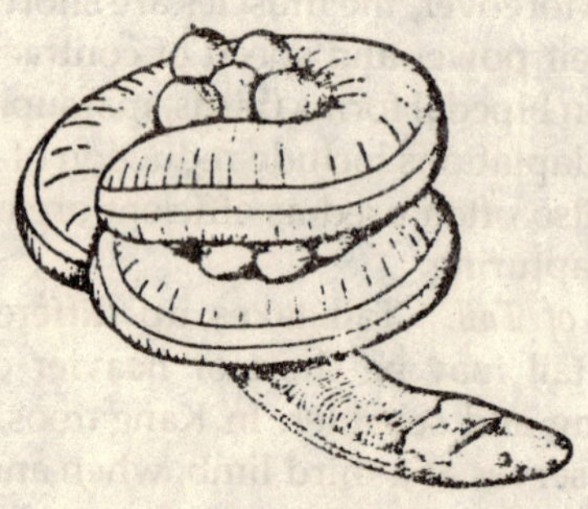

Fig. 7.2 Ichtyophis

2. *Reduction of tail.* As a long tail is inconvenient for subterranean life, it is short is hedge-hog, ratel and wood chuck. It is vestigial in the wombat and several moles. Tail serves as a valuable tactile organ.
3. *Loss of eyes.* In the fossorial animals, the eyes tend to become vestigial as they are of no use and if present will be injured. That is why are vestigial. Eyes are small in pocket gophers

(*Geomyidae*). In mole rats they are simply black specks among the muscles having complete structure. In Marsupial mole (*Notorcytes*) the eyes are functionless; and are concealed with skin in golden mole.

4. *Disappearance of ears or pinnae.* The pinnae are obstructions to burrowing life, the pinnae are disappeared. (e.g. moles, monotremes etc.)
5. *Digging mechanisms.* For digging mechanism following modifications in body occur :
   (i) *Snout.* The snout forms an important organ for digging and is truncated and upturned at the tip (e.g. *Heterodon*). In Talpa a prenasal bone develops at the tip of the cartilage of the nose.

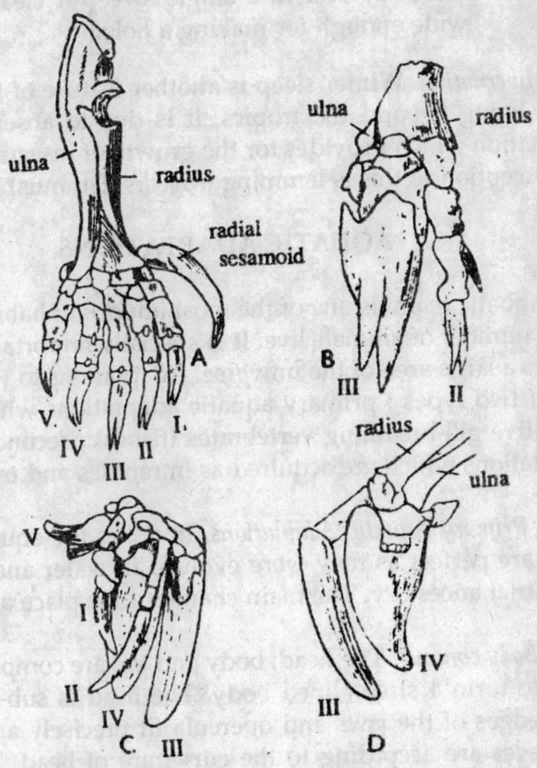

Fig. 7.3. Hands of Moles. A=a common mole, B=golden mole, C=palmer mole, D=marsupial mole ; I-V digits.

(ii) *Incisor and canine teeth.* The incisor teeth particularly and sometimes canines form very adequate fossorial organs. The incisors are forwardly directed as in pocket gophers. In swine the canine teeth are the digging organs.

(iii) *Fore limbs.* These are the most important fossorial organs. The fore limb and limbs are short and stout, as they are unnecessary not only in speed but in average burrowing. The hand is broad and stout with long claws suitable for loosening the earth. Foot serves to drive the creature ahead and to resist the backward thrust received from the hands. In common mole, *Condylura* and hand is so broad as the entire height of the body and in a single sweep it cleans the space wide enough for making a hole.

Hibernation. Winter sleep is another feature of fossorial animals living beyond the tropics. It is due to absence of green vegetation which provides for the growth of insects and worms. An exception to this is lemming (*Myodes* lemmus)

AQUATIC ADAPTATIONS

Aquatic realm is one of the most important habitat. Where a large number of animals live. It is specially important because it covers a large area of the universe. Adaptations to water habitat are of two types : primary aquatic adaptations which includes primitive gill-breathing vertebrates (fishes) ; secondary aquatic adaptations which are acquired as in reptiles and mammals.

I. *Primary Aquatic Adaptations.* In fishes the aquatic adaptations are perfect as they were evolved in water and never had terrestrial ancestory. The main changes took place are :

1. *Body contour.* The head, body and tail are compressed so as to form a streamlined body. The head is sub-conical, the edges of the jaws and opercula fit precisely and even the eyes are according to the curvature of head. These is no protuberance over the body which would hamper the swift movements of the animals through water.

2. *Locomotion.* Locomotion is effected by undulations of the flexible body, having fins. The fins are paired or unpaired extension and serve as accessory locomotary organs.
3. *Swim bladder.* Presence of *air bladder* or *swim bladder* in bony fishes serves as accessory respiratory organ as well as hydrostatic organ. It is a hollow structure and filled with gas or air and maintains the fish at a certain depth of flotation.
4. *Gills.* Occurrence of ctnedial respiration as gills are well suited for gaseous exchange in water.

II. SECONDARY AQUATIC ADAPTATIONS

Secondary aquatic forms are lung breathers which under stress of circumstances were forced to return to water and readapted themselves to aquatic habitat. They, however, retained higher brain and effecient methods of aeration of blood.

Class-Amphibia includes the amphibious forms who spend part of their time on land and part is the water. They show only partial adaptations in webbed feet, laterally compressed swim-

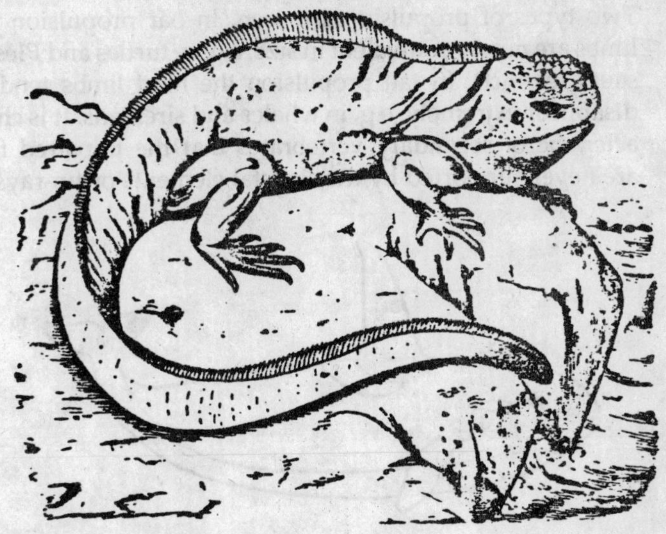

Fig. 7.4. Amblyrhynchus cristatus (Sea Lizard)

ming tail and gills. In reptiles marine turtle, crocodiles and alligators show semi aquatic adaptations with respiratory aids. But for the egg-laying female has to come to land. *Ichthysauria* (extinct reptile) were fully aquatic. Among birds quite a few forms are amphibious such as *Pelican,* flamingo, ducks, geese etc. The penguins are aquatic. Among mammals some forms are amphibious like sea-otter, otter, mink, hippopotamous etc. and other like cetacean and sirenian are aquatic.

Following adaptations are seen in secondary aquatic adaptations:

1. *Body contour.* It is also streamlined ; neck shortens or disappears, tail enlarges, a fish-like form is developed. Several modifications viz., skull modification, neck shortening vertebrae are biconcave as in fishes, sacrum is more or less reduced, bones become light and spongy, loss of external ears, external nostrils or nares move towards the apex of head, eyes shift higher on face etc., (as in hippopotamous).
2. *Locomotive mechanism.* Fleshy fin like expansions of the body wall without skeletal support occur in the whales and Ichthyosaurs (extinct). These fins may be dorsal and caudal. Two types of propulsion are seen. In oar propulsion the limbs are nearly equivalent in size, e.g. in turtles and Plesiosaurs (extinct). In tail propulsion the hind limbs tend to disappear extremely, e.g. in whales and sirenians. It is characteristic of secondary vertebrates that the unpaired fins are never supported by the skeletal elements or fin-rays.

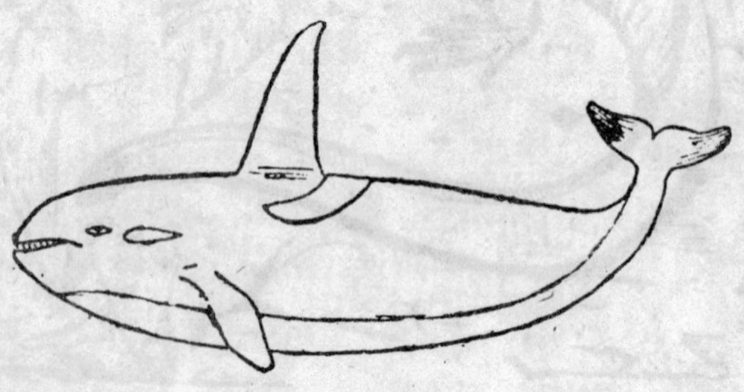

Fig. 7.5. Killer Whale

3. *Limbs.* Webbed feet is another aquatic adaptation in aquatic forms, they develop into paddles in which there is a loss of mobility of the various joints so that a flexible paddle of great aquatic utility is formed. As a further modification, the individual phalangeal bones increase in number.
4. Integument. Skin is naked i.e. there is the reduction of armouring of hair, skin glands, muscles and nerves. The loss of hair is characteristic of marine mammals. The whales and sirenians have lost all the traces of hair except of few bristle around the mouth, but most of them are well covered with partial hair before birth. As a compensation of the loss of hairs a layer of fat or subcutaneous tissue develops beneath the skin called *blubber* for the retention of bodily heat.
5. Mouth armament. Except in sea-cows and walrus the jaws are not used for mastication but only for the prehension of feeble prey. Teeth become simplified, increase in number or total loss from one jaw (sperm whale) or both (baleen whale). The reptiles have simple prehensible teeth fitted for the retention of slippery prey.
6. *Mental precocity.* It is a necessity for the aquatic animals and they soon show ability to keep up with the mother. The new born young of whales, much smaller to their parents, is capable to maintain its position.
7. *Speed.* Some aquatic animals have a very fast speed in water. This speed is maintained with the vibrations of highly efficient propelling tail.

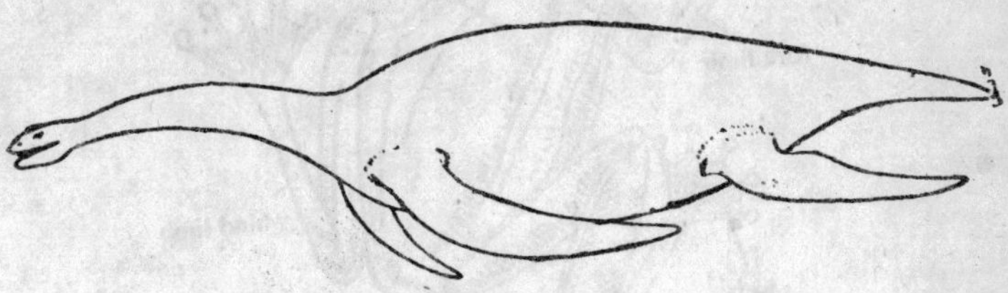

Fig. 7.6. Plesiosaur

8. *Size.* Water-borne animals are larger in size. The largest terrestrial animals is elephant measures 3.5 meter in length while the aquatic sulphur-bottom whale (*Balaenoptera mus-*

culus) is about 26.10 meter is length several times bigger than the largest elephant.

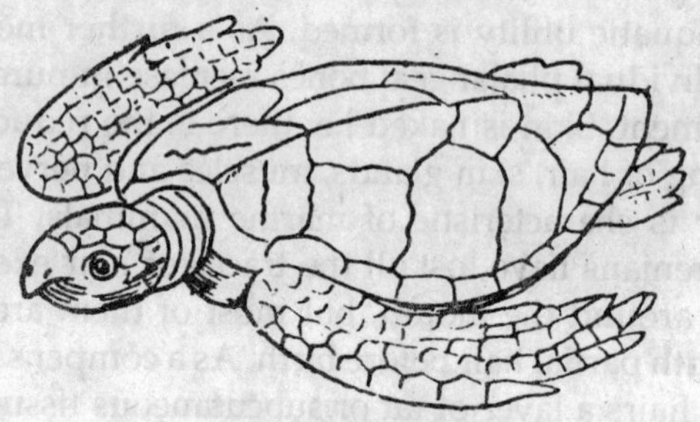

Fig. 7.7. Marine Turtle (Chelone)

SCANSORIAL OR ARBOREAL ADAPTATIONS

Only a few animals take to trees for safety, retreat and for abundant and easily procured food.

Climbers can be of three types (a) *Wall and rock climbers* (b) *Terrestrio-arboreal forms* (c) *Arboreal forms.*

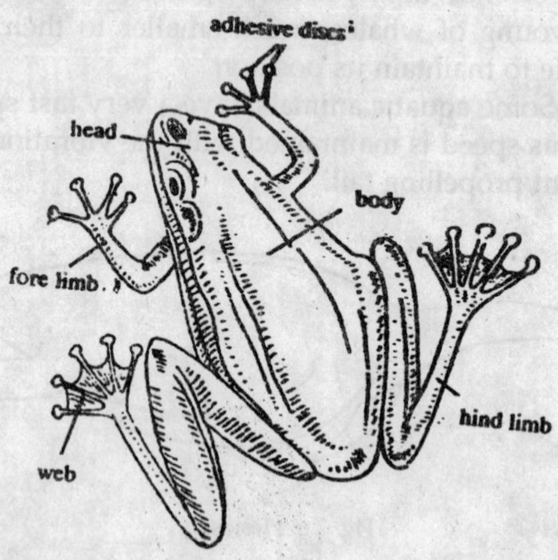

Fig. 7.8. Tree frog Hyla

(a) *Wall and Rock Climbers*. These are well-suited for climbing on the walls of building as well as on similar surfaces in nature.

Examples are : gecko-lizards. Among mammals, the example is that of flying squirrels.

(b) *Terrestrio-arboreal forms*. These are capable for climbing but they feel at home beneath the grounds. Examples are : a number of carnivores, rodents and insectivores.

(c) *Arboreal forms*. These make the trees their home and some occasionally descend to the ground. The forms include some primates and on the basis of locomotion they can be divided into following three subdivisions :

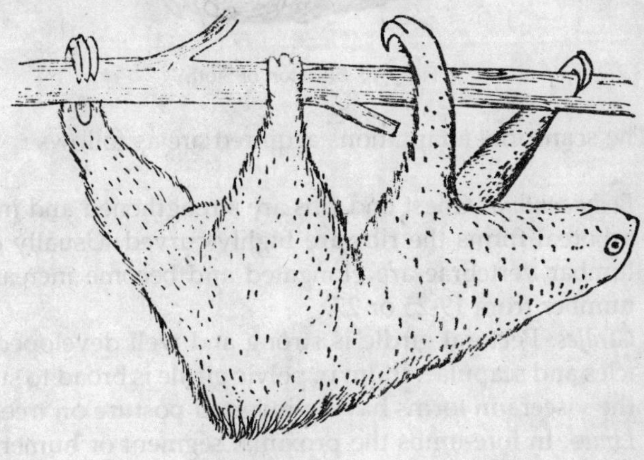

Fig. 7.9. Sloth (*Choloepus*)

(i) *Branch runners*. Various squirrels, lemurs, chameleons etc. are the examples of this subdivision. They live and move on the upper surface of branches by their four legs.

(ii) *Suspended forms*. Bats, sloths and flying lemurs (Galeopithecus) etc. are the examples. These animals rest and move suspended on the trees etc. by their powerful recurved claws of their limbs.

(iii) *Brachiator forms*. These forms swing by their forelimbs. Examples are monkeys, man-like apes etc.

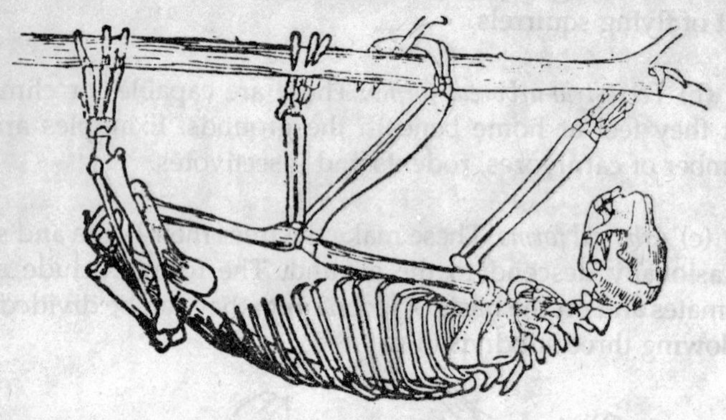

Fig. 7.10. Skeleton of Sloth

The scansorial adaptations acquired are as follows :

1. *Body contour*. Chest and ribs are strengthened and in more arboreal forms the ribs are highly curved. Usually dorso-lumbar vertebrae are elongated and become increased in number from 19-25 or 27.
2. *Girdles.* Pectoral girdle is strong and well developed clavicles and scapulae. Ilium in pelvic girdle is broad to support the viscera in forms having inverted posture on trees.
3. *Limbs.* In fore-limbs the proximal segment or humerus becomes elongated in suspending form. In sloths the humerus is very long. In gibbons, arms are very long so that the hands touch the ground when it stands erect.
4. *Syndactyly and zygodactyly in limbs.* The feet are prehensile. If the feet are non-prehensile, the digits possess claws e.g. squirrels, cats etc. Adhesive pads on the tips of digits or on the soles of feet occur in *Hyla, geckoes* (lizard) and *Dendrohyrax* (mammal) etc.

   If the feet are prehensile, *syndactyly* (union of digits) is common. The well known example is that of chameleons. Here syndactyly is marked in both the fore-limbs and hind-limbs. On the hand first three fingers are opposed to outer bundle formed by the fusion of 4th and 5th fingers. In foot the condition is reverse, outer bundle is of three fingers and inner bundle of two fingers. In parrots, woodpeckers etc.

the outermost toe becomes rotated backward in such a way that 4th toe and hallux become opposed to the 2nd and 3rd toes. This type of foot where the outer toe rotation is permanent is called *zygodactylous*.

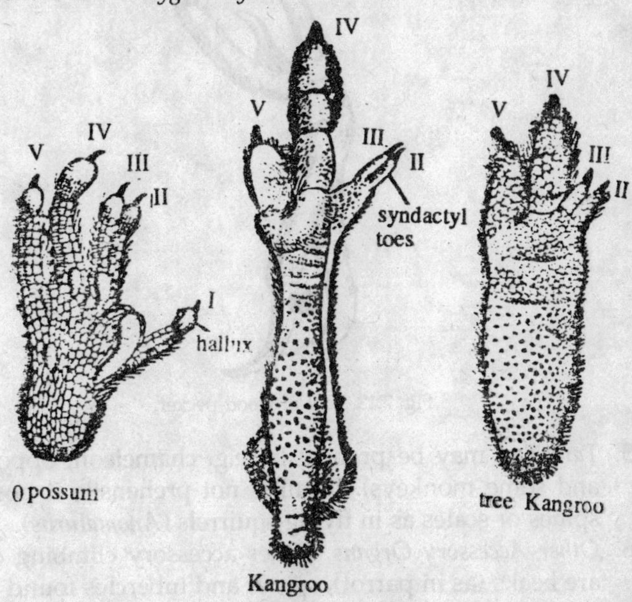

Fig. 711. Hind feet of marsupials

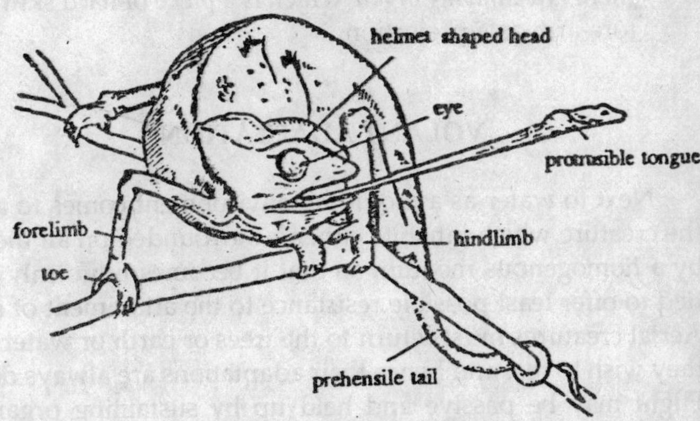

Fig. 7.12. Chameleon

Syndactyly is seen in marsupials, primates, birds, reptiles etc.

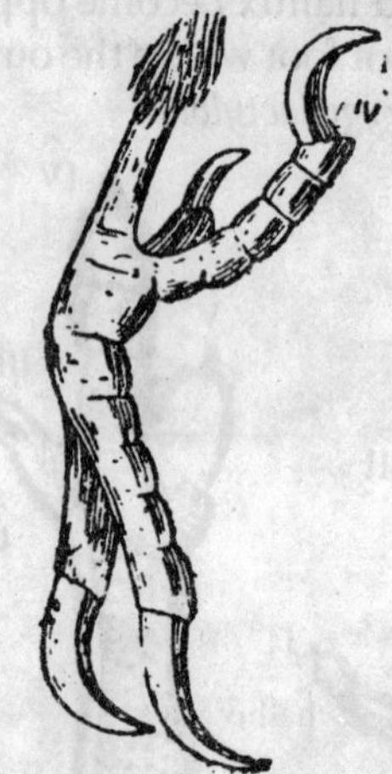

Fig. 7.13. Foot of wood-pecker.

5. *Tail.* Tail may be prehensile (e.g. chameleon, oppossums and some monkeys). If tail is not prehensile it possesses spines or scales as in flying squirrels (*Anomalurus*).
6. *Other Accessory Organs.* Other accessory climbing organs are beaks (as in parrot), spines and tubercles found on the fore-arms in some lemurs (*Hapalemur grisous*). In *Lemur cetta* there is a *climbing organ* which is a piece of hard skin on the fore-arm as a projection.

VOLANT ADAPTATIONS

Next to water as a moulding environment comes to air, for the creature which inhabits either is surrounded on all the sides by a homogenous medium so that it becomes uniformly modified to offer least possible resistance to the attainment of speed. Aerial creatures must return to the trees or earth or water when they wish to rest and hence their adaptations are always double. Flight may be passive and held up by sustaining organs the creature merely glides from a higher level to a lower level without any locomotive force. *True flight* implies power and there is a sustained movement through the air. It has evolved three times in the vertebrates-in pterodactyles (Reptilla), birds (Aves) and bats (Mammalia).

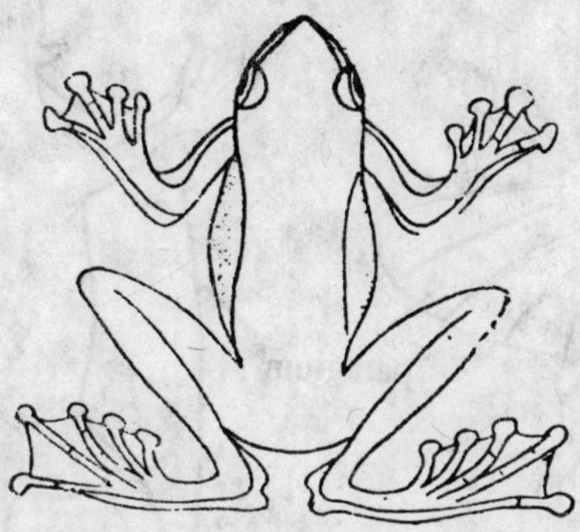

Fig. 7.14. Flying Frog Rhacophorus

The following adaptations are noteworthy :

Adaptations for Gliding. The gliding flights are performed by fishes (*Exocoetus*) amphibians (*Rhacophorus*), reptiles (*Draco*) birds (*Ostriches*) and mammals (*lemurs*).

The following adaptations are noted :

(i) *Development of Patagia.* Except in fishes, the patagium is a fold or series of folds of skin supported by ribs. In *Draco*, there is a pair of large wing-like membranes, which extends outwards from depressed body and each supported by 5 or 6 ribs. In flying lemur (*Galeopithecus*), the patagium extends from the back of the neck to the tip of tail even including digits.

(ii) *Enlargement of Pectoral Fins.* In the flying fish (*Exocoetus*) large pectoral fins are present, which serves as organ of flight. Pelvics are smaller while the lower lobe of tail is longer. *Exocoetus* flies upto 200-300 meters. Another examples are *Pantodon*. (African flying fish). *Gigantopterus* (Extinct flying fish) etc.

(iii) *Webbing of Feet.* The tree frog, *Rhacophorus* is the only amphibian in which volant adaptations is found. It has webbed feet by which it has long prolonged leaps. The digits terminate in adhesive pads. Rudiments of patagia in front and behind the arms are also present.

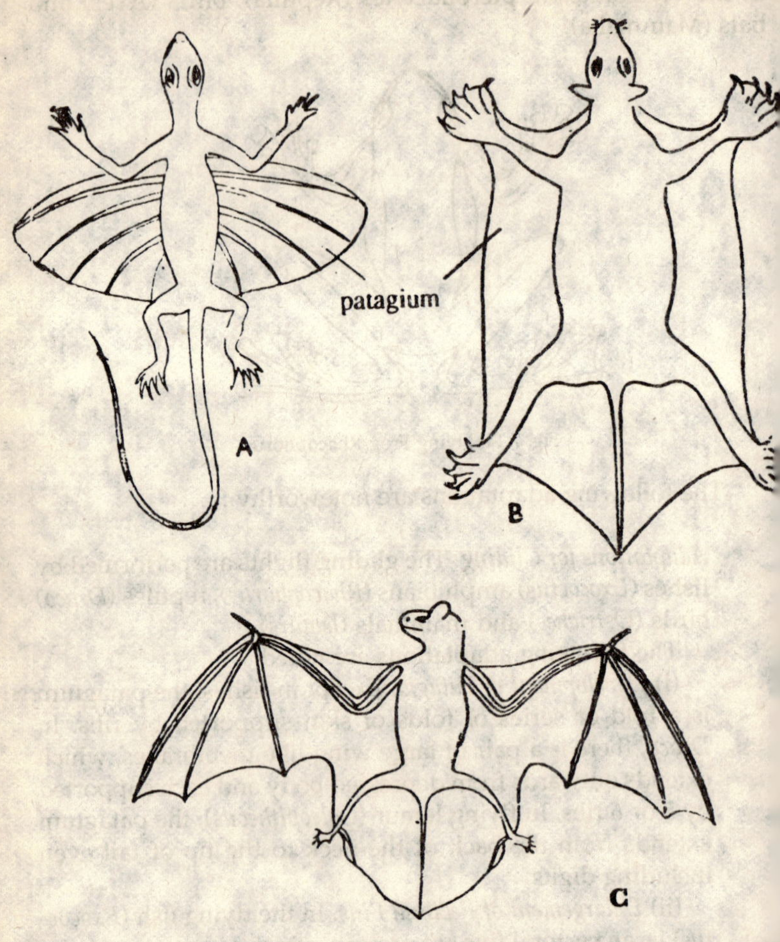

Fig. 7.15. Volant adaptation A=Draco, B=Galcopithecus, C=Vespertilio

2. *Adaptations for True Flight.* True flight is seen in birds, i sects and few mammals like bats and flying squirrels e Following modifications are seen here.

(i) *Feathers.* Birds develop peculiar structures known feathers which shows an extreme adaptation for flight. Ea feather consists of a *quill* or *calamus* and the *rachis* or *sha* On the rachis a double series of *barbs* are developed carr ing a double series of *barbules* which in their turn give ri to *barbicels,* these terminate distally into hooklets. These catch in the folded margins of the next proximal row, thus producing a firm surface.

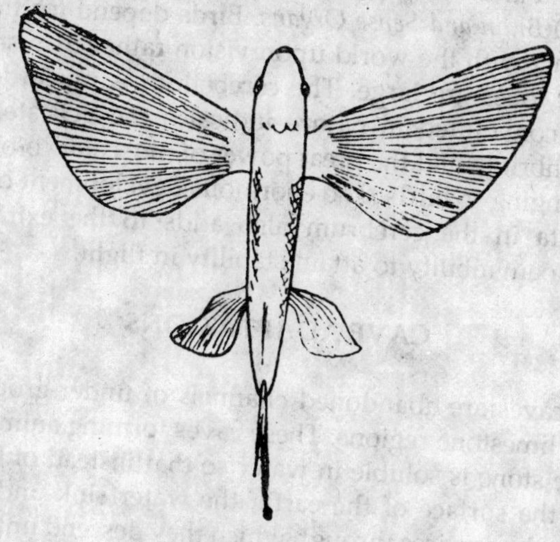

Fig. 7.16. Flying fish, *Exocoetus*

(ii) *Wings.* There are three types of wings : (a) *bat wings* (b) *pterodactyle wings* and (c) *bird wings* (a) In bat-wing humerus is well developed, radius is long and ulna is *vestigial.* The *polex* is free and clawed. In micro-chiropetra, second finger is distinct but not free from the third and is attached distally, to support the anterior margin of the wing. Fourth and fifth digits are also well-developed (b) In *Megachiroptera,* the second digit is free from third and possess a claw like the first. In pterodactyl wing, radius and ulna are more or less equal while the former or radius is somewhat smaller. The wing is flexed between the metacarpal and proximal phalynx rather than the wrist as in birds and bats. (c) In bird-wings, digits are reduced to three but they are more or less fused and their main function is flight.

(iii) *Pneumatic Bones.* Hollow air filled bones are found in birds and pterodactylas. In birds, air-sacs not make them light but act as accessory respiratory organs.

(iv) *Sternum and pectoral Girdle.* Sternum or breast bone is well developed bearing a keel or carina for the attachment of pectoral muscles which support the wings. Pectoral girdle is rigid and develops clavicles.

(v) *Brain and Sense Organs.* Birds depend for their main contact with the world upon vision rather than small. The optic lobes are large. The cerebellum is much developed and convoluted in nature indicates the delicate sense of equilibrium and the great power of muscular co-ordination belonging to birds. The enormous development of corpora striata in the cerebrum also adds to the extraordinary manoeuvrability to attain stability in flight.

CAVE ADAPTATIONS

The caves are abandoned channels of under-ground rivers found in limestone regions. These caves forming animal habitat. This lime stone is soluble in water so that instead of being confined to the surface of the earth, the water sink underground, enlarging the cervices through which they descend until the level of ground-water is reached, when the movement becomes lateral and subterranean channels of considerable magnitude are formed.

Distribution of Caves. In North America there is a large cave area extending through parts of Indiana, Kentucky, Tennessee and Missouri, embracing the so-called Mammoth cave region. In Edmonson country, Kentucky, there are said to be at least 4000 sink holes or pipes through which surface water pass under ground and 500 caves are known. Wyandotte cave in Indiana, Luray Cavern in Virginia and Carlsbad Caverus are noted. In Cuba there are extensive caves in communication with the sea. In Europe there are other caves. Few caverns exist in the glaciated regions of Europe or N. America, almost all of them lying south of the great terminal moraine.

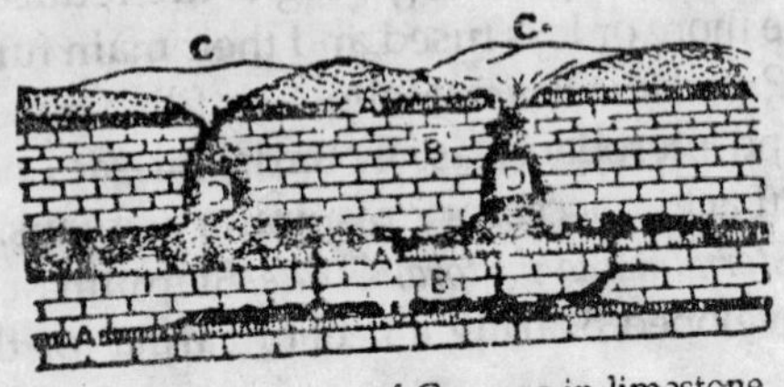

Fig. 7.17. Formation of Caverns in limestone.

Cave regions : The caves can be divided into three regions :

(i) *Twilight* (Transitional region). It is the region lying within the mouth of the cave between the outer world and the real cave. Therefore, in this region, conditions vary.

(ii) *Region of Fluctuating Temperature.* Here, the diurnal or sea sonal variations of heat and cold can be felt.

(iii) *Inner Cave Region.* In this region, light is absent and the temperature remains constant. The moisture is uniform here.

The Fauna of Caves can be divided into two types :

(a) *Temporary Fauna.* These show little or no special adaptations to deep cave life as they are temporary visitor. Viz. *Myotis lucifugus* of the brown bat.

(b) *Permanent Fauna.* This includes those animals which permanently live in the caves. Among fishes a large number of cave dwellers are there e.g. cave catfish (*Gronias nigrilabis*), Dismal swamp fish, *Chologaster cornutus, Ambloyoposis spelaeus. Typhlichthys subterraneus* etc. In Amphibia only the Salamanders are cave dwellers (*Spelerpes maculicauda, S. Stejnegeri* etc.) In Reptiles and birds there is no example of permanent cave-dweller. Besides bats only one mammal called white footed mouse *Peromyscus leucopus* is a truely cave-dweller.

Following are cave adaptations in cave dwellers;

1. *Loss of pigmentation.* A general effect of the lack of light is the bleaching of the skin of cave dwellers, examples are *Stygicola* (fish) and *Proteus* (Amphibian).
2. *Reduction of eyes.* Eyes may become reduction or degenerate, may be covered by other tissues or become entirely obsolate. Blind forms are never the less sensitive to light. *Gronians* is partially blind fish. *Typhlichthys* is an another animal in which eyes are functional in the young but become defective in the adult. *Amphyopsis* is a totally blind fish. Among amphibians, the blind form is a *Proteus* and

Typhlomolge with degenerate eyes. To compensate the loss of vision, tactile organs or sense of small is highly developed.

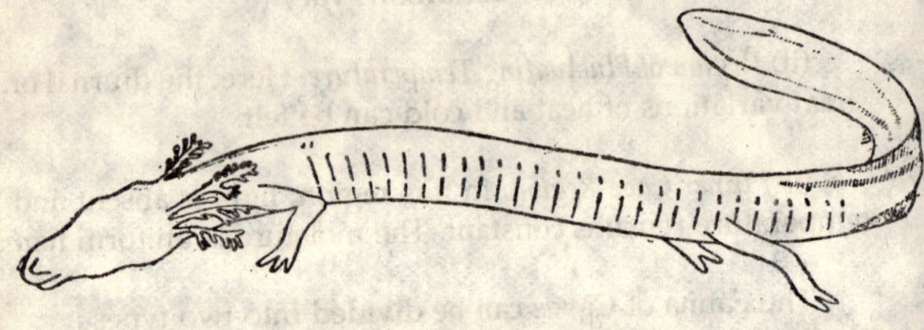

Fig. 7.18. Proteus anguinus

3. *Organ of digestion.* The absence of light means very poor vegetation and hence, there is scarcity of food. The organs of digestion so modified that they completely utilize the food which the animal takes.

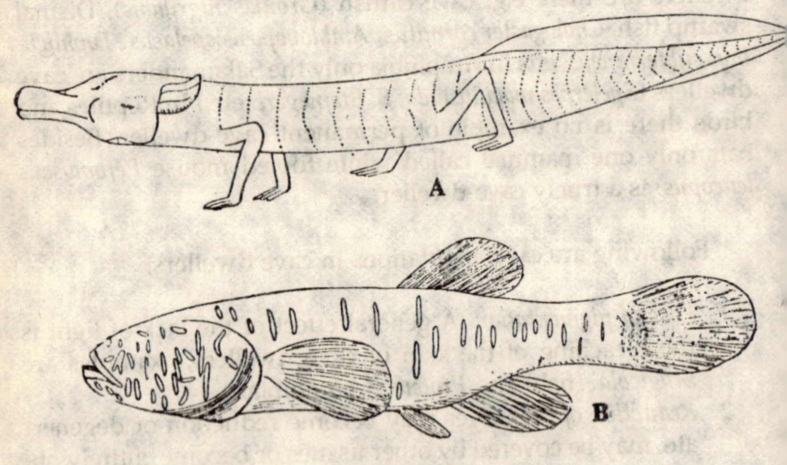

Fig. 7.19. A = Cave Salamander, B = Cave fish

4. *Slender bodies.* Cave dwellers have slender and attenuated appendages e.g. *Proteus* etc.

DESERT ADAPTATIONS

A desert is a vast level stretch of drifting sand, devoid of vegetation except in the rare cases and peopled by camel and the venturous of humidity. The desert does not imply sterility but simply the possession of a rainless climate, where drought may be said to be almost continuous.

In desert the struggle for existence is exceedingly severe because food, safety and continuity of generation three great needs of organic race are in danger of being lost in open fields with adverse climate. In desert the prime conditions of life for existence are :

1. *Moisture getting.* The prime requirement of the desert form is to have sufficient supply of moisture. In the desert, there is scarcity of water, therefore, there is need of not only water-getting but also of effectively conserving it. Animals get their water supply mainly from the juice of the food, whether plant sap or blood of prey. Many desert forms entirely depend on such a source and they never drink water, even if it is available. The skin of some of the animals such as Australian Lizard (Moloch) absorbs water like blotting paper. Its surface is covered by thorn-like scales.
2. *Moisture Conservation.* In animals there are various ways of water conservation. In camels, developed water cells in its walls. There are closed by a sphincter muscle. When the animal drinks water then the cavities are filled and this water is used later.
3. *Avoidance of Evaporation.* Animals conserve water by non-perspiring.
4. *Defence.* The desert animals unprovided with additional garment to protect them from sun, seek out shadow of a great rock or if non is available, it must burrow and thus escapes the extreme of heat and cold. In digging species of reptiles, the nostrils are directed upward instead of forward. The nostrils of snakes are provided with valves or they reduced to pin holes. The nostrils of camel are capable of being closed like eye-lids.

The eye-lids are greatly enlarged or may be modified into windo-like window which cover the eye. The eyes of camel are guarded by long eyelashes. The eyes of *Typhlops* (burrowing snake) are overhung by head shields.

The *ear* openings are either small or protected by fringes or scales or they may be abolished.

Hard surface and spinoscence are as characteristic of desert reptiles (*Molach, Phrynosoma* etc.).

Venom is a desert adaptations. Almost all the reptiles have poison in fang or sting. All the spider family are poisonous and almost everyone of them is represented here.

Speed is characteristic of the dwelling in arid climate far the have to travel far and wide for food and drink or to pursue o evade pursuit. In camel, the broad pad and secondary retrogres sion to digitigrade are fitted to move on sand.

Sense of sight, hearing and smell are highly developed.

Intelligence is also an important characteristic of desert adapte animals.

Gazelle resembles the general colouring of the surroundin

DEEP SEA ADAPTATIONS

Deep sea extends to about one half of the entire globe a includes all waters below a depth of 200 meters which is the lin of effective sunlight and green plant life. It is divisible into tw regions; from a depth of 200 to 1000 meters it is known *archibenthal* and below 1000 meters as abyssal benthal. The ch acteristics of the deep sea are intense cold, utter absence movement, profound darkness and enormous pressure. Th characteristics gradually increase with depth and hence, ther naturally a transitional zone.

The deep sea forms are adapted migrants from the pelagic realm and show convergent evolution as follows :

1. *Fragile and Weak Body.* The animals are fragile and weak having this and feebly flesh and with very little lime in their bones that is why the skeletons are weak and fragile. They possess relatively great jaws and cruel mouth ornaments e.g. Silver sharks (*Gastrostomus*). The other examples are glass sponges (Hexactinellida), long legged crab (*Kacmpferia*), fishes (*chimaera*) etc.
2. *Colouration.* It is more or less uniform. As a rule colours are simple, and common being brown or gray. In *Macrurus* the belly is black and the top is silvery.
3. *Tectile Organs.* Long feelers, slender attenuations of the fins are present.
4. *Photoreceptors.* In archibenthos, which is a transitional zone the eyes are enlarged e.g. in *Pandalus, Cyrtisome longipinnis* and *Regalecus* (fish). Next below this zone (dimlight the eyes though telescopic show enlargement of the lens; examples being the fished *Argyropelecus* and *Gignatura.* Here the retina of the eye possesses specialized rods and no cones. In abyssal benthos, eyeless animals and those with reduced eyes are numerous. Examples of eyeless forms are *Eulima* and *Ipnops.*
5. *Presence of Luminescent Organs.* It is common among the curstaceans, cephalopods and fishes. Luminescent organs are found either over the entire body or in the belly or localized on highly modified organs. Teeth and mouth may also be luminous. The function of bioluminiscence may be of attractions of prey in the benthic forms. It may be possible that it helps in sex differentiation. Examples are *Ipnops Oneirodes, Photostomias* etc.
6. *Loss of Power of Mastication.* The power of mastication is lost in many deep-sea fishes e.g. *Cetomimus.*
7. *Parental Care.* Parental care is shown by many deep-sea fishes while some other produce youngs in large number.

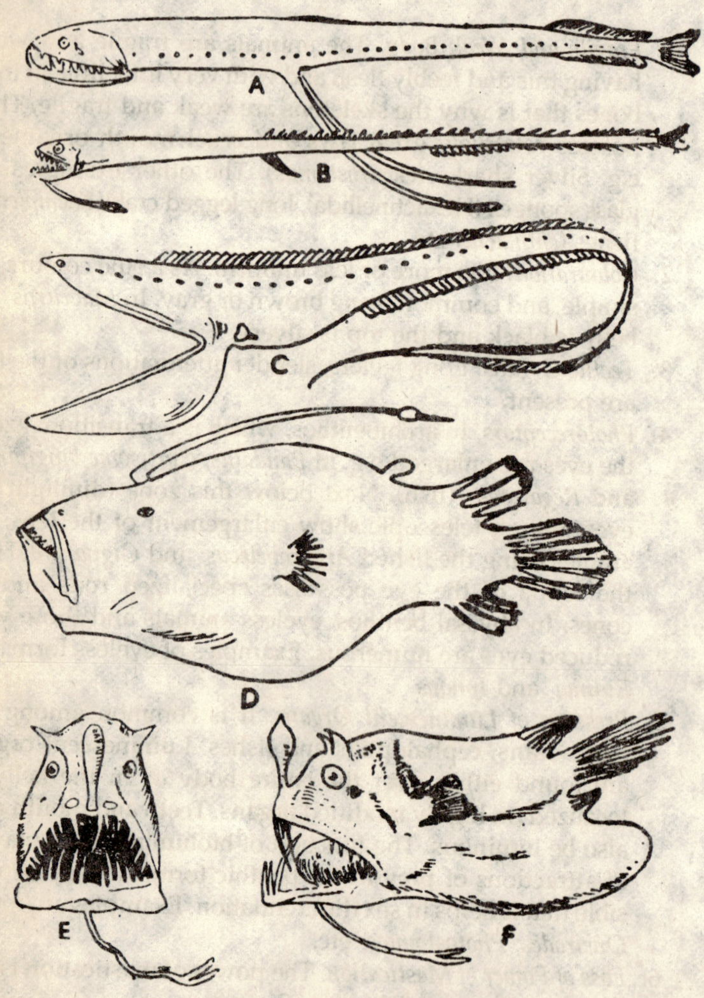

Fig. 7.20. Deep sea fishes. A= Photostomias, B=Idicanthus, C=Gastrostomus, D = Cryptopsaras, E & F = Linophryne.

II. PHYSIOLOGICAL ADAPTATIONS

The physiological adaptations are changes in the functions of animals to adopt themselves to the changed condition of life. In some organisms, there is competition for food, therefore, there is mutation which enables the animal to utilize a new food ; temperature tolerance ; adaptation to certain ranges of pressures are also physiological adaptations.

III. PROTECTIVE ADAPTATIONS

Adaptations, which protect the animal from its natural enemies are called protective adaptations. Colouration and mimicry is one of them. For detail see the chapter colouration and mimicry.

IV. ANIMAL ASSOCIATION ADAPTATIONS

Some species-to-species adaptations are so exact that one cannot live without other. There can be :

1. *Socialism.* Some insects like bees, termites ants, wasps etc. live together forming colonies. In honey bee the individuals are distinguished into queen which is modified to lay eggs, the drones are fertile male and workers are modified for collecting honey, pollen etc.
2. *Commensal adaptations.* In this association of two individuals at least one gets benefited and other neither benefited nor harmed. An example is seen in *Eupagurus* (hermit crab) and *Metirdium* (sea anemone).
3. *Symbiotic Adaptations.* In this association two different animals live together in such a way that both are beneficial to each other. Association between termite and flagellate (*Trichnympha*) offers an example of symbiotic adaptations. Another example is that of *Hydra* and *Zoochlorallae.*
4. *Parasitic adaptations.* In this association the animals live together in such a way that one gets benefited, other is harmed.

PARASITIC ADAPTATIONS

Parasitism is an association of two organisms of different species in which one is benefited and other is harmed. The benefited organism is called *parasite* and other is the *host*. The parasitism is seen in invertebrates.

Following adaptations are seen :

1. *Loss of organs.* The locomotory, digestive and sense organs are usually lost or reduced.
2. Usually the body of endoparasite becomes flat, leaf-life.
3. The adhesive organs are developed like suckers, hooks etc. (Helmenth worms).
4. Epidermis is lost and the body is covered by a very thick cuticle.
5. Pharynx becomes suctorial.
6. Secretion of anti enzymes and mucous.
7. Reproductive system extraordinary developed.
8. Life-cycle becomes complex. (*Fasciola, Taenia* etc.)
9. In ectoparasites the mouth parts are modified for required purposes.

8

VARIATIONS

There are various factors which are responsible for evolution. The most important are variation, isolation, adaptation heredity and natural selection. Variation is the first and most fundamental factor of evolution. It is a characteristic of all living organisms. No two individuals are exactly alike. Differences and dissimilarities may be apparent in any character, which an organism displays. The differences and dissimilarities may be between *sibs* (related by common descent), between individuals or groups of individuals (such as populations, races or sub-species) of a species or between species. It provides raw material for evolution.

All the variations are not alike and only some of them are heritable. The effects of variations may be morphological or physiological or both. In the former case variation effects size, shape and pattern of organism. In the phylogical case variations may effect all the physiological processes including reproduction and other metabolic activities. The variations may occur along positive or negative lines, i.e. they may be useful, useless or harmful.

KINDS OF VARIATIONS

Variations are grouped into three pairs of contrasting type.

1. Germinal or acquired, 2. Continuous or discontinuous, 3. Determinate or indeterminate.

1. Blastogenic or Germinal variations

These are intrinsic which ; apart from the external influences, arise in the germ plasm of the animals and plants. These may be caused by the recombinations of genes which results into a group of new combination, or it may be caused due to mutation which is the result of some radical change in the gene complex. These changes do not depend on external conditions for their origin. Such conditions may hinder or arrest their development for cannot cause them. Germinal variations may occur at any period of life from the beginning of life to the death of the organism. Examples are : occasional occurrence of supernumery digits in man, domestic cat, horse and other animals.

2. Somatogenic or Somatic variations

The variations in the soma and the body cells caused by the factors of environment such as food, heat intensity of light, pressure etc. are called somatogenic variations. These are also called the acquired variations as they are acquired by the individual during its life-time. They are lost with the death of the individual. They are neither inherited from the parent nor transmitted to the future generation.

For examples, the long neck of giraffe, well developed muscles of an athlete, sometimes there is loss of dight in men etc.

3. Continuous variations

If the variations occurred very small, abundant and in a graded series then such variations are called continuous variations. These are usually qualitative. If these variations occurred accidentally (fortuitous) they are called Darwanian variations, or fluctuations which are acted upon by natural selection. Examples of continuous variations are : gradation in stature, height and intelligence in man ; skin colour, weight and milk production in cow etc.

4. Discontinuous variations

These variations appear suddenly without any known reasons. They show wide deviations from the normal condition and are not linked with intergrades. This discontinuous variations are also called saltations, or sport or mutations.

For example : in vertebrates often 6, 7 or even 8 digits have been observed. Such variations may also occur in the segments of worms ; vertebral column, ribs, muscles and in the number of appendages. These variations are quantitative.

5. Indeterminate variations

Variations which are not governed by any law but take place in some imaginary or thinkable direction of change. Thus these variations depend on chance only variation of size in closely related organisms is an example of indeterminate variation.

6. Determinate variations

These variations are governed by some unknown force and are imposed to occur in one line or certain lines, usually in an adaptive direction. These are also known as *orthogenetic variations*. This type of variation is seen in the evolution of overgrown anthers of Irish deer or tusks of Jefferson mammoth.

Besides the above variations these are *numerical* or *meristic variations*.

Meristic variations

When an organism possesses additional similar part than the normal number, it is said to have undergone meristic variation. The development of an extra digit on the hand or foot of a man, the occurrence of six instead of the normal five arms in a starfish.

SOURCES OF VARIATION

Sources of acquired variation are apparent. Any external condition, influencing of organism, produces this type of variation. The external factors may be light, heat, cold, feed etc. These variations, because they are somatic, may not be inherited. The cause of evolution, really speaking, comes from the germinal variation which is inheritable.

1. *Light*

When two animals or plants of the same species are grown under different conditions of light intensity, they show mark variations in their form. *Cuuningham* proved experimentally that the flat fish, Solea developed pink colour on its ventral surface, which is normally white, when exposed to light. The upper surface, which is normally pink, turns white when the animals are kept in shed.

2. *Temperature*

A number of variations can be observed by lowering or increasing the temperature. *Tower* and *Agar* by their experiment an mice have shown, that mice reared in a warm room at about 21°C were found to differ considerably from those reared in a cold room at 5°C.

3. *Water*

It is also an important factor for normal growth. Plants growing in dry and arid soils undergo conserve water, while plants of moist areas show luxurious growth.

4. *Nutrition*

Nutrition, like water, is another very important factor for the growth of an organism.

5. *Endocrine glands*

The hormonal secretions of endocrine glands, which influences the development and differentiation of various physical and mental characters are also responsible for causing variations. For example Axolotl larva of *Ambyostoma*. Due to thyroxine deficiency it remain as larva.

6. *The use and disuse of organs*

Use and disuse of organs also produce variations. The organs which is put to continuous use shows better development than less used. The constant disuse of an organ leads to atrophying of that organ.

7. *Cytological basis*

The cytological or genetic sources of variation may be due to three reasons.

(i) Difference in the number of chromosomes
(ii) Change in the structure of individual chromosomes
(iii) Gene mutations

The first two are collectively called chromosomal aberrations.

(i) Differences in the number of chroinosomes. It is also called heteroploidy. It is of two types :

(A) Changes involving entire sets.

(a) Haploidy. Having are genome only (n).

(b) Polyploidy. Each genome is represented more than twice like triploidy (3n), tetraploidy (4n) and so on.

(B) Changes involving the number of chromosomes in one genome.

(a) *Monosomic.* Loss of one chromosome from diploid set (2n-1).

(b) *Nullisomic.* Loss of both the homologous chromosomes from diploid set (2n-2)

(c) *Trisomic.* Increase of one chromone in a diploid set (2n + 1)

(d) *Tetrasomic.* Increase in one pair of homologous chromosomes (2n + 2)

(ii) Change in the structure of chromosomes :

(a) *Delation.* Loss of one or more genes.

(b) *Dupliction.* Addition of one or more genes.

(c) *Inversion.* A chromosomal segment is inverted at 180°C.

(d) *Translocation.* Exchange of parts between non-homologous chromosomes.

(For detail see the chapter - *Mutation theory*).

SIGNIFICANCE OF VARIATION

Germinal variations are more important because they are inherited to the offsprings and they are regarded as the raw material of adaptation and evolution. Somatic variation is of no importance for evolution, as such differences are not in general transmissible to offsprings and, therefore, are not the basis for evolutionary adjustment. Some genetical changes represent only a breakdown of genes and genetic mechanisms and they cause drastic changes unfitting in their effects on the individuals showing them, therefore, tend to be weeded out by natural selection. As a result, they appear as rare abnormalities in a population and are present mainly because they continually reappear through mutations.

Continuous variations is most important in relation to evolution. From variation, Darwin's adaptive change is deduced. The continuous variation is also concerned to plant and animal breeders and is mainly of great significance.

9

SPECIES AND ORIGIN OF SPECIES

The entire course of evolution depends upon the origin of new populations having greater adaptive efficiency than their ancestors. The study of *speciation* or populational divergence is therefore crucial to an understanding of evolution. At one time, even at present, the process of speciation was thought to be synonymous with evolution. As most biologists now realize that evolution is not a simple process involving only the origin or divergence. The factors for race and species formation are considerably different from those operating to produce sequential micro evolution, and evolution above the species level also entails a different complex of processes. Evidences have accumulated to the point where it is no longer proper to speak of a single origin of species, since we know that species may originate in several very different ways.

The term *species* was originally used as a *Latin* equivalent to *'kind'*. The precise meaning of species has been a subject of much discussion but now most of the biologists are agreed on what a species is : According to them *a species is an assemblage of animals which do not differ from one another and which interbreed freely with one another to produce fertile offsprings.* They usually inhabit geographical areas (niches) distinct from those inhabited by the nearly related species. According to *Ross* (1962) the species is the total of the individuals forming its population. Now it is regarded that a population, which is morphologically different is taken as a separate species.

According to *Mayr* (1940), "species is a group of actually or potentially interbreeding natural population that is reproductively isolated from other such groups". According to *Dobzhan-*

sky (1950), "A species is the most inconclusive Mendelian population". *Merrell* (1962) mentioned, "The species is a natural, biological unit, tied together by the bond of mating and sharing a common gene pool. For this reason it has objective reality."

However, there is difficulty with biological species definition, it is limited to sexually reproducing species. *Mayr* (1963) enumerative three important characters of a species as follows :

(i) Species form reproductive community.

(ii) It is an ecological unit as it interacts as a unit with other species which it shares the environment.

(iii) Species is a genetic unit consisting of large intercommunicating gene pool.

Polytypic species. A species which has two or more sub-species, are known as polytypic species. The species that is not subdivided into sub-species is known as *monotypic species.*

Sub-species. Mayr (1969) defined a sub-species as a geographically localized sub-division of species that differs generally and taxonomically from other sub-divisions of a species. The sub-species are fertile in crosses and intergrade between adjacent sub-species at the meeting place of their ranges.

Clines. A cline is formed by a series of continuous populations in which given character changes slowly. Such geographical character gradients are called clines. The term was introduced by *Huxley* (1939). They are of two types (a) Intergroup or stepped cline in which changes in characters are constant, (b) Internal cline in which no such variations in the rate of change in characters is seen. The gradient is more or less constant throughout.

Race. A category which is used in the taxonomy of organisms that consists of a group of individuals within a species that are geographically, ecologically and physiologically distinct from other members of the species. The term is also used in the same sense as sub-species.

Supraspecies. It is the collection of sub-species, which replace one another geographically or physiologically and in which intrinsic isolation has taken place.

Clone. It is a group of individuals all derived from a single individual without sexual combination.

Linage. It is a radial complex of several lines of descent, which forms a mesh network of evolution within the species.

Many groups of related population live together in the same area and remain distinct from each other without exchanging genaes. These are the entities which we usually recognise as *sympatric* (overlapping) *species* as opposed to *allopatric species* which inhabit different areas. However, there are examples of related species which are allopatric in some parts of their distributional range but sympatric in others. A distinct species is one which pass the test of sympatry i.e. retain their identity even though they live close enough together so that cross fertilization between them is possible. A good example of sympatry is provided by three species of *Rana, R. pipiens, R. sylvatica* and *R. eatesbiana* found together in streams and lakes of U.S.A.

ORIGIN OF SPECIES

Evolution depends upon the origin of new populations and species. There are two distinct ways in which new species arise from pre-existing ones.

I. Speciation.
II. Transformation in time.

I. Speciation

This causes increase in the existing number of species. Multiplication of species by major mutations was supported by *De Vries* and recently by *Goldschmidt*. Mutational speciation is not supported by modern geneticists because observed drastic mutations are highly deleterious. The second method of speciation in *sympatric speciation.* The sympatric speciation is the establishment of a new reproductive isolated species population within the normal cruising range of reproductive individuals of the parental species. According to *Mayr* this method does not explain the genetic repeating of species. There are a number of evidences that speciation is usually done by *geographic speciation.*

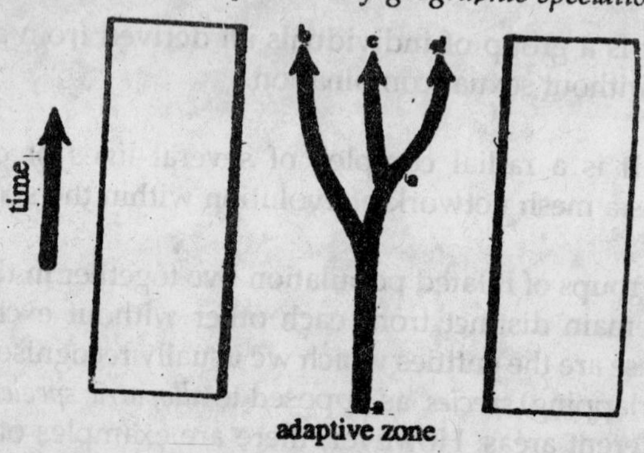

Fig. 9.1. Showing Speciation

Geographic speciation

A single population in a homogenous environment spreads to adjoining areas. This migration to new environment produces racial differentiation. In this way a polytypic species is evolved consisting of many races and sub-species. The sub-species may diverge from the parental population in such a way which decrease or prevent their ability to exchange of genes have been strongly developed, the sub-species rank as distinct species. Changes in the environment again permit geographically isolated population to exist together in the same region as sympatric species.

Sometimes it has been seen that two differently adapted populations or sub-species of a polytypic species can come together reproductive isolation between them. In such case they can exchange to a limited degree results in hybrid. The hybrids are adapted to environments different from those occupied by either of the parental populations. In animals the hybrids are most often unsuccessful because of their weakness or sterility. But some of them may give rise to a new population. The process of speciation occurs only in allopetric populations. It cannot action sympatric population inhibiting the same area. The sympatric species can arise either due to change in the chromosome number or due to introgressive hybridization and polyploidy. By hybridization and polyploidy a number of species can be formed in plants and a few in animals. For examples : Diploid old world cotton (*Gossypium herbaceum*) having 13 pairs of chromosomes (26). Tetraploid New world cotton (*Gossypium hirsutum*) having 26 pairs of chromosomes (52). Similarly different species of *Drosophila* have different number of chromosomes. *Drosophila melanogaster* have 4 pairs of chromosomes (8) : *Drosophila willistoni* have 3 pairs of chromosomes (6) : *Drosopnila virilis* having 6 pairs of chromosomes (12). *Drosophila persimilis* possesses 5 pairs of chromosomes (10)

Introgressive hyberdization may form hybrid swarm which is a population in which F_1 and F_2 and late generations of hybrids segregation are intermingled with backcross progeny of various degrees. A backcross progeny will contain genes derived principally from one of the parental species and thus, it is most likely that it is well adapted to a habitat already present. The best documented example of introgression is found in *Raphanobrassica*. In 1927, *G.D. Karpechenko* performed across between radish (*Raphanus sativum*) and cabbage (*Brassica oleracea*), and got F_1 sterila hybrid as well as few fertile plants. Radish and cabbage each have 18 chromosomes (2n) while the *Raphenobrassica* has 36 chromosomes (4n). These hybrid tetraploids shared characters of both the parents ; and were unable to interbreed with either of parent. Thus naturally formed a new species.

Generally hyberdization can give rise only to populations which are intermediate between and share characteristics of the parental populations.

II. Transformation of a Species in Time

Transformation of a species into a new species in due course of time is the second mode of evolution. In this type only one species exists at a time. Say for example from adaptive zone 'a' species evolved into 'b' ; 'b' into 'c' ; and 'c' into 'd'. According to *Simpson* there are two types of transformation.

1. Phyletic evolution.
2. Quantum evolution.

1. *Phyletic evolution*

In the phyletic evolution there is a gradual change in the average characters of a species to achieve suitable adaptation to the existing environments. This is caused either due to adaptations to a shifting environment or due to increasing specialization for a particular environment or improved adaptations in a constant environment. This causes origin of new species from an existing one but there is no increase in the number of species. The paleantology provides many evidences of such type of evolution.

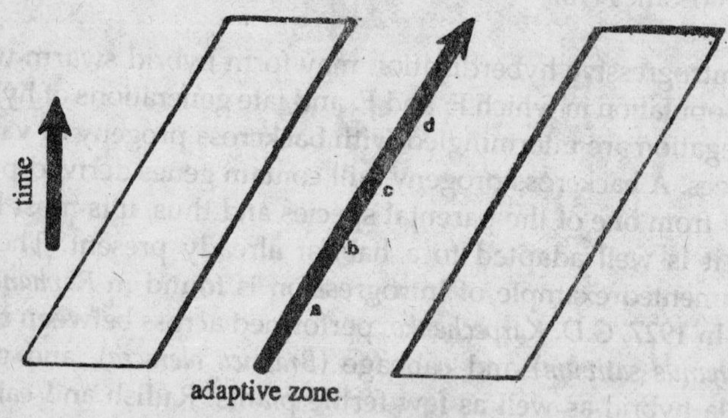

Fig. 9.2. Showing phyletic evolution.

2.*Quantum evolution*

It causes the evolution of higher taxonomic groups such as new orders and classes. Here there is a rapid change in the character of a population. In fossil records, new orders and classes generally appear without intermediate stage. Therefore, it is regarded that higher taxonomic groups originate by a different methods. The quantum evolution is *macro-of mega-evolution* as they are originated by macromutations, which are rare but produce widely different individuals. The individual becomes adapted to new mode of life.

The quantum evolution can be explained by conceiving preadaptation. The organism is modified in such a way that it is also by chance adapted to some other conditions. The organism, then, shifts to new adaptive zone. In this way many preadaptations may be present in a population. The organism evolves rapidly by mutation, selection and genetic drift.

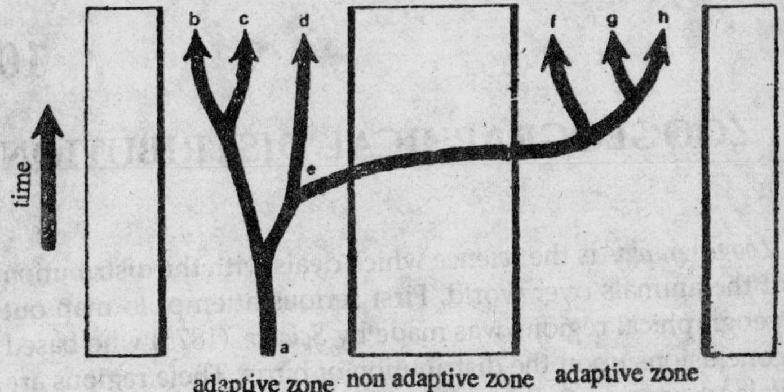

Fig. 9.3. Showing Quantum evolution.

10

ZOOGEOGRAPHICAL DISTRIBUTION

Zoogeography is the science which deals with the distribution of all the animals over world. First serious attempt to map out the geographical regions was made by *Sclater* (1875) who based his conclusions upon the distribution of birds. Theie regions are : 1. Palaertic region, 2. Ethiopian region, 3. Indian region, 4. Australian region, 5. Neotropical region, 6. Neartic region. There are, however, very apparent objections to utilizing vagrant and barrier defying creatures like birds for this purpose. Accordingly, *Murray* in 1866 and more in detail *Alfred Russel Wallace* in 1876, divided the surface of earth into zoological regions based chiefly on the distribution of mammals.

Many other regional classifications have been made, based on either discontinuous distribution of one particular class or upon the distribution of temperature, variations and similar climatic factors. None of these is satisfactory. Therefore, *Wallace* combined Sclater's system. *Blanford* (1896), *Lydekk* (1896), *Heilprin* (1887), *Gudow* (1913), *Schmidt* (1954) etc. and also took their contributions for the study of zoogeography.

Karl P. Schmidt (1954) divided the earth into three zoogeographical realms :

1. Arctogaean,
2. Neogaean, and
3. Notogaean.

Arctogaean includes two regions the (a) Holarctic with subregion: Arctic, Nearctic, Caribbean and Palearctic, (b) Paleotropical with subregions : Oriental, Ethiopian and Malagasy.

Neogaean includes a single sub-region the Neotropical. *Notogaean* consists of regions : the Australian having the Australian and Papuan sub-regions and the Oceanian, which is formed of the New Zealandian, oceanic and Antarctic sub-regions.

Wallace's classification is generally considered to be accepted system.

The Indian region of *Sclater* is termed as Oriented region in the classification of *Wallace.*

Thus, six zoogeographical regions have been distinguished as follows :

1. *Palaearctic Region.* It includes Europe, temperate Asia, North Africa and Arabia.
2. *Nearctic Region.* It includes whole of north America and Greenland.
3. *Ethiopian Region.* It includes whole of Africa, Arabia, South of the tropic of Caneer, and Madagascar.
4. *Neotropical Region.* It includes whole of South and Central America and West Indies.

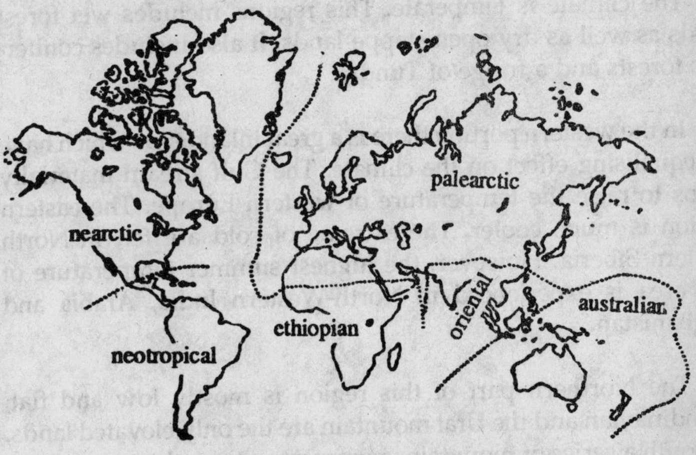

Fig. 10.1. Zoogeographical region of world.

5. *Australian Region.* New Guinea and neighbouring islands.

6. *Oriental Region.* It includes India, Sri Lanka, Indochina and Malaya.

The exact boundaries of these regions are very difficult to recognize. The fauna of these regions are described only with reference to the vertebrates, although they form only 3-4% of animal kingdom.

PALAERCTIC REGION

Extent

This, the largest of the six regions, is estimated to cover an approximate area of 14,00,000 sq. miles. It includes the whole of Europe, Iceland, the Azors, Maderia, Canary Island Cape Verde Islands, all the portion of Africa and Arabia which lies to the north of the tropic of Cancer, Asia Minor, Persia, Afghanistan and Baluchistan and the whole of Asia north of a line which runs up to valley of the Indus, along the great Himalayan range, thence eastwards to the Nanling Mountains, south of the Yang-tse-kiang and out to sea just south of the Japanese islands.

Climate

The climate is temperate. This regions includes wet forest lands as well as dry open steppe lands. It also includes coniferous forests and a fringe of Tundra.

In the western portion there is a great inland seas which have an equalising effect on the climate. The Gulf stream materially helps to raise the temperature of western Europe. The eastern region is much cooler. The extreme of cold are felt in North Eastern Siberia. However, the highest summer temperature of the area is experienced in North-Western India, Arabia and Afghanistan.

The Northern part of this region is mostly low and flat, Scandinavian and the Ural mountain are the only elevated lands. In South a series of mountains ranges run across the region from west to east, including in Europe the Alps, Balkans, Caucasus etc., in Asia the Tian shan, Altai Himalayan range etc.

Zoological Characteristic

The fauna of this region as a whole is very similar to the Nearctic region, that is why *Heilprin* proposed a great region, *Holarctic Realm* for both palaearctic and Nearctic regions.

The region possesses representatives of 135 families of terrestrial vertebrates, namely 33 of mammals, 68 of birds, 24 of reptiles and 10 of Amphibia. None of these, however, is peculiar to this regions but 9 are common and confined to the Palaearctic and Nearctic Regions. The nine families are the Talpidae (Moles) Ochotonidae (Picas) and Castordae (Beavers) among mammals, the Regulidae (Gold-crests), Colymbidae (Divers) and Tetraomide among birds ; the Proteidae Protous, Salamanders and Amphiuma among Amphibia. The fresh water fisthes also support the union of the two regions, for five families namely the perches, stickle backs, Pikes, sturgeons and Polyodontidae are distinctly Holoarctic.

The palaearctic region is sub-divided into four sub-regions ;

1. European sub-region,
2. Mediterranean sub-region,
3. Siberian sub-region,
4. Manchurian sub-region.

1. *European sub-region*

It comprises Northern and Central Europe. In this sub-region only 85 families of terrestrial vertebrates are represented and of these the reptiles and Amphibia number only 6 each. Only one from of mammals are peculiar namely Myogale but such animals as the wolf, Hedgehog, shrew, mole and Darmouse are very characteristic as are also the wag tails, Pipits, Tits, Thrushes and many other birds.

2. *The Mediterranean sub-region*

It includes the rest of Europe, all the African and Arabian portion, Asia Minor, Persia, Afghanistan and Baluchistan. This is the richest region possessing representatives of 120 families of terrestrial vertebrates. the Fallow-Deer, Elephant Shrew, Civent, Ichneumon, Haena, Hyrax, Porcupine are all characteristic mammals.

3. *Siberian sub-region*

It embraces all Northern Asia, southwards to the Himalayas. It possess representatives of 94 families of the terrestrial vertebrates. Four genera of mammals i.e. the Yak, Musk deer and a mole are almost confined to this sub-region but also ranges into the Oriental region. One of the most important members of the Siberian fauna is the fresh water seals, *Phoca ibirica* which inhabits the great fresh water lake-Baikal.

4. *The Manchurian Sub-region*

It includes China, Mongolia, Manchuria and Corea together with the whole of Japan. It has a rich and varies fauna with representatives of 102 families of terrestrial vertebrates. At least a dozen genera of mammals including Tibetan Langur, Great Panda etc. are peculiar.

NEARCTIC REGION

Extent

It includes the whole of North America and extends south as for as the middle of Mexico. It includes Greenland in the east and Aleution islands in the west.

Climate

It has a great range of temperature. The chief physical features of the regions are (1) Large lakes and inland sea in the north eastern portion and the important ranges of high mountains in the west. (2) In the east are smaller ranges, constituting the so called Appalachian high land. (3) In the centre of this great continent is a vast extent of plain which in the north is frozen and hence barren, between attitudes 50° and 60° covered with forest, and in the south dry treeless desert.

Zoological Characteristics

The number of families of terrestrial vertebrates represented in the Nearctic Region is 120 viz. 26 of Mammals, 59 of birds, 21 of Reptiles and 140 of Amphibians. The Nearctic Region possesses five peculiar familiar ; viz. the Haplodontidae and Antilocapridae among Mammals ; the Chamaeidae among Birds ; the Aniellidae among Reptiles and Sirenidae among Amphibians.

The Nearctic differs from the Palaerctic region, in the possession of several characteristic Mammals, such as oppossums (Didelphyidae) and Racoon etc., many birds such as the Blue-jays, and Turkey-buzzards etc., Reptiles such as Rattle snakes and Igunanas : Amphibia including Axolotl, Nectures, Siren and other large Urodeles.

There are, several peculiar genera of importance of which Scalops (web-footed Moles), Toxidae (American Badger), *Haplocerus* (Rocky mountain Goat) and Musk may be taken as examples.

Wallace has divided nearctic Region into four sub-regions :

(1) California sub-region,
(2) Rocky Mountain sub-region,
(3) Alleghany sub-region,
(4) Canadian sub-region.

1. ***California sub-region*** embraces a narrow strip of country between Sierra Nevada and the Pacific. In the North it includes island of Vancouver and the Southern part of British Columbia and in the South it extends up to the head of the Gulf of California. It has 86 families of terrestrial vertebrates and of which 21 are mammals, 49 of birds, 8 of reptiles and 8 of amphibians. These families are peculiar to this region, namely Haplodontidae, Chamaeidoe and Aniellidae. Vampires and free tailed Bats are characteristic of this region.
2. ***Rocky Mountain sub-region.*** It lies immediately to the east of California and includes the whole of the dry and elevated area covered by the mountains. It is the richest portion of nearctic region. It has 107 families of terrestrial vertebrates out of which 25 are mammals, 55 of birds, 18 of reptiles and 9 of amphibians. Although there are no peculiar families but are several characteristic genera like prongbuck (Antilocapra), Rocky mountain goat (*Haplocerus*), Prairie dog (*Cynomys*), American Bison and poisonous lizard (*Heloderma*).
3. ***Alleghany sub-region*** comprises the United States east of

the Rocky mountain sub-region and South of the Great Lakes and includes Novo Scotia. Some 99 families of terrestrial vertebrates including, mammals 8, birds 53, reptiles 16 and amphibia 12 are represented in this sub-region. The peculiar animals are : oppossum, starnosed moles, vampire bats etc. Turkeys and Sirenids (mud eel) are the other two families.

4. ***Canadian sub-region.*** All the remaining portion of North America and Greenland constitute the great Canadian sub-region. In this sub-region are to the found the representative of only 75 families including 20 of mammals, 44 of birds, 3 of reptiles and 8 of amphibian, thus it is the poorest region. But there are characteristic families including Deer, Rein-deer, Elk, Bison, Sheep, Gluttons, Lemmings, the polar deer etc.

ETHIOPIAN REGION

Extent

The Ethiopian region consists of the whole of Africa and Arabia, south of the tropic of Cancer, together with Madagascar and the small adjacent islands. *Darlington* (1957) has not included Medagascar but has considered it as separate region on account of its distinctive fauna.

Climate

This region is mainly tropical. It is a large block of rain forests and isolated mountains. The eastern part has wide grassy plains. Its southern part is warm temperate with mixed vegetations.

Zoological Characteristics

The fauna of Ethiopian region is rich, varied and well marked. There are about 161 families of terrestrial vertebrates. Out of these 30 are peculiar.

Among mammals 12 families are peculiar which are ; Chiromyidae (Aye Aye), Chrysochloridae (Golden moles), Centetidae (Tenress), Potamogalidae (Potamogale), Protelidae (Earth wolf), Battryergidal (African mole rats), Lophimyidae (crested rats),

Pedetidae (African Jamping Hares), Anomaluridae (African flying squirrels), Giraffidae (Giraffes), Hippopotamidae (Hippopotamus) and Orycteropodidae (Aard-Varks).

Among birds 13 families are peculiar ; a Promeropidae (Promerops) Acerocharidae (Helmet Birds), Vangidae (Vangidal), Philepittidae, Musophagidae (Plankton eators), Coliidae (Colies), Serpentariidae (Secretary birds), Scopidae (Hammer-head bird) Mesoenatidae, Numididae (Guinea fowl) and Balaenicipitidae (Whale head).

Among reptiles following families are peculiar : Rhachiodontidae (Egg-eating snakes), Gerrhosauridae, Zonuridae (Girdled lizard) and Uroplatidae.

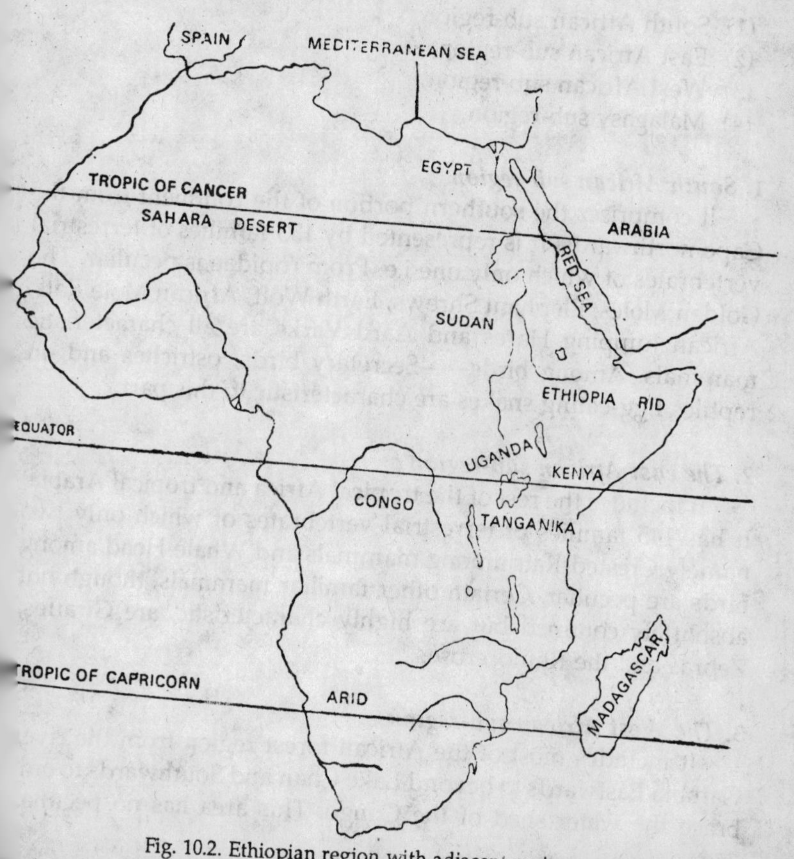

Fig. 10.2. Ethiopian region with adjacent regions.

Among amphibian family Dactylethridae (clawed toads) is peculiar.

In addition to these families, a large number of important genera are confined to this region, some of them are ; Macroscelidae (Elephant shrews), Hyaenidae (Hyaena) Elephantidae (Elephants), Rhinocerotidae (Rhinoceroses), Procavidae (Hyraces), Equidae (Horse etc.) Manidae (Pangolins) ; and among Birds the Ploceidae, Nectariniidae (Sundbirds), Zosteropidae (White Eyes); Indicatoridae (Honey Guides), Capitonidae (Barbets), Bucerotidae (Hornbills) and Struthionidae (Ostriches).

The Ethiopian Region is divided into four sub-regions.

(1) South African sub-region,
(2) East African sub-region,
(3) West African sub-region,
(4) Malagasy sub-region.

1. *South African sub-region*

It comprises the southern portion of the continent from the Cape northwards. It is represented by 133 families of terrestrial vertebrates of which only one i.e. Prom ropidae is peculiar. The Golden Moles, Elephant Shrews, Earth Wolf, African Mole Rats, African Jumping Hares and Aard Varks are all characteristic mammals. Among birds——Secretary birds, ostriches and, in reptiles Egg-eating snakes are characteristic to this part.

2. *The east African sub-region*

It includes the rest of the tropical Africa and tropical Arabia. It has 145 families of terrestrial vertebrates of which only two namely Crested-Rats among mammals and Whale-Head among birds are peculiar. Certain other familiar mammals, though not absolutely confined but are highly characteristic, are Giraffes, Zebras and the Rhinoceroses.

3. *The West African sub-region*

It includes most of the African forest region from the river Gambia Eastwards to beyond Lake Chan and Southwards to embrace the water shed of the Congo. This area has no peculiar families although 134 occur in this sub-region. The most characteristic mammals are the Gorilla, Chimpanzee, the Monkeys, Potamogal, the African flying squirrel and Okapi.

4. *Malagasy sub-region*

It includes Madagascar, Mauritius, Secychelles and neighbouring islands. The fauna of this sub-region is one of most interesting in the whole world. 86 families of terrestrial vertebrates found here, no fewer than 8 are absolutely confined to it. These includes two of mammals Chiromyidae (Aye Aye) and Centetidae (Trenecs) ; 5 of birds i.e. Aerocharidae (Helmet Bird), Vangidae, Philepittidae, Mesoenatidae and Leptosomatidae ; and one of reptiles i.e. Uroplatidae.

The most characteristic feature is that all the 35 known species of sub-family lemurinae of Family-Lemuridae are confined to this sub-region. Of birds 55 families are represented, 15 families of reptiles occur here, presence of 2 genera of guanidec is of special interest, since this is an essentially New World group. Chamaelions are very characteristic of Madagascar because they are more abundant than in any other part of the world.

NEOTROPICAL REGION

Extent

It embraces South America, most of Mexico and West Indies. It is joined to the Nearctic Region by Central American isthmus and Separated from other regions by sea.

Climate

Neotropical region is mainly tropical but southern south America continues into south temperate zone. From the west to the east runs the river Amazon with its hundred of square miles of evergreen forests. In the west the long range of the Andes has high mountain forests, plateau land and gentle slopes.

Zoological Characteristics

155 families of terrestrial vertebrates found here and not less than 39 families are absolutely confined to it.

Along mammals 10 families are peculiar : Cebidae (American Monkeys), Callitrichidae (Marmosets), Solenodontidae (Solenodonts), Dasyproctidae (Agouties), Chinchillidae (Chinchaillas), Caviidae (Cavies), Dinomydidae (Dinomys), Bradypodidae (Sloths), Calnolestidae (Selvas) and Myrmecophagidae (Ant-eaters).

Among birds 23 families are peculiar viz. Coerebidae (Honey Creepers), Phytotomidae (plant Cutters), Pipridae (Manakins), Oxyrhamphida, Dendrocolaptidae, Cononpophagidae, Formicarridae, Pteroptochidae, Galbulidae, Bucconidae, Rhamphastidae, Tinamidae, Steatornithidae, Momotidae, Todidae, Palamedeidae, Psophiidae, Aramidae, Cariamidae, Eurypygidae, Thimocorythidae, Opisthoconidae and Rheidae.

Among reptiles two families are peculiar viz. Xenosauridae and Dermatemydidae.

Among amphibians, 4 families are peculiar——Dendrobratidae, Dendrophryniscidae, Hemiphractidae and Amphignathodontidae.

Neotropical Region is divided into four sub-regions.

1. Chillian sub-region
2. Brazilian sub-region
3. Mexican sub-region
4. Antilean sub-region

1. *Chillian sub-region*

It includes Western coast of South America and embraces the summits of Andes of Peru and Bolivia. This region does not contain any peculiar family but characteristic forms are Chinchillas, Llamas, Rheas etc.

2. *Brazilian sub-region*

It includes all the rest of South America teminating Northwards at the Isthmus of Panama. This is the richest of the Neotropical sub-regions, containing representatives of 133 familiar of which 27 are of mammals, 71 birds, 23 reptiles and 12 amphibians. This sub-region is the great home of rearly all the arboreal vertebrates

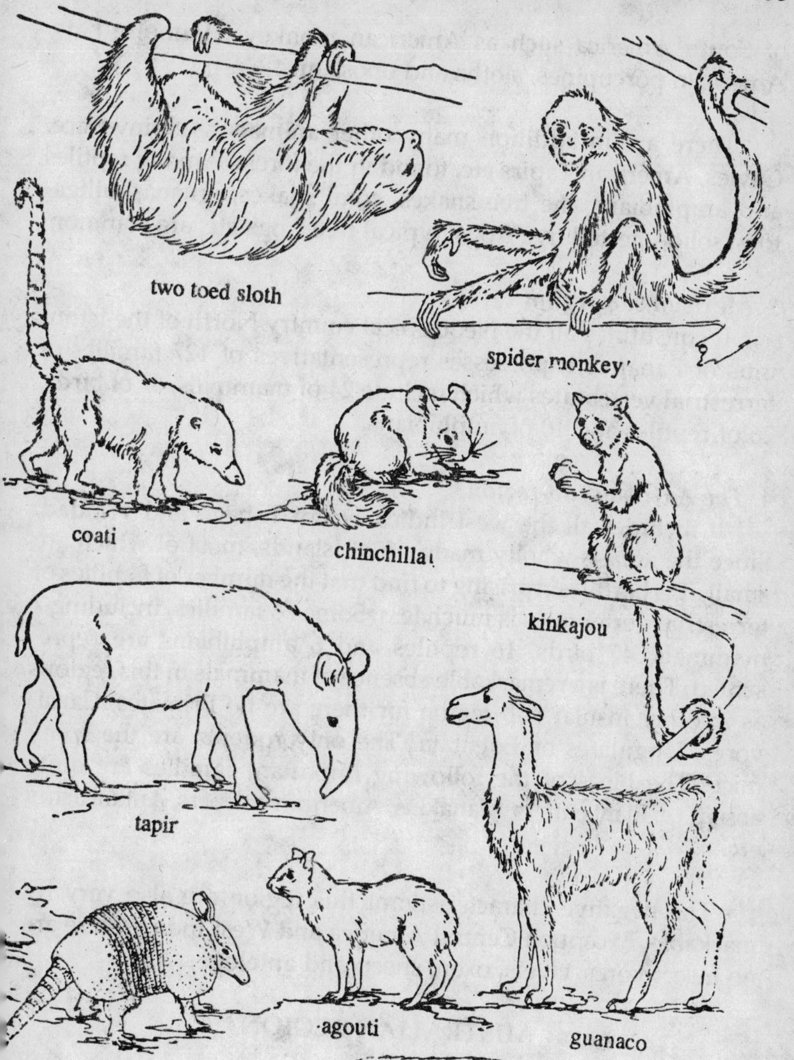

Fig. 10.3. Typical South Americal placental mammals.

of South America such as American monkeys, Vampire bats, American porcupines, sloths and opossums.

There are in addition many other animals as Spiny-mice, Cavies, American Tapirs etc. found in the forest. Among reptiles and amphibians, the tree snakes, coral snakes, iguanas, alligators, solid-chested tree frogs, typical tree frogs etc. are common.

3. *Mexican sub-region*

It constitutes all the Neotropical country North of the Isthumus of Panama. It possesses representatives of 127 families of terrestrial vertebrates which include 24 of mammals, 67 of birds, 26 of reptiles and 10 of amphibians.

4. *The Antilean sub-region*

It includes all the west Indies except Tobago and Trindad. Since the area is wholly made up of islands, most of which are small, it is hardly surprising to find that the number of families of terrestrial vertebrates is much less. Some 76 families, including 7 mammals, 47 birds, 16 reptiles and 6 amphibians are represented. There is a remarkable absence of mammals in this regions as in other insular sub-region for there are no Primates, Carnivores, Ungulates or Edentata. The only rodents are the spiny mice. The birds of the following important families are quite absent i.e. Plant cutters, Manakins, American creepers, Ant thrushes etc.

The negative characteristic of this región are also very remarkable. Except on Central America and West Indies, there are no insectivores, civets, oxen, sheep and antelopes.

AUSTRALIAN REGION

Extent

The Australian Region includes the whole Australia, New Zealand, New Guinea, the Molluca and other neighbouring islands, and practically the whole of islands in the Pacific ocean. Its boundary on the west is a line drawn between the islands of Bali and Lombok (Wallace's line), thence to the east of Celebes or the Philippine Islands. The line then due eastward along the tropic of

Cancer to include the Sandwick Islands, thence curves round to the south of New Zealand and Auckland Islands, Tasmasnia and Australia.

Climate

The northern part of the Region, North Australia and New Guinea, lies within the tropics with high summer temperature and much of the area is covered by rain forest. The interior of the Australia continent is also hot, but dry, while further south are climate becomes mainly temperate.

Zoological Characteristics

There are 134 families of terrestrial vertebrates about 30 families are peculiar.

Among mammals 8 families are peculiar viz. Macropodiae (kangaroos), Phalangeridae (Phalangers), Phascolomyidae (Wombats), Peramelidae (Bandicoots), Notoryctidae (Marsupial), Dasyuridae (Dasyurus), Echidnidae (Echidna) and Ornithorhynchidae (Ornithorhynchus).

Among birds 17 families are peculiar namely : Paradiscidae (Birds of Paradise), Ptilonorhynchidae (Bower Birds), Meliphagidae (Honey Eaters), Drepanididae (Drepanis), Artichornithidae (Scrub Birds), Cyclopsittacidae, Stringopidae (Own-Parrots), Phinochaetidae (Kagu), Gonuidae (crowned pigeons) Didunculidae (Tooth-billed pigeon), Apterygidae (Kiwis), Dromaeidae (Emus) and Casuariidae (cassowaries).

Among reptiles 3 familiar are peculiar : Pygopodidae (scale footed Lizards), Hatteriidae (Tuatra) and Carettchelydidae (fly-River turtle).

Among amphibians 2 families are peculiar : Cerato-batrachidae and Genyophrynidae.

The Australian Region is also characterized by the absence of certain important groups. Thus, only few mammals are there except marsupials and monotremes. The other order being represented by some bats and small rodents. Apes and monkeys, insectivores, carnivores, ungulates and edentates are entirely absent. Among birds the finches, buntings and wood packers are absent.

The Australian Region has been divided into four sub-regions.

(1) Australo-Malayan sub-region
(2) Australian sub-region
(3) Polynesian sub-region
(4) New Zealand sub-region.

1. *Australo-Malayan Sub-region*

It comprises all the islands of the Malaya Archipelago not included in the Oriental Region together with New guinea, the Moluccas and the Solomon Islands. In this sub-region, there are 113 families of terrestrial vertrebrates of which 4 are peculiar. These are crowned-region and Fly-River Turtle, both confined to New Guinea and two little known Amphibian families Ceratobatrachidae and Genyophrynidae from the Solomon Islands and Sudest Island respectively. Since most of this area consists of small islands, a large number of peculiar genera and species exists. In New Guinea, three marsupial genera are peculiar. The Babirussa is another remarkable and peculiar member of the Austro-Malayan fauna occurring in Celebes, Buru and the Sulu Islands. Among birds, Birds of Paradise, Bower Birds, Honey-Eaters, White eyes, Frog mouth, Lories and Megapodes attain their highest development in this area ; while Honey-peckers, Cuckoo-Shrikes, Fly catchers, Pittas and Fruit-pigeons are very numerously represented. Lastly in New Guinea and the neighbouring islands, the amphibian families Narrow-mouthed Toads and the Tree frogs are characteristic.

2. Australian sub-region

It consists of the whole of Australia and Tasmania. In the sub-region 98 families of terrestrial vertebrates are represented namely 15 mammals, 67 birds, 13 of reptiles and 3 of amphibians. Of these about half a dozen, which include wombats, marsupial mole Duck-Bills, Scrub-Birds, Lyre-Birds and Emus are confined to this region. This area is notable as being the great home of

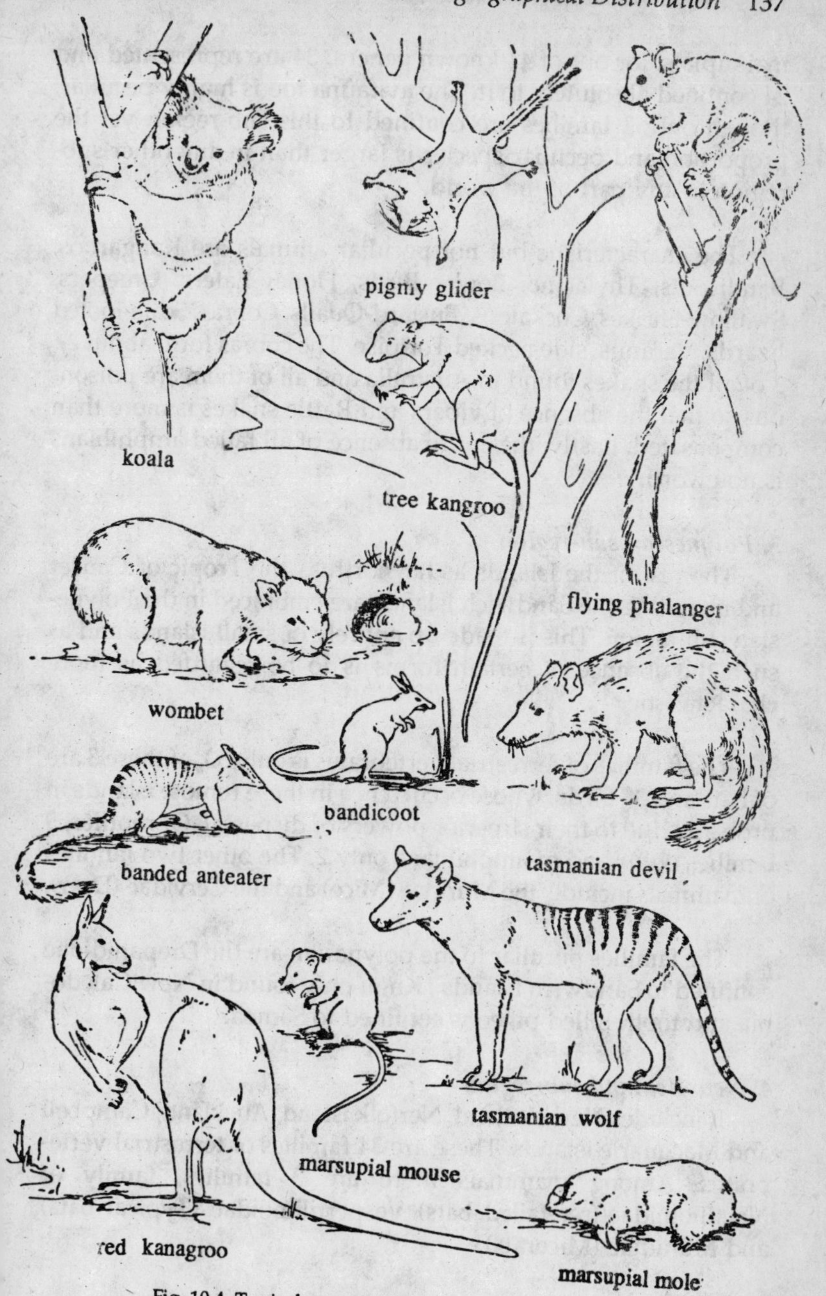

Fig. 10.4. Typical marsupials of Australian Region

marsupials, for out of 41 known genera, 34 are represented and 24 confined absolutely to it. The avifauna too is highly peculiar; though only 3 families are confined to this sub-region yet the proportion and peculiar species is larger than in any other sub-region in any part of the world.

The characteristic but not peculiar animals are Kangaroos, Bandicoots, Thylacine, Bower Birds, Honey-Eaters, Creepers, Swallow-Shrikes, Cockatoos, Bustard-Quails, Cobras, Scale-footed lizards, Varanus, side necked Tortoise. The cobras form about 2/3 of all the snakes found in Australia and all of them are poisonous so that the absence of vipers and Rattle snakes is more than compensated. Lastly, the entire absence of all tailed amphibians is noteworthy.

3. *Polynesian sub-region*

The rest of the Islands as far north as the Tropic of Cancer and including the Sandwich Islands are embraced in the Polynesian sub-region. This is made up entirely of small islands and as such the absence of certain forms is to be regarded as more characteristic.

The families of terrestrial vertebrates is only 53, of these 3 are of bats and 37 birds, whose occurrence in these remote islands in probably due to their superior powers of dispersal. Of reptiles, 9 families occur and of amphibians only 2. The other two families of mammals include the Muridae (Mice) and the Cervidae (Deer).

The families peculiar to the polynesian are the Drepanididae confined to Sandwich islands ; Kngu only found in New Caledonia and tooth-billed pigeons confined to Samoa.

4. *New Zealand sub-region*

It includes New Zealand, Nerfolk island, Auckland, Campbell and Macquarie islands. These are 34 families of terrestrial vertebrates. Among mammals there are 3 families, family of Noctiliomidae(free-tailed bats) Vespertilimoidae (Typical bats) and Muradiae (Micerats).

Among birds 5 families namely the Xeicides, Nestorids (nestor parrots), Stringopids (owl-parrots), Apterygids (Kiwis) and Hatterids are confined to this sub-region.

Among reptiles 13 families are peculiar. Snakes are absent. The amphibian is only represented by one frog, *Liopelma*.

The peculiar animal known as Tuatra (*Sphenodon punctatus*) belonging to family Rhynchocephalidae (class-Reptilia). It is commonly known as living fossil.

ORIENTAL REGION

Extent

This region includes those portions of continental Asia which are not comprised in the palaearctic and Ethiopian Region together with the Malaya Archipelago as for east including Bali, Borneo the Philippine islands and Formosa.

Climate

The Indian sub-region is in its northern portion, chiefly composed of plain and desert, more particularly in the watersheds of great rivers Indus and Ganges. Its fauna as a whole shows a desert affinity to that of the Ethiopian Region ; while the desert in the north-west is debatable ground, and may be regarded as a transitional tract between the Oriental and Palaearctic Regions. The southern portion of India is more luxurient than the northern one, and is largely covered with tropical forest, with a series of elevated tracts culminating in Western and Eastern Ghats. Ceylon, the Indo-Chinese sub-region and most of the Malayan islands are almost entirely covered with tropical forests of the most luxurient character and possess varied and extremely rich fauna.

Zoological Characteristics

The terrestrial vertebrates are represented with 153 families of which 10 are peculiar.

Among mammals 4 families are represented by Hylobatidae (Gibbons), Tarsiidae (Tarsiers), Galeopithecidae (Flying lemures), Galeopithecidae (Flying lemures) and Tupaiidae (Tree-shrews).

Birds are with only one family——i.e. Eurylaemidae (Broad Bills).

Among reptiles 5 families are peculiar they are Elachistodontidae, Uropeltidae (Shield Tails), Lanthanotidae, Gavialidae (Gavialis) and Platysternide (Big Head Tortoise).

In addition to the above, several well known species and genera are quite characteristic. Among Mammals the Orangutan (*Simia satyrus*) the Macaque monkeys (*Macacus*), the Tiger (*Felis tigris*) and Indian elephant (*Elphas maximus*), Malayan Tapir (*Tapirus indicus*), and three out of the five known species of Rhinoceros are nearly or quite confined to the Region, while families Tragulidae (Chevrotains) and Manidae (Pangolin) are very characteristic. Although only one family of Birds is given above as peculiar, yet many other have their monopolies in the Oriental Region. They are Starlings drongos, Orioles, Honey Peckers, Bulbuls, Pittas and many others. Reptiles and Amphibians are very well represented in this region for besides the five peculiar families above enumerated, the following are characteristic Illysiidae (Cylinder Snakes), Xenopeltidae, Acrochordidae (Wart snakes) and pitvipers etc.

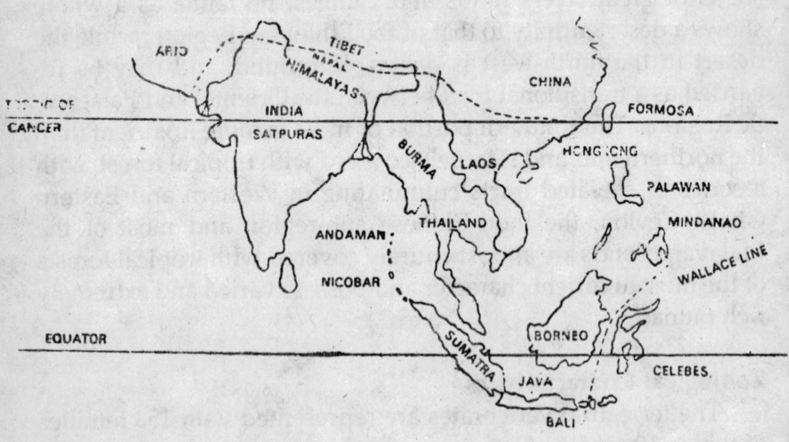

Fig. 10.5. Oriential region

Wallace divided Oriental region into four sub-regions :

(1) Indian sub-region
(2) Ceylonese sub-region
(3) Indo-Chinese sub-region
(4) Indo-Malayan sub-region

1. *Indian sub-region*

It consists of Central and Northern India, from the river Indus and the foot of the Himalayan southwards to Goa and the River Krishna, the line of demarcation taking a southward bend nearly as far as Mysore. It is inhabited by 123 families of terrestrial vertebrates of which only one is peculiar i.e. Elachistodontidae which include a single species of Colubrine Snake. There is no other peculiar feature. Indeed by *Sclater* and other, the first two of the Wallace's sub-regions which together include the whole of Indian peninsula are regarded as one.

2. *Ceylonese sub-region*

It includes the remaining portion of Indian Peninsula, not included in the Indian sub-region and the island of Ceylon. The main peculiarities of this area are the exclusive possession of the curious family of snakes known as Shield-Tails and the presence of Loris which does not occur in Northern India, though recorded from Eastern Burma. The genera Platacanthomys (Spiny-Rat) is also characteristic, only occurring elsewhere in Cochin, China. On the whole, 122 families of terrestrial vertebrates are represented and are indentical to the fauna of Indian sub-region.

3. *Indo-Chinese sub-region*

It includes China, south to the Palaeartic region, Burma, Thailand and the islands of Hainan, Formosa and Andamans. It contains as many as 138 families.

Among mammals three genera i.e. Takin, Hapalomys and Panda are confined to this sub-region. It also contains Gibbons, Flying lemurs, Java Rhinoceros, Malayan Tapir etc.

Among birds wrens are common. One family of tortoise i.e. Platysternidae is peculiar. Among amphibians salamander and disc-tongued frogs occur.

4. *Indo-Malayan sub-region*

It includes the Malayan Peninsula and all those islands of the Malaya Archipelogo which fall with Oriental Region. In this region occur 132 families of terrestrial vertebrates of which one, the Lanthonotidae is peculiar and another i.e. Tarsiidae is practically so. In addition, several genera of mammals are peculiar. Among these may be mentioned Orang-Utan, Proboscis-monkey, Heringale, Cynogale, Malayan Badger and some small Rodents. The green Tupaia (Tree-shrews) is well represented and characteristic while the Gibbons, Flying lemurs, two species of Rhinoceros, the Malayan Tapirs and the Broad-bill are peculiarly Oriental forms which this region shows with the Indo-Chinese. The typical Australian Cockatoos are represented by a single species in the Phillipines while the Magapodes another essentially Australian group occur in the Phillipines, Borneo and the Nicobar Islands.

ZOOGEOGRAPHY OF INDIAN SUB-REGION

Blanford (1901) in *Phil. Trans Royal Soc. London* discussed the geographical distribution of animals on the earth in British India. In his discussion he included India, Pakistan, Kashmir, Gilgit, Ladak, Nepal, Bhutan, Sikkim, other Cis-Himalayan states, Assam, countries between Assam and Burma such as Garo, Khasi and Naga Hills, Manipur, Burma with Karenni, Tenasserim and the Mergui Archipelago, Andaman and Nicobar Islands *B. Prasad* (1942) added Laccadive and Maldive islands.

Sub-regions of India

Owing to the heterogeny nature of the faunas of the different parts further divisions of Indian sub-region is not an easy task. Its divisions has been attempted by a number of scientists. A brief history of such attempts is as follows.

Jorden (1862) divided it on the basis or birds ; *Gunther* (1864) on the basis of reptiles ; *Blanford* (1876) on the molluscs ; *Wallace* (1876) considered the distribution of all the groups of animals. *Blanford* (1888) on mammals, *M. Smith* (1931) based his findings of reptiles and amphibians ; *B. Prasad* (1921) sub-divided Indian sub-region into 5 division. *Mahendra* (1942) divided Indian sub-region into 10 sub-divisions on the basis of distribution of reptiles and amphibians these are :

1. The arid and semiarid province of North India.
2. The western Himalayans.
3. Southern Burmese Province.
4. Trans-gangatic province.
5. Gangatic plain and adjacent part as for far south as 20° latitude.
6. South India below 20° latitude excluding Travancore.
7. Travancore province.
8. Ceylon
9. Andaman Islands.
10. Nicobar Islands.

1. *The arid and semiarid province of North India*

It consists of W. Pakistan, Punjab, Western Rajasthan and Cutch. The fauna is allied to that of the countries to the west of present W. Pakistan and also almost all genera and species are characteristic.

Among lizards are *Teratoscincus, Stenodactylus, Alsophylax, Agamura, Pristurus Eremias* etc. Among snakes are *Leptotyphlops, Contia, Lytorhynchus* etc. are present. Many species are endemic. Very few turtles occur but none are endemic or peculiar to it.

Amphibians are rare the only genera found being the cosmopolitan *Rana* and *Bufo*.

2. *Western Himalayas*

It embraces Kashmir, Simla, Kumaun and Garhwal Districts, adjacent mountainous regions of Western Tibet Alapine and Punjab etc. This zone is poor in amphibians and reptiles. There are certain endemic species e.g. *Gymnodactilus fasciolatus, G. lawderanus, Japalura major, J. Kumaonesis* and *Phynocephalus theobaldi* and *Leiolopisma ladacense.*

3. *The Trans-genetic provice*

It consists of the northern part of Bihar and undivided Bengal, the whole of Assam, Burma north of 20° latitude Nepal,

Himalayas to the east of Nepal, Sikkim and Bhutan. The herpetological fauna is both rich and characteristic. Amongst the endemic genera are *Ptyctoaemus, Mictopholis, Oriocalotes, Stolizteaia, Tylotriton* etc.

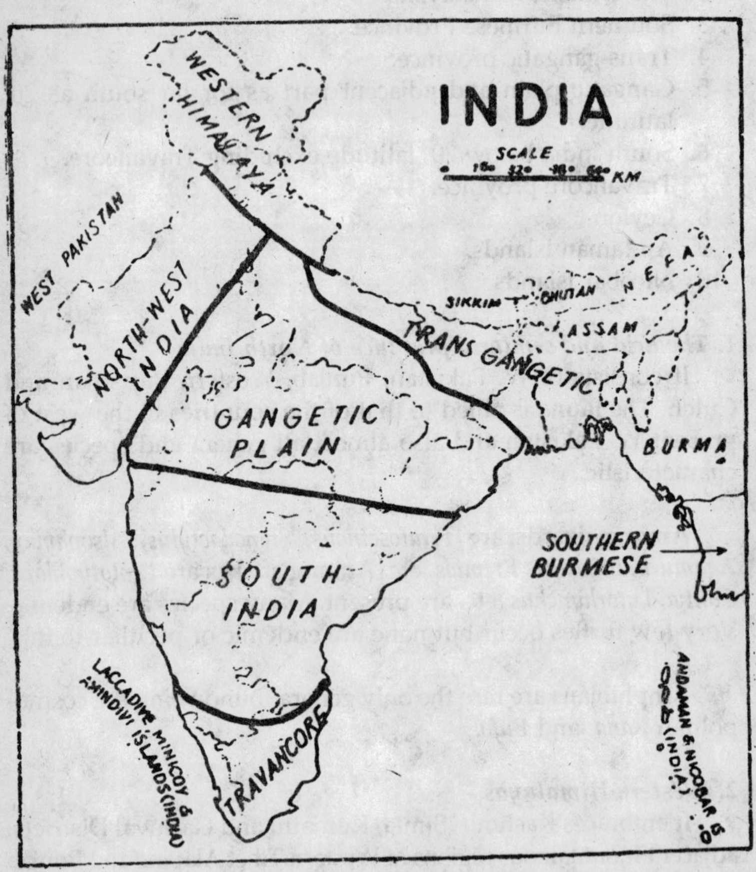

Fig. 10.6. Indian Sub-region.

4. *Southern Burmese Province*

It comprises southern Burmese province including Burma approximately south of 20° latitude. It includes certain characteristic snake species and some endemic amphibians.

Among snakes are *Gymnodactylus oldhami, G. Consobinoides, Riopa anguina, Bungarus flaviceps, Doliophis intestinalis, Coluber melanurus.* Among turtles are *Platysternum megracephalum, Triony cartilagineus, Geoemyda grandis* etc.

Among amphibians *Kaloula macrodactyla, Glyphoglossues molossus, Callulla guttulata* are characteristic of this region.

5. *Gangatic plain and adjacent Region as far South as 20° lat*

The southern boundary is very vague and approximate. This sub division is characterised by the extreme poverty of fauna and has no endemic species. There is complete absence of house gecko. The Indian gharial, *Gavialis* ranges as much as in the Indus system as in Ganges, Brahmputra and Mahanadi.

6. *South India below 29° lat. excluding the Travancore Province*

This province is faunistically characteristic and has *Riopa lineala, Barkudia insularis, Gomnodactylus dekkanenois, Hemidactylus subtriedrus* and *Hemidactylus reticulatus.*

Only a few wide spread species of fresh water turtles are found.

7. *The Travancore*

Consisting of the hilly country south of Lat. 12° or 13° on the west, and south of the Coleroon river in the east. The distinctness of this division is well recognised, the fauna being extremely rich in endemic forms. The number of characteristic genera and spp. is too large.

8. *Ceylon*

It forms a distinct zoogeographic province, with clear affinities to the Travancore sub-region.

9. *Andaman Islands*

Besides having a few endemic forms, which differentiate the fauna of this region as separate from others, the Andaman are faunistically allied to the Burmese sub-region on one hand, and to Nicobars on the other. There are hardly any endemic genera owing evidently to the fauna being imported from the continent in comparatively recent times.

The endemic species are *Gymnodactylus rubidus, Phelsuma andamanesis, Caslotes andamansis, Typhlope andamansis, Boiga andamanesis* etc. There are no amphibians (except 2 spp. of *Rana*) and no fresh water turtles.

10. *Nicobar Islands*

Its fauna has affinities with Andaman Islands. It has fauna like Calotes mystaceus, Mabuya andamanesis, Goniocephalus suberistatus. The endemic species are few in number like Mabuya rugitera, Calotes jubatuo, Leiolopisma macrotis and some other.

WALLACE'S LINE

The Wallace's line is the supposed boundary between the Oriental and Australian faunas. The faunas of the Oriental and Australian Regions are extra-ordinarily different. What happens where they meet in the Indo-Australian Archipelago has long fascinated Zoogeographers. As first drawn by *Wallace* (1860), the line ran between Bali and Lombok, between Borneo and Celebes and between the Philippines and Sangi and Taland islands. Later authors debated the position of the line especially the northern part of it. *Huxley*, for example, who named Wallace's line, thought it should split the Philippine putting Palawan in the Orient and rest of the Philippine in the Australian region. Still later even th existence of the line was debated.

Later zoogeographers doubted the validity of Wallace's line Majority of the scientists thought it be imaginary, some regarde that such as sharp boundary could not be drawn between an two faunal regions. Now Wallace's line is no longer accepted a the boundary between the two regions, as there is great diffe ence between the faunas of Bali and Lombok, that are separate by only about 32 km. The rich fauna of Borneo and compar. tively poor faunas of Celebes and the Philippines cannot l denied. The difference is regarded due to impoverished your fauna in one area and an older richer fauna in the other.

WEBER'S LINE

In 1904, *Weber* draw another line between the Oriental and Australian regions. It demarcates fauna to the west as predominntally oriental and to the East Australian. However, one problem is that Australian elements for one group of animals, it may not be the same for another group. Majority of the zoogeographers do not recognize Weber's line and prefer a broad belt as a separate zone. This is due to the difference in motility of different kinds of animals. A further proof of these differences is that the flora of New Guinea is mainly Oriental while its fauna is strictly Australian.

Dickenson and others (1923) gave the term 'Wallacea' to separate eastern boundary of the Oriental region at or near Wallace's line and western boundary of the Australian Region just west of New Guinea. In that the intervening area may be regarded as a separate subtraction transition area. *Darlington* (1957) also recognized that this is an appropriate and useful term. Wallacea bounds the Oriental and Australian regions.

11

GEOLOGICAL DISTRIBUTION

To understand the complete evolutionary changes in the organisms (plants and animals), one has to study the organisms of the distant part which are now extinct. The extinct forms of life, with primitive forms and recent forms, are preserved in the rocks as *fossils*. The study of these fossils constitutes the subject matter of *palaeontology*.

A number of estimates have been proposed from time to time about the age of earth. For examples, *Archbishop Ussher* of Ireland in 1645 declared that the creation of earth took place on 26th October 4004 B.C. at 9 o'clock in the morning. This was the adopted version of the *Bible* for a long time. *James Hutton* believed that geological time was unimaginable long. *Lord Kelvin* (1877), from a study of the flow of heat from the interior to the surface of earth, estimated the age of earth from 20-40 million years.

The most accurate method of determining the age of a rock is by radioactive decay studies. Certain radioactive elements like uranium and thorium, found in certain rocks, decay into lead. The rate of this radioactive disintegration is constant and is unaffected by external physical conditions like temperature, pressure, etc. The formula may be written as $U^{238} = Pb^{206} + 8He^{4} +$ heat. It has been determined that one gram of uranium gives or decay 1/7,600,000 gram of lead in one year. The lead : uranium ration in a rock would thus give the age of the rock. The maximum age of the earth has thus been estimated to be around 5500 m.y. (million years). Other methods of dating e.g., potassium argon method, radiocarbon methods, etc. are also known today

GEOLOGICAL TIME SCALE

By studying the fossils, present in the rocks, the geologists have divided the earth's past history into *Era* which are major divisions. The eras are divided into *Periods*. The periods are subdivided into *Epochs*. These eras, periods and epoches are arranged on the time scales in an order of their age, and this arrangement is called, *geological time scale.*

The first geological time scale was developed by *Giovanni Avduina*, an Italian scientist, in 1760.

Eras

Based on the nature of the forms of life preserved as fossils in the rock, the earth's past history is divided into six eras:

I. Azoic
II. Archaeozoic or Eozoic (Primal life or dawn of life)
III. Proterozoic (Early life)
IV. Palaeozoic (Ancient life)
V. Mesozoic (Mediaeval life)
VI. Cenozoic (Recent life)

Periods

These are the fundamentals units of the standard geologic time scale. There are 12 periods :

I. *Periods of Palaeozoic Era.* There are 7 periods in palaeozoic era.

1. Cambrian
2. Ordovician
3. Silurian
4. Devonian
5. Mississippian
6. Pennsylvanian
7. Permian

II. *Periods of Mesozoic Era.* There are three periods :

8. Triassic

9. Jurassic
10. Cretaceous.

III. *Periods of Cenozoic Era.* There are two periods :

11. Tertiary
12. Quaternary

Epochs

There are seven epochs. The epochs of Cenozoic's period are:

I. *Quaternary period* : There are two epochs

1. Recent
2. Pleistocene.

II. *Tertiary Period.* It is sub-divided into five epochs.

3. Pliocene
4. Miocene
5. Oligocene
6. Eocene
7. Palaeocene.

I. AZOIC ERA

This was the time, in which life was not present on the earth. During this time, earth was formed, cooled and underwent many changes. These charges made favourable conditions for the appearance of living organisms. The rock of this time are igneous type without any fossil.

II. ARCHAEOZOIC ERA

The manner in which life originated is not known. It is probable that sometime in early Archaeozoic Eras the earliest living matter that could reproduce itself, got generated under very favourable conditions of temperature, humidity, light etc. by the combination of certain chemicals. The first living matter may have been very similar to protoplasm. Filterable viruses which represent an intermediate stage between living and non-living entities, may have been the first to appear on the surface of the globe in the early Archaeozoic Era. Unicellular Protozoa and Protophyta may have been also present.

According to *Stirton* (1959), the oldest known fossils are blue-green algae, fungi, and probably a flagellate described from Ontrario, Canada. The age of the rock in which these algae occur has been estimated to be about 200 m.y. (million years) by radiometric methods.

III. PROTEROZOIC ERA

It may be called the '*Age of Primitive Invertebrates*'. Life was in the form of algae, precipitations, siliceous sponge spicules, remains of radiolarians, impression of jelly fishes, a simple brachiopod (*Lingullela montana*) as well as deposits of graphite. These first organisms were quite possibly soft bodies. Reducing bacteria must also have been predominant during this era because the chief iron-ore deposits of the world are found in the Proterozoic era.

The fossil record from the rocks is much less probably due to absence of hard parts in the organisms to be preserved as fossils. The fossils which were formed must have been destroyed due to effect of pressure and high temperatures.

This era is estimated to have lasted 3.5 billion years.

IV. PALAEOZOIC ERA

The fossil record in this era are very extensive. Almost all the major invertebrate phyla are represented even in the early Palaeozoic era. The fossils of vertebrates also present late in the era because the early chordates were soft-bodies and could not be preserved as fossils.

Palaeozoic era is divided into following periods :

1. Cambrian Period

The name cambrian was proposed by *A. Sedgwick* in 1835. It is taken from *cambria* the Latin name of city of Wales.

This period started by the melting of glaciers, slow rise of sea-level and warm climate.

Almost all the main invertebrate phyla had existed during this Period as also the main phyla of plants. Trilobites were the most dominant forms of life, the important genera being *Olenellus, Redlichia* in the early Cambrian times ; *Paradoxides* in the middle Cambrian and Crepicephalus in late Cambrian. Small primitive brahiopods and gastorpods with simple shells are found in early Cambrian rocks. Some foraminifers and radiolarians have also been found. A few graptolites are recorded in the Cambrian rocks. Echinoderms have been recorded from Cambrian rocks of Australia while some bryozoans from Russia and Canada.

The first land plants also appear in the Periods.

2. Ordovician Period

The name Ordovician was proposed by *Charles Lapworth* in 1897, on the basis of the ordovies, and ancient tribe, that formerly inhibited the city of Wales.

During the period, conditions became more favourable as the climate was uniformly warm with glacial activities in certain regions.

This was the "Age of Giant Mollusca". Graptolites, which started in late Cambrian, show their maximum development during Ordovician. They infact serve as index fossils in Ordovician rocks. Trilobites were still abundant and reached the climax of their evolution. First ostracods appeared on the scene and brachiopods developed harder shells. Cephalopods, both straight-shelled and coiled type were abundant. Echinoderms appeared in large numbers and show diversification, the starfish being very common.

Ordovician is also characterised by first appearance of conodonts which are very important marine environment indicators. Land plants are meagre. First appearance of fish-like animals Ostracodersm is also recorded in Ordovician rocks. This period probably marks the first appearance of vertebrates.

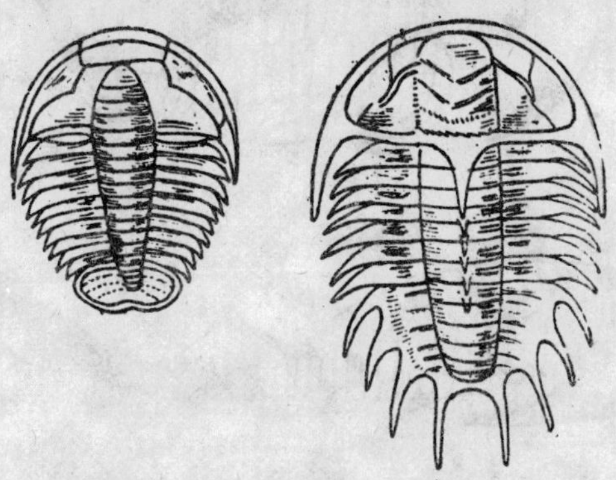

Fig. 11.1. Few Trilobites.

3. Silurian Period

The term Silurian was proposed by *Murchison* in 1835 to designate the rocks present on the borders of Wales and England. This area was inhibited by Silures, an ancient tribe, inhibited Wales.

The climatic conditions were mild and some areas were arid. Land elevation at places caused formation of deep continental seas. Rise of *Caledonian Mountain* in British Isles, Scandinavia and N. Greenland and in N. Africa and East. Central Asia.

The first air-breathing invertebrates on the earth were scorpions which appeared in the Silurian period. Trilobites now started waning. Bryozoans were extremely abundant. Brachiopods continued their development and first *Spirifer* appeared in Silurian Period. Graptolites also started a decline at the end of Silurian Period.

The fish is found to have developed lower jaws in the Silurian Period. The organisation of the Silurian fishes is similar in many respects to that of the fishes of today.

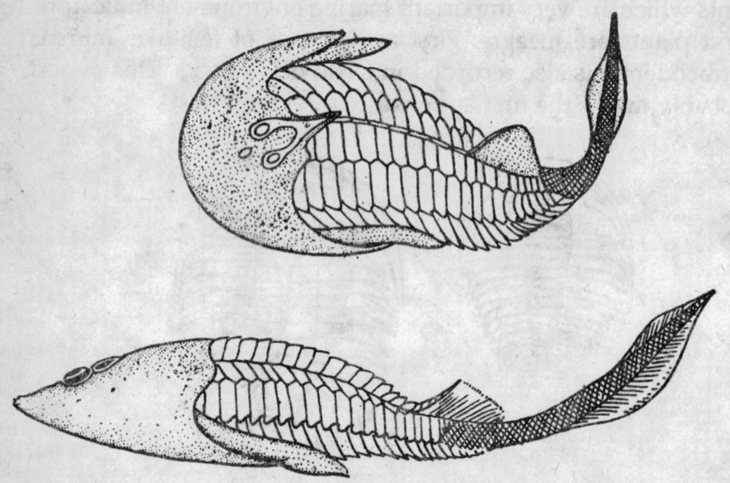

Fig. 11.2 Cephalapsis (an Ostracoderm)

Although algae were still dominant but some terrestrial primitive ferns also evolved.

4. Devonian Period

The name Devonian was proposed by *Sedgwick* and *Murchison* in 1839 after Devonshire, a country of south-Western England, where rock formation of this period were first found.

The land elevation continued. Consequently larger seas were further divided into smaller seas. Due to fall of temperature, climate remained cold and dry. This period was marked by great volcanic activities and the formation of coal, oil and gas.

During this period, branchiopod developed wonderfully. Corals and bryozans were also abundant.

The Devonian Period called the '*Age of Fishes*, because of their great number. Plate-skinned fishes, sharks and bony fishes were common. The Devonian ancestors of modern lung fish, Choanichthyes, were able to survive dry period by burrowing in the moist beds of streams or lake. The lobed-fin fish, crossopterygians were characterized by the presence of lobed rounded bases of the paired fins. These were on the direct line of evolution from fish to terrestrial vertebrates. They became extinct at the closer of Palaeozoic except *Latimeria* and *Melania*.

From the late Devonian Rocks of Pennsylvania, the footprint named, *Thinopus antiquas* grave the evidence of first amphibian life.

Tall terrestrial Psilophytes, club-mosses and horse-tails occur in the rock of Scotland. First wingless insects also appeared in this period.

5. Mississippian Period

The name Mississippian was given by *Alexander Winchell* in 1869 to designate the area in eastern Mississipi basin where rock formation of this period were found.

The climatic condition were hot and damp which caused formation of widespread swamps.

During this period, sharks were the dominant firshes in the seas and oceans. They were of many kinds but consisted principally of the more ancient shell-feeding types which were subsequently almost wholly blotted out.

This period is called *Age of Crinoids* because they were most abundant and diversified. Amphibian spread and the insects evolved wings during Mississipian period.

No evolutionary change in terrestrial plants in comparison to those of Devonian period is observed in this period.

6. Pennsylvanian Period

Term 'Pennsylvanian' was proposed by *H.S. Williams,* in 1819 which refers to the state Pennsylvania.

The climate conditions were disturbed so that the forests burried under the swamps and turned, in due course of time, into present-day coal mines. For this reason, Mississipian and

Pennsylvanian Periods are often combined together under a head, *Carboniferous period* (i.e. coal bearing).

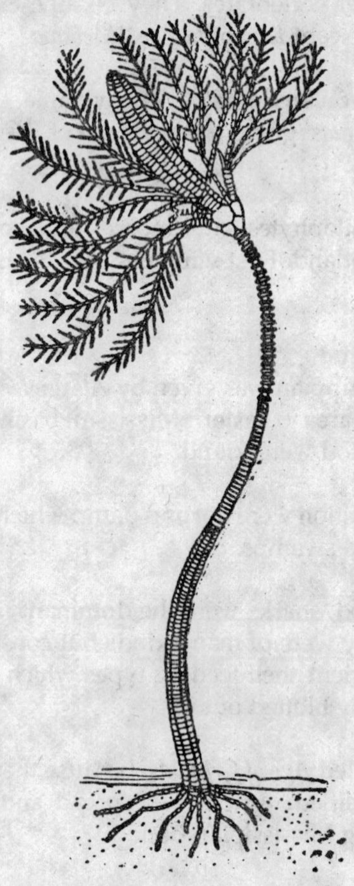

Fig. 11.3 Crenoids or sea-illies

Amongst animlas, insects developed abundantly both in size and diversity. Cockroaches reached such a large number that some times this period is called the '*Age of Cockroaches*'. Dragon flies were also abundant. Among vertebrates, amphibians showed maximum diversity and specialization during this period. True sharks and sea-lilies were common. Towards the close of this period appeared the first animal *Tuditanus punctulatus*, showing the reptilian affinities, from stegocephalians.

Among plants, ferns dominated and bryophytes also appeared.

7. Permian Period

The term 'Permian was given by *Murchison* in 1941, because fossil record of the period were found in Russian province Perm.

The cold and dry condition caused widespread galciation. Extensive land elevation caused the formation of high mountains. Consequently, shallow seas were emptied and their bottom became exposed as salty deserts. Melting of glaciers gave rise to rivers upon the land.

Great diversification in reptiles took place and first mammal like reptiles appeared in the Permian times. Many important groups of marine invertebrates now dwindled. Permian marks the complete extinction of Trilobites which were very important and dominant during the early Paleozoic. Due to the cold climates, the insect developed larval adaptations seen in the metamorphosis of present day insects.

Among terrestrial animals spiders, scorpions, centipedes, snails etc. were present.

Among plants swampy trees declined and were replaced by tall gymnosperms. The true conifers and cycads became most abundant and trees somewhat similar to date palms appeared.

V. MESOZOIC ERA

In contrast to the dominance of marine animals throughout palaezoic era, the Mesozoic Era is characterized by the dominance of land animals, the most spectacular of which were giant dinosaurs which ruled the earth for thousands of years. That is why this era is known as *'Age of Reptiles'*. This era is divided into three Periods.

1. Triassic Period

This name was given by *F. Von Alberti.*

This period was characterized by hot and dry climate and land elevation which helped in expression of deserts and continents.

Snails, bivalved molluscs, insects and sea-urchins diversified and spread. This period is characterized by the diversification of reptiles. Dinosaurs spread upon land; Ichthyosaurs (fish-like) in water; lizard-like Plęsiosaurs in water; and bird like Pterosaurs in air. The egg-laying mammals also made their appearance.

During this period horstails, club-mosses and seed fern declined, Gymnosperms progressed fast.

2. Jurassic Period

The name was given by *A. Von humboldt* in 1799. This period has been named after the Jura Mountains of Switzerland and France. The climates during this period were mild throughout the world. Consequently both invertebrate and vertebrate fauna thrived. Among the invertebrates, belemnites and ammonites were most abundant; the latter, in fact, served as a basis for division of Jurassic rocks into eighty stages and thirty-three zones by *Oppel.*

Jurassic is the age of giant dinosaurs like Ichthyosaurs which were more than 50 ft. long and whose skill alone measured more than 8 ft. The first bird *Archaeopteryx*, which is the connecting link between reptiles and birds has been found in the Solnhofen limestone of Jurassic Period. Similarly the first mammals are recorded in Jurassic Period. Among plants gymnosperms continued spreading. Advanced seed ferns gave rise to the first Angiosperms which were dicotylednous.

3. Cretaceous Period

The term was given by *J.J. d' Omalus d' Halloy* in 1882 derived from latin word Creta=chalk.

The climate was warm and somewhat uniform over the most earth surface, but became cooler later on. The seas spread widely over the continents in the earliest part of this period. The Larmide Orogeny changed the surface relief of the earth which affected the climates. The changed climates accelerated the evolution of mammals, birds, flowering plants etc. while caused complete extinction of certain groups of animals like the dinosaurs, ammonites and rudistids.

In the sea, sharks and bony fishes flourished. Snakes first appeared in this period. New varieties of birds appeared. Mammals were still small and less numerous. Marsupials diverged from the archaic forms. Placental mammals appeared.

During this period the dinosaurs became extinct. Because of their heavy body and small brain, lack of adaptability, cld bloodedness, berbivours food etc.

Among plants, the gymnosperms declined. Dicot angiosperms flourished and tall oak, maple etc. formed thick forests. The first monocots appeared.

VI. CENOZOIC ERA

It is known as "Age of mammals". It was marked by great adaptive radiation in bird, insects and flowering plants. Wide variety of animals got food protection as a result of development and spread of deciduous trees, herbs and grasses.

The cenozoic era is divided into two periods, and each period into epochs.

1. Tertiary Period

This period includes five epochs.

(i) *Palaeocene Epoch.* In the beginning the climate was fairly warm but gradually it became colder.

After complete extinction of dinosaurs, nine new orders of terrestrial mammals evolved. Among these were the first primitive carnivores, lemurs, tarsiers etc. Modern group of birds evolved. Plants also underwent a corresponding evolutionary change.

(ii) *Eocene Epoch.* Climate remained less hot. There was a widespread erosion of mountains.

All the modern orders of mammals were present. The first horse *Eophippus* or *Hyracotherium* evolved also first camel which were originally of the size of a dog or even smaller evolved during this period. The horse had progressed to the *Epihippus* stage by this time. Pigs, rats, monkeys, whales and seals appeared.

Angiosperms spread and evolved, giving rise to several modern types. Heavy forests and limited grass land characterized this period.

(iii) *Oligocene Epoch.* Climate remained hot. The level of land decreased.

Most of the families of mammals were recognizable by this time. Larger brontotheres reached their climax in early Oligocene Period and suddenly died out before middle Oligocene Period. The true flesh-eaters like dogs, cats sabertoothed cats and other small animals, as well as rodents and insect-eating animals became most abundant. The horse had reached the *Miohippus* stage. It was of the size of a sheep with three toes in each foot. Tortoise of medium size were abundant. Hawks and vultures hovered in the sky and the 'American pigs' on the ground. Near the end of the Oligocene Period the first New World monkeys appeared.

Among plants tropical and subtropical forests, flowering plants and monocots became widespread.

(iv) *Miocene Epoch.* In miocene epoch, the Alps reached their highs and Himalayas were pushed up. So the climate remained somewhat cold. New mountain ranges such as Cascade, Sierra etc., formed upon American continent.

This Period was the rise and rapid evolution of grazing mammals, long slender-limbed camels, *Oxydactylus*, bear dogs, small foxes, American pigs etc. were particularly abundant. The horse had reached *Parahippus* stage a major step in evolution towards modern horse. A free interchange of old and new world terrestrial mammals took place among which cats, dogs, horses and mastodonts were especially common. In late Miocene Period, the horse had reached *Merychipps* stage of evolution in North America. In Eurasia, the Miocene Epoch is marked by the appearance of hyenas, deer, giraffes, and true antelopes.

Terrestrial plants were more progressive.

(v) *Pliocene Epoch.* This period started with subsidence of land in many places and ended with the beginning of one or two Ice Ages. The climate became still cooler..

The mammals became more specialized and reached their peak of evolution. Camels, horses, rhinoceroses, etc. were abundant during this period. Camels had grown larger in size, and the horse had evolved into several genera. *Pliophippus,* which ultimately gave rise to modern horse, evolved during this period from tis Miocene ancestors. *Hipparion* fauna was typical of Pliocene Period in Eurasia and was distributed from Western Europe and North Africa to South western Asia, India, Burma and China. Characters found in the fossil jaws and teeth of *Dryopithecus,* found in Siwalik rocks of India, showed affinities with chimpanzee, gorilla and modern man. the lack of a land bridge between North and South America in early Pliocene period inhibited the free migration and dispersal.

Thick forests declined due to cold. Tall and woody plants were replaced by soft monocot plants.

2. Quaternary Period

This period is divided into two epochs :

(i) *Pleistocene Epoch.* There are evidences of four *Ice Ages* alternating with warmer intervals. Widespread glaciation during this epoch lowered the sea level. Land connection between Europian continent and Britain, and Siberia and Alaska were established. Due to these land connections dispersal of horses, camels, deer, cats, saber, dogs, rodents etc. took place.

The modern horse, *Equus* originated. The first evidence of a primitive man Homo *heidelbergensis,* recognised by a massive mandible, was found in the middle Pleistocene rocks of Heidelberg, Germany. The Peking man, *Pithecanthropus pekinensis,* lived in the mildy cooler climates in parts of China and adjoining areas. The ape man of Java, *Pithecanthorpous erectus,* found among Pleistocene fauna of Java, attests to the evidence of a land bridge between Java and mainland of Asia. The entire Pleistocene Period shows dominance of man.

(ii) *Recent Epoch*. The climate has again become hot. Supremacy of man as the wiser and dominant species has been established, with increasing mental development, gradually he got control over water, air and land. He is trying to get control over planets other than earth. Thus we can say that this epoch is the *'Age of man'*.

Table11.1
Geologic Time-table

Era	*Period*	*Epoch*	*Duration in million of years*	*Time from beginning of period to present (millions of years)*	*Geologic conditions*	*Plant Life*	*Animal Life*
Cenozoic (Age of Mammals)	Quaternary	Recent	0.025	0.025	End of last ice age; climate of warmer.	Decline of woody plants; rise of herbaceous ones.	Age of man
		Pleisto-cene	1	1	Repeated glaciation; 4 ice ages	Great extinction of species	Extinction of great mammals; first human social life
	Tertiary	Pliocene	11	12	Continued rise of mountains of western North America; volca-nic activity.	Decline of forests; spread of grasslands; flowering plants, monocotyledons developed.	Man evolving, ele-phants, horses, camels almost like modern species.
		Miocene	16	28	Sierra and Cascade mountains formed; volcanic activity in north-west U.S., cli-mate cooler.		Mammals at height of evolution; first manlike apes.

Era	*Period*	*Epoch*	*Duration in million of years*	*Time from beginning of period to present (millions of years)*	*Geologic conditions*	*Plant Life*	*Animal Life*
		Oligocene	11	39	Lands lower; climate warmer	Maximum spread of forests; rise of monocotyledons, flowering plants	Archaic mammals extinct; rise of anthropoids; forerunners of most living genera of mammals.
		Eocene	19	58	Mountain eroded; no continental seas; climate warmer.		Placental mammals diversified and specialized; hoofed mammals and carnivores established.
		Paleocene	17	75			Spread of archaic mammals.
Mesozoic (Age of Reptiles)		Cretaceous	60	135	Andes, Alps, Himalayas, Rockies formed late; earlier, inland seas and swamps; chalk, shale deposited.	First monocotyledons, first oak and maple forests, gymnosperms declined.	Dinosaurs reached peak became extinct, toothed birds became extinct, first modern birds, archaic mammals common.
	Jurassic		30	165	Continents fairly high, shallow seas over some	Increase of dicotyledons, cycads and	First toothed birds, dinosuars larger and

Era	Period	Epoch	Duration in million of years	Time from beginning of period to present (millions of years)	Geologic conditions	Plant Life	Animal Life
					of Europe and western U.S.	conifers common	specialized, insectivorous marsupials
		Triassic	40	205	Continents exposed widespread desert conditions, many land deposits.	Gymnosperms dominant, declining toward end, extinction of seed ferns.	First dinosaurs, pterosaurs and egglaying mammals, extinction of primitive amphibians.
Paleozoic (Age of Ancient Life)		Permian	25	230	Continents rose, Appalachians formed, increasing galciation and aridity.	Decline of lycopods and horsetails	Many ancient animals died out, mammal-like reptiles, modern insects arose.
		Pennsylvanian (Carboniferous)	25	255	Lands at first low, great coal swamps	Great forests of seed ferns and gymnosperms	First reptiles, insects common, spread of ancient amphibians)
		Mississippian (carboniferous)	25	280	Climate warm a and humid at first, cooler, later as land rose	Lycopods and horsetails dominant gymnosperms increasingly wide spread.	Sea lilies at height, spread of ancient sharks

Era	*Period*	*Epoch*	*Duration in million of years*	*Time from beginning of period to present (millions of years)*	*Geologic conditions*	*Plant Life*	*Animal Life*
		Devonian	45	325	Smaller inland seas, land higher, more arid, galciation	First forests; land plants well established first gymnosperms	First amphibians; lung-fishes, sharks abundant.
		Silurian	35	360	Extensive continental seas, lowlands, increasingly arid, glaciation	First definite evidence of land plants; algae dominant.	Marine arachnids dominant, first (wingless) insects, rise of fishes.
		Ordovician	65	425	Great submergence of land, warm climate even in Arctic.	Land plants probably first appeared; marine algae abundant.	First fishes, probably freshwater, corals, trilobites abundant, diversified molluscs.
		Cambrian	80	505	Lands, low, climate mild, earliest rocks. with abundant fossils.	Marine algae.	Trilobites, brachiopods, most modern phyla established.
Archeo-Zoic			???	???	Great volcanic activity, some sedimentary deposition, extensive erosion.	No recognizable fossils,	Indirect evidence of living things from deposits of organic material of rocks

12

EVOLUTION OF HORSE

One of the best evidence in the favour of organic evolution is furnished by our knowledge of the evolution of horse. The physogeny of the horse is most thoroughly known. The history of horse is of about 60,000,000 years starting from the Eocene period and involving 20 genera and several species. These fossil horizons furnish a remarkable record through the time of the progressive evolution of horses.

The progressive trends that characterized the evolution of horses through the Cenozoic Era may be listed as :

1. Increase in size.
2. Lengthening of legs, feet and development of cannon bone.
3. Reduction of lateral toes with emphasis on the middle toe.
4. Widening of incisor teeth.
5. Molarization of the premolars.
6. Increase in height of the crowns of the check teeth.
7. Complicated development of crown patterns in teeth.
8. Deepening of the front portion of the skull and of the lower jaws to accommodate the high-crowned cheek teeth.
9. Lengthening of the face infront of the eye, to accommodate the high-crowned cheek teeth.
10. Reduction of canine teeth.
11. Straightening and stiffening of the back.
12. Increase in the size and complexity of brain.

PLACE OF ORIGIN

The first ancient known horse *Hyracotherium* of the Old World has been found from the London clay, an Eocene formation of Europe. While in the Wasatch rocks of Western North

America, the earlier american genus *Eohippus* has been found.

Horse in Eocene

In Eocene several generic names have been given to Eocene horses, among them *Eohippus* and *Orohippus* are best known.

Eohippus

The Eohippus are dawn horses found from the lower Eocene. *Eohippus* is 4 toed and represents the first stage of equine evolution. It is 12" or 3 hands in size, with arched back, short head and neck. The limbs were of moderate length showing digitigrade character of feet, beginning of cursorial adaptation. The four feet had 4 complete toes each terminating in nail with no trace of first digit or pollex, Hind foot had 3 complete in a nail with no trace of first digit or pollex, Hind foot had 3 complete and one vestigial remnant of the 1st and 5th toe. Both ulna and fibula were slender separate and complete. Complications begin to occur. The originally separate cusps fuse and 4th premolars were tending to become molariform.

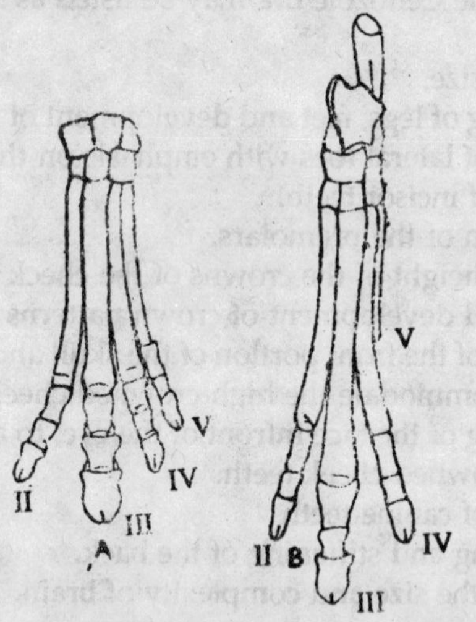

Fig. 12.1 Eohippus A = Hand, B = Foot

Orohippus

The second stage is Orohippus of the Middle (Bridger) Eocene, of which several species are partially known. They were small in size but the fore feet had the third toe slightly large and the vestiges of the first and fifth toes had disappeared from the hind feet. The third and fourth premolar were more advanced and the molar pattern was more pronounced.

Epihippus

It is the third stage recorded from upper Eocene. It was even slightly larger than *Orohippus*. The fore feet were with 4 digits and hind feet with 3 digits. Last two premolars were molar-like in appearance.

It complete skeleton could not be traced and hence is not regarded as the ancestor of the oligocene horse.

Horses of Oligocene

Oligocene was a time of increased aridity due to continental uplift. The broad meadows and dry prairie developed due to dwingling of streams and lakes. These conditions gave rise to several diverging lines of evolution, some of which terminated in the struggle for existence and other gave rise to Pliocene horses. *Meso* - and *Miohippus* are 4th and 5th stages of equine development.

Mesohippus

The fourth stage-*Mesohippus* occurs in the Lower and Middle Oligocene, and the fossil remains of several species are rather common. The size ranged from that a coyote to a sheep. The cranium was still proportionately large and the face small with shallow jaws. The eyes were not far back and the bony orbits were opens behind. The legs were slender; the ulna, although still complete, had become very slender, and the fibula was greatly reduced and partially coalesced with the tibia. All of the feet were three toed. The third or central, toe was largest. The cheek teeth had increased in complexity but were still relatively low crowned and not adapted to hard food.

Miohippus

This was the horse of the upper Oligocene. Its average size was large than *Mesohippus*, about 0.60 m., in height. *Miohippus* cannot be easily distinguished from *Mesohippus*. The low-crowned

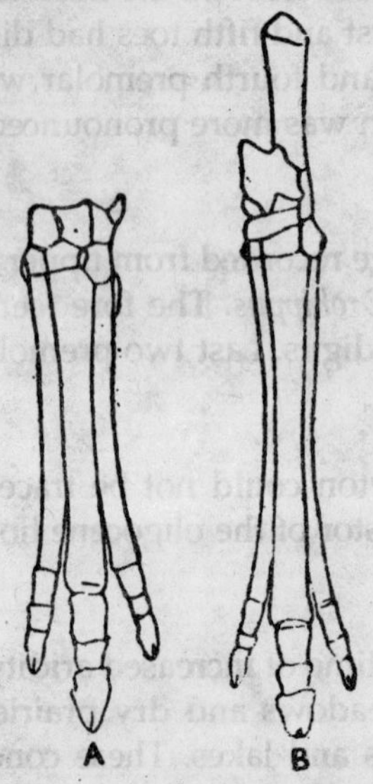

Fig. 12.2 Mesohippus A = Hand, B = Foot.

teeth and the spreading three-toed feet suggested that this animal lived in forest on soft vegetation. It was a three-toed browser, feeding on leaves and shoots, like his ancestor, *Hyracotherium*.

Miohippus regarded as the ancestor of several radiating lines.

Horses of Miocene

Miocene was a time of great continental elevation and prairies expanded. The forests further diminished. Many browing animals could not withstand and died while grazing types of animals like horses, camels etc. survived.

Parahippus

The next stage is *Parahippus* which was abundant during the lower Miocene. A considerable number of species are known of various sizes. Some are conservative, and other progressive in either tooth or foot structure. The teeth, in general, became more complicated with the Pliocene horses and the valleys between the crests of the molars began to contain cement.

Merychippus

It is the 7th stage from middle Miocene. It was horselike with short crowned uncemented teeth. Therefore it was thought to be the reminiscent to its ancestry. It was 3 toed and often vestige of outermost digit on hand was seen. Only the functional toe in foot was present. Ulna was slender and fused with radius.

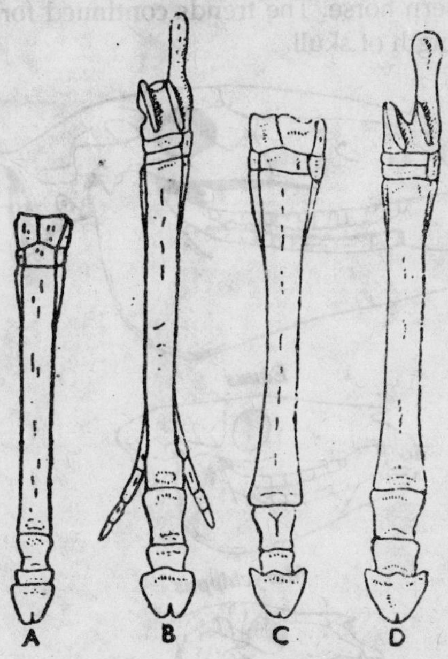

Fig. 12.3 Hands and feet of A, B = Merychippus; C, D = Eqqus

At the close of Miocene period two lines of horses arose from *Merychippus* ancestry. One of them was the direct line of evolution which has included genus *Pliohippus*. The other was an assemblage of closely related genera, of which *Hipparion* was typical. *Hipparions* were lightly built horses, progressive in the development of skull and the very high-crowned teeth, but conservative in the retention of three toes feet. These horses continued through the Pliocence Epoch, and a few stragglers held on it to the Pleistocene epoch, when they became extinct.

Horses of Pliocene

It was the time of great unrest. The conditions were severe

and land bridges were formed result in migration of fauna.

Pliohippus

It had a shoulder hight of 40", about the size of a modern poney. This was first one-toed horse and both fore feet and hind feet were one toed. The crowns of the upper molars were similar to those of modern horse. The trends continued for increase in the preorbital length of skull.

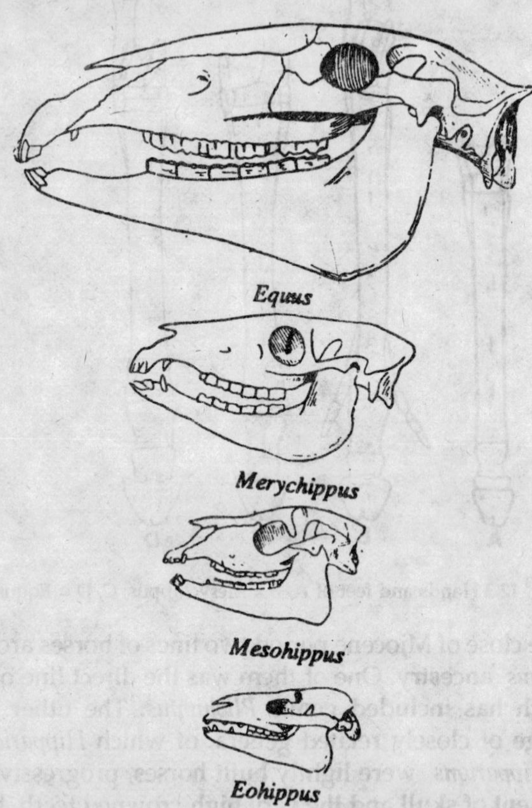

Fig. 12.4 Diagram, showing skull of horses.

Plesippus

The next stage-*Plesippus* is in the direct line of evolution and belongs to pliocene Period. It was about the size and proportions of a modern horse but with smaller hoofs and shorter back. The teeth were high and straighter and prophetic of those of *Equus*.

The feet were like those of modern horses, with the side toes reduced to splints, the skull had lengthened the face and was also more like the skull of a modern horse.

Hippidion

It is South American Pliocene house and is derivative of *Protohippus*. Teeth are like *Pliohippus*. It became extinct in Pleistocene.

Equus

It is the modern horse of Pleistocene and of Recent epoches. It is about 60" in height and has lost the first and fifth digits entirely and the second and fourth digits are represented by splins so that the entire body weight is balanced on the third digits. It bears well developed hoof. The molars possess much elongated crowns and complicated enamel ridges, adapted to feed on dry and harsh grass.

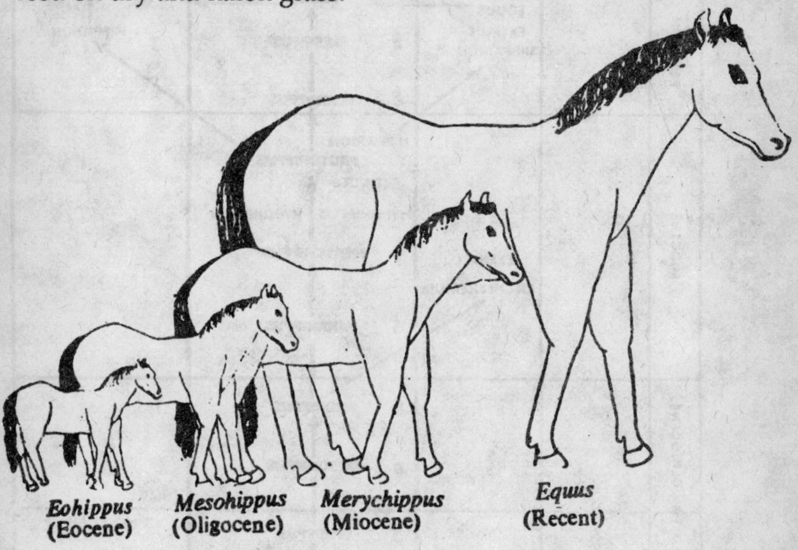

Fig. 12.5. Showing pedigree of horse.

At present time true wild type of horse are present only is Asia (*Equus hemionus*, the Asiatic wild ass and *E. prezewalskii*, the Przewalisky's horse) and Africa (*E. asinus*).

Simpson concluded that from *Eohippus* to *Equus* there must have been at least 15 million generations. The actual increase in size between these stages is 8-40 mm. divided into 300-steps increase per minute being 0.1 mm.

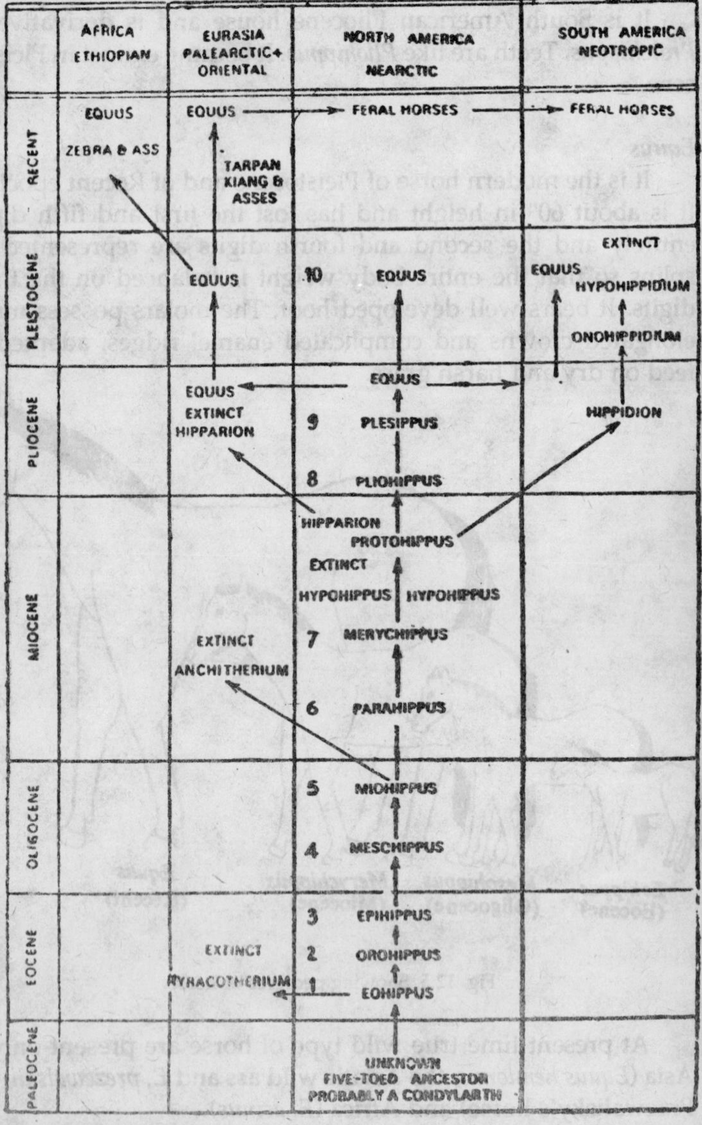

Fig. 12.6. Phylogeny of Horse.

13

EVOLUTION OF MAN

Man is the crowning achievement of evolutionary history. He surpasses all other animals in mental development, a phenomenon unique in the history of life on the earth and which has made him ruler of the world and arbiter of his destiny. It is therefore, natural that enquiry into his ancestory has attracted the attention of scientists throughout the world. The fossil records of man's ancestory are very incomplete. However, the search is continued and the gaps are being filled.

Man as a primate

Homo sapiens, or the modern man is a member of the order Primata, class Mammalia, along with the prosomians, monkeys and apes. As a primate his characteristics are : one pair of mammary glands, nails instead of claws, eyes directed anteriorly, proportionately great development of brain.

In the Late Mesozoic, there were only two main groups of mammals : The marsupials and placentals. The placental mammals were collected from the fossils in Mongolia and these were insectivores. These insectivores are regarded that they gave rise to other orders of placental mammals including the primates. The insectivore was somewhat similar to the modern tree shrew which lived between 75 and 60 millions years ago. Two evolutionary lines diverged from the ancestral stock of primates including the tree-shrews. They were (a) *Prosimian* and (b) *Anthropoid*. The prosimian ancestors gave rise to the Lemurs and Tarsiers. The Lemurs are small, tree-living animals mainly found in Medagascar. The Tarsiers are found on some of the islands of East Indies. These are also small primates with long tail but snout is reduced. The Anthropoid ancestors gave rise to the old world monkeys, new world monkeys, apes and man. New world monkeys placed in the family Cebidae diverged from ancestral stock later on in the Eocene or early Oligocene. These are flat nosed, hairy, widely separated nostrils in contrast to other higher primates. Tail is prehensile.

The old world monkeys placed in the family Cercopithecidae which diverged from ancestral stock in the early Oligocene. They are characterized by non-prehensile short tail.

The two other superfamilies which arose are : (a) Pongidae and (b) Hominidae. Pongidae includes Apes (Gibbons, Orangutans, Chimpanzees and Gorilla). The Hominidae includes man.

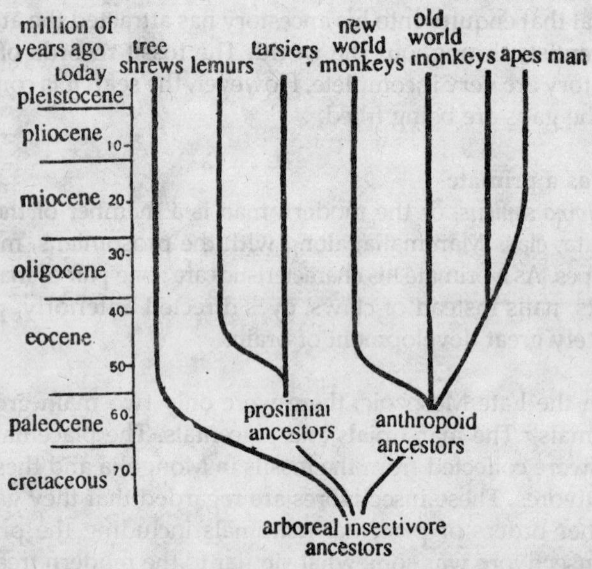

Fig. 13.1. Showing the Probable evolutionary relationship among man and other Primates.

The Gibbons (genus *Hylobates*) and Siamangs of Southern China and Indomalaya are small sized apes. The Gorilla and Chimpanzee (genus *Pan*) are large and heavy, semiarboareal apes found in the forests of Africa. The orangutan (Genus *Pongo*) of Malayas, Sumatra and Borneo are also large and heavy apes.

The apes are differed from the old world monkeys principally in their teeth and mode of locomotion. Being mostly large-sized, these were incapable of walking on the tree branches. They swing by their arms which are grasping type, longer than the legs.

A close phylogenetic relationship of apes with man is revealed by the characteristics given below :

1. Absence of tail.
2. Head is larger : the neck and limbs are longer.
3. The chest is broad due to flat sternum.
4. Lumbar region is short due to the presence of 4-5 lumbar vertebrae.
5. Prominent bowridges above the eyes.
6. Molar teeth with 5 cusps instead of four.
7. Large brain and cranial cavity or cranium.
8. Capable of sound production.
9. Highly developed facial musculature for expressions (like surprise, pleasure etc.)
10. Manstruation in females.

On the basis of such resemblance between apes and man, it has been presumed that the apes and man are cousins. These resemblances occur between Orangutan and Gibbons. The Gorilla and Chimpanzee and regarded as less distinct cousins due to semiopposable thumbs of apes.

Ancestral Apes : The earliest and the most primitive ape, of which we have any fossil remains dates back to Oligocene Period (40 million years ago). It has been called *Parapithecus* and is known only from a lower jaw found in Egypt approximately 60 miles from Cairo, a region which was then covered by tropical forests. From the reconstruction it is clear that is was small ape of the size of squirrel monkey and possessed a dental formula of present day apes and man. Another large ape in Oligocene of Egypt is known by a fossil jaw. It has been named *Propliopithecus* and shows a stage higher than *Parapithecus* in being of the size of a gibbon. These two fragmentary fossils show clearly that apes descended from primitive lemurs without the intervention of a phase of evolution which included the monkeys. Fortunately only a few years ago a complete skull and lower jaw with teeth present, have been unearthed in the same region belonging to the same period. This extraordinary fossil has been named *Aegyptopithecus.* Since it comes from a higher and therefore, a later level than the horizon in which Parapithecus was found, is more advanced toward the typical ape adaptations. *Aegyptopithecus* about the size of a modern gibbon, had a somewhat expanded cranium, large forwardly directed eyes adapted to binocular vision and depth perception, a face that was appreciably longer than in the later apes, a deep jaw, teeth in a continuous series but with the canines of large size, two spatulate like incisors, two premolars, and three low crowned molars with five cusps. Such an ape could very well have been derived from *Propliopithecus* and in turn could be nicely antecedent to the Miocene apes exemplified by the genus *Dryopithcus,* which comes in line of the evolution towards man. *Dryopithecus* is the name given to forms represented by fragmentary remains of large primates of the Miocene Period (30 million years ago) found in Asia and Europe. Indian finds of the Siwalik hills (*Ramapithecus* and *Sivapithecus*) consist entirely of teeth and jaws and are dryopithecines. It has been concluded that these apes were about the size of modern chimpanzee and were very agile. They were however not specialized for arboreal habitat as is evident from their slender limb bones and short arms. Jaws and teeth were also less specialised as compared to the modern apes and were more human in appearance. 'Simian' shelf was not present and the canines not very large.

ORIGIN OF MAN

Place of Origin

The fossils of prehuman and ancestral human forms are obtained from widely diverged areas of Africa, Asia and Europe. This indicates that the main centre for the origin of man was probably in Asia and Africa.

Time of Origin

The time of the desent is not later than early pliocene nor early than Miocene time when the terrestrial ape-man became what we would call human.

Impelling Causes

The Pliocene epoch was characterized by continental elevation and subsequently increased aridity of climate, especially to the northward of the Himalayas. With this increased aridity and tempering of tropical heat came the dwindling of the forest areas. the dwindling of the forests would have an effect upon the tree dwellers. They get down from the trees. Once upon the ground, they rapidly acquired such adaptations as were necessary to ensure survival. These changes framed out individuals which are called human.

Significance of the descent from trees

As a result of the descent from the trees, certain definite factors were called into play. These are (1) Assumption of the erect posture (2).Liberation of the hands from their ancient locomotor function to become organs of mind. (3) Loss of the easily obtainable food of the tropical forests, necessitating the search for plant and animal and man became hunter (4) Need of clothing with increasing inclemency of the weather, especially during the long winters (5) Freedom from climatic restrictions-man was no longer limited to one definite habitat and the result was dispersal (6) The development of communal life.

Evolutionary Trends

The human evolutionary changes which are recorded as follows :

1. More erect posture due to development of lumbar curve.
2. Shortening of the fore-arms and the perfection of thumb opposability into the organs of manipulation.
3. Reduction in the size of incisors and canines because of omnivorous diet.
4. Development of chin prominence.
5. Loss of jaw power.
6. Reduction in the size of eyebrow ridges and loss in simian shelf.
7. Increase in the size and complaxicity of brain, especially the frontal lobes.
8. Broadening of iliac bones of pelvic girdle.
9. Development of articulated speech.

10. Increase in the cranial capacity.
11. Bipedal locomotion.
12. Loss of opposability of great toe in hind limbs.

Fossil men

Well authenticated fossils are as follow :

1. *South African Apeman or Australopithecus africanus*

It was discovered in 1925 by Raymond Dart. Several specimens were found. It is regarded that these creatures were of small stature, about 1.20m. tall. It is definite that they walked upright. Brain-case was small with large jaws and teeth. Teeth resembled those of man. Cranial capacity was from 450 to 600 cc. Till recently, this fossil was considered to be of ape but recent investigations proved it to be of *apeman*. Its ape-like characters are: grasping hands, binocular and stereoscopic vision. Its man-like characters are upright posture and teeth similar to man. Brain was also larger than that of apes. Most of the anthropologists regard that *Australopithecus* represents the line of human ancestory at the beginning of Pleistocene or the end of the Pliocene.

2. *Homo habilis*

Its fossils were discovered by *Leaky, Tobias* and *Napier* in Tanzania in the year 1964. *Homo* habilis was like *Australopithecus* about 1.2 to 1.5 m. tall and weighed 40-50 kg. It lived in open grassy land, moved erect and was omnivorous, but had a larger brain than that of *Australopithecus* with a 660 c.c. cranial capacity. The lower jaw was lightly built. The devtition was more like that of modern man.

3. *Homo heidelbergensis*

It was discovered from Heidelberg in Germany in 1907 in the form of fossil jaw.

4. Jawa Ape man (*Homo erectus erectus*)

It was excavated in 1891 by *Dubois* from the rocks in central Java. This fossil was found to belongs to a prehistoric man closely related by to *Homo Heidelbergensis*. Its name was proposed *Pithecanthropus erectus* by *Dubois*. *Mayer* (1950) proposed the present name *Homo erectus erectus*. The Java ape man was about 1.50 m. in height. He walked erect. The skull cap is thick and heavy, flattened infront. Cranical capacity was 800-1000 c.c. He lead slanting fore head and heaving brow ridges. He had no chin but jaws and teeth were large. He used tools.

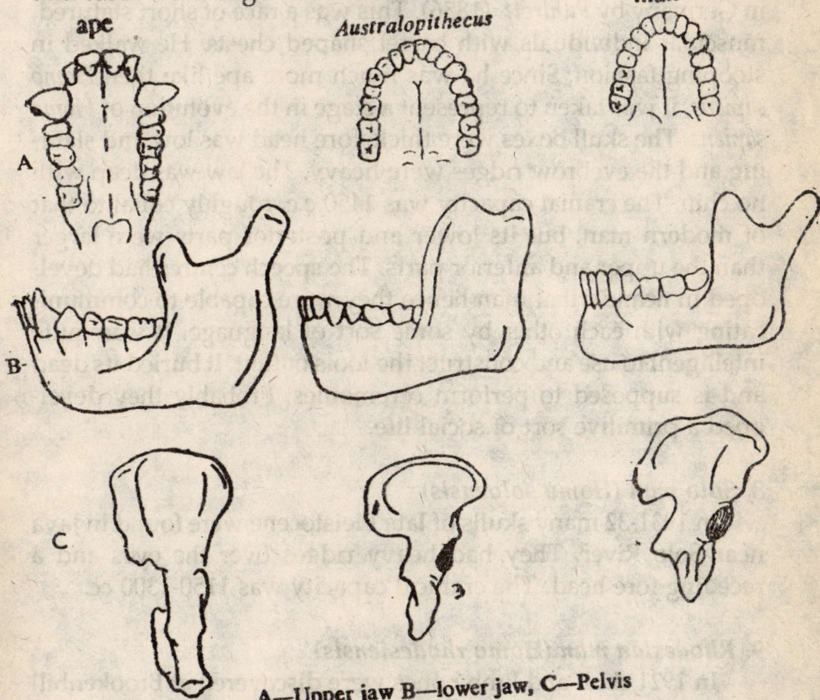

Fig. 13.2. Salient skeletal features of Ape, Australopithecus and man.

5. *Peking man (Homo erectus pekinesis)*

Their fossils were discovered near Peking (China). *Davidson Black* (1927) concluded that these belonged to the different species of *Homo* quite similar to Java ape man. *Black* named it *Sinanthropus pekinesis*. *Mayer* (1950) considered it to be a subspecies and named as *Homo erectus pekinesis*. They do not differ significantly from Java ape man. The cranial capacity was 850-1200 c.c. with an average 1075 c.c. He also used tools and fire. He was cannibal. He was better developed for control of speech.

6. *Atlantic or Tenifier man (Homo erectus mauritanicus)*

It was excavated from Africa in 1954 and 1955 in the form of three jaws.

7. *Neanderthal man (Homo neanderthalensis of Homo sapiens neanderthalensis)*

The fossils of Neaderthed man were collected from Europe and west Asia. Its first fossil was obtained from Neander Valley in Germany by *Fuhlrott* (1856). This was a race of short statured, muscular individuals with barrel shaped chests. He walked in stooping fashion. Since he was much more ape like then *Homo sapiens*, it was taken to represent a stage in the evolution of *Homo sapiens*. The skull boxes were thick, fore head was low and slanting and the eyebrow ridges were heavy. The jaw was deep with no chin. The cranial capacity was 1450 c.c. roughly equal to that of modern man, but its lower and posterior parts were larger than the upper and anterior parts. The speech centres had developed in neanderthal man hence they were capable to communicating with each other by some sort of language. It was quite intelligent to use and construct the tools of flint. It buried its dead and is supposed to perform ceremonies. Probably they developed a primitive sort of social life.

8. *Solo man (Homo soloensis)*

In 1931-32 many skulls of late Pleistocene were found in Java near Solo River. They had heavy ridges over the eyes and a receding fore head. The cranical capacity was 1150-1300 cc.

9. *Rhodesian man (Homo rhodesiensis)*

In 1921 skull and limb bones were discovered at Brookenhill in Northern Rhodesia. The skull had a cranial capacity of about 1300 c.c. with receding forehead and heavy eye brow ridges. The teeth were set in a finely arched palate and the 3rd molars were smaller than other teeth.

10. *Piltdown man*

Skull fragments of piltdown man were found by *Charls Dawson* in 1908 and 1911 near Piltdown Common, Sussex, England. In 1912 *Dawson* and *Sir* Arthur Smith-Woodward discovered a large piece of skull. *Smith-Woodward* gave it the name *Eoanthropus dawsoni* ("Dawson's Dawn-man"). The skull bones are thick and cranial capacity lies near 1350 c.c. The lower jaw showed a combination of man and ape as the molars are alike those of modern man and the canine is interlocked with its opposite as in apes. The chin was retreated.

11. ***Cro-magnon man (Homo sapiens fossilis)***

It was discovered by *MacGregor* in 1868 from the Cro-Magnon Rock of France. Later on its fossils were recorded from Germany, Czechoslovakia, Africa and other parts of France. The males were about 1.8 m. in height while females were about 1.60

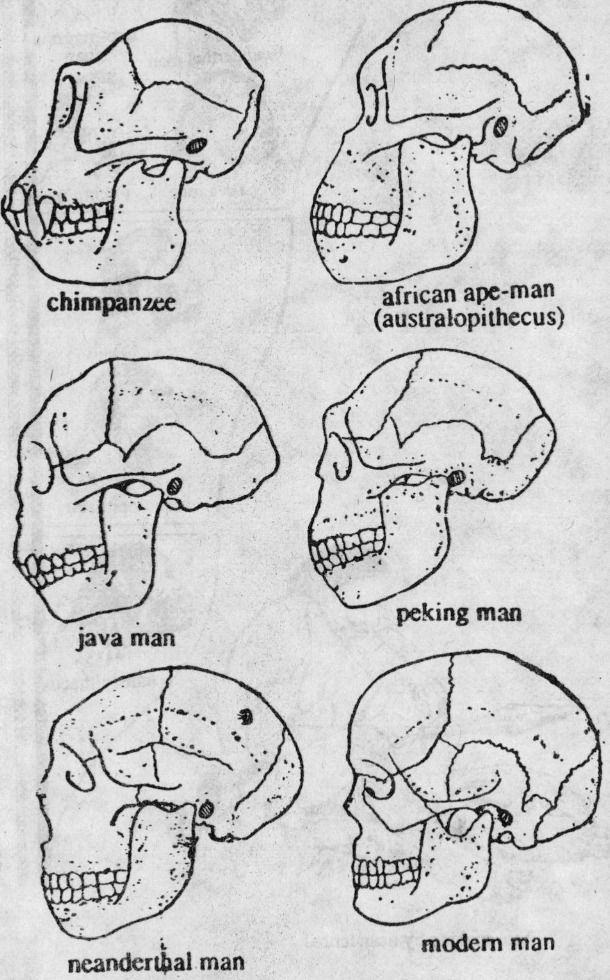

Fig. 13.3. Skulls of five hominids with an anthropoid ape.

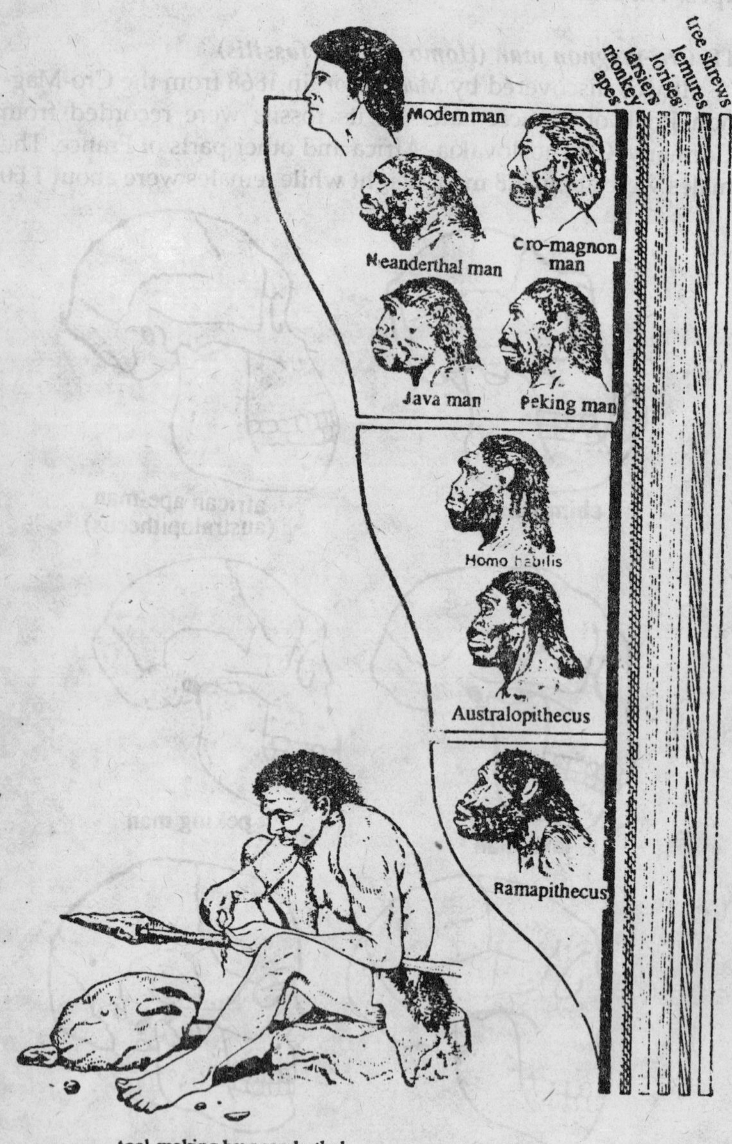

Fig. 13.4. Stage of human evolution